Cram101 Textbook Outlines to accompany:

Human Diseases:A Systemic Approach

Mulvihill, et al..., 5th Edition

An Academic Internet Publishers (AIPI) publication (c) 2007.

Cram101 and Cram101.com are AIPI publications and services. All notes, highlights, reviews, and practice tests are prepared by AIPI for use in AIPI publications, all rights reserved.

You have a discounted membership at www.Cram101.com with this book.

Get all of the practice tests for the chapters of this textbook, and access in-depth reference material for writing essays and papers. Here is an example from a Cram101 Biology text:

When you need problem solving help with math, stats, and other disciplines, www.Cram101.com will walk through the formulas and solutions step by step.

With Cram101.com online, you also have access to extensive reference material.

You will nail those essays and papers. Here is an example from a Cram101 Biology text:

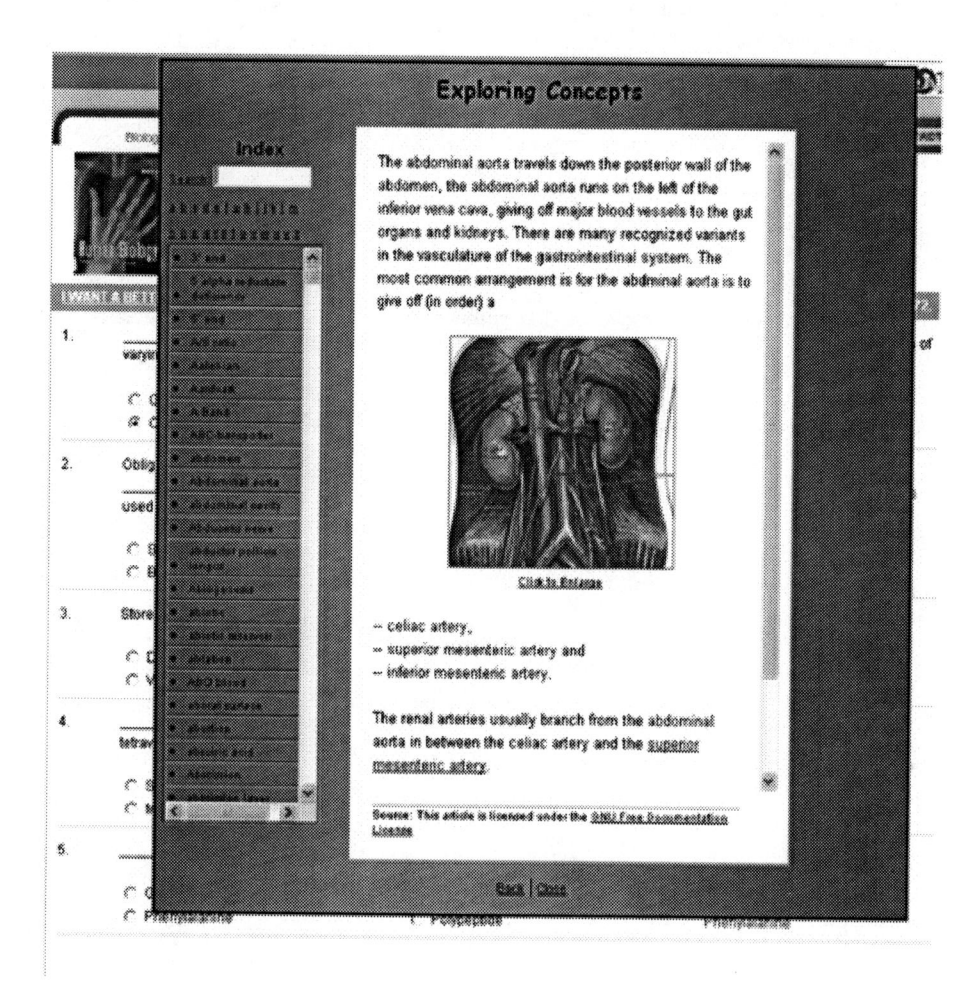

Visit **www.Cram101.com**, click Sign Up at the top of the screen, and enter DK73DW3456 in the promo code box on the registration screen. Access to www.Cram101.com is normally $9.95, but because you have purchased this book, your access fee is only $4.95. Sign up and stop highlighting textbooks forever.

Learning System

Cram101 Textbook Outlines is a learning system. The notes in this book are the highlights of your textbook, you will never have to highlight a book again.

How to use this book. Take this book to class, it is your notebook for the lecture. The notes and highlights on the left hand side of the pages follow the outline and order of the textbook. All you have to do is follow along while your intructor presents the lecture. Circle the items emphasized in class and add other important information on the right side. With Cram101 Textbook Outlines you'll spend less time writing and more time listening. Learning becomes more efficient.

Cram101.com Online

Increase your studying efficiency by using Cram101.com's practice tests and online reference material. It is the perfect complement to Cram101 Textbook Outlines. Use self-teaching matching tests or simulate in-class testing with comprehensive multiple choice tests, or simply use Cram's true and false tests for quick review. Cram101.com even allows you to enter your in-class notes for an integrated studying format combining the textbook notes with your class notes.

Visit **www.Cram101.com**, click Sign Up at the top of the screen, and enter **DK73DW3456** in the promo code box on the registration screen. Access to www.Cram101.com is normally $9.95, but because you have purchased this book, your access fee is only $4.95. Sign up and stop highlighting textbooks forever.

Copyright © 2008 by Academic Internet Publishers, Inc. All rights reserved. "Cram101"® and "Never Highlight a Book Again!"® are registered trademarks of Academic Internet Publishers, Inc. The Cram101 Textbook Outline series is printed in the United States. ISBN: 1-4288-1902-9

Human Diseases: A Systemic Approach
Mulvihill, et al..., 5th

CONTENTS

1. Introduction to Disease 2
2. Inflammation, Immunity, and Allergy 12
3. Infectious Diseases 34
4. Neoplasms 48
5. Hereditary Diseases 66
6. Dietary Deficiencies and Excesses: Malnutrition, Obesity, and Alcoholism 86
7. Diseases of the Blood 116
8. Diseases of the Heart 132
9. Diseases of the Blood Vessels 152
10. Diseases of the Urinary System 172
11. Diseases of the Digestive Tract 194
12. Diseases of the Liver, Gallbladder, and Pancreas 216
13. Diseases of the Respiratory System 234
14. Diseases of the Endocrine System 254
15. Diseases of the Reproductive Systems and Sexually Transmitted Infections 286
16. Diseases of the Nervous System 322
17. Diseases of the Bones, Joints, and Muscles 356
18. Diseases of the Skin 378
19. Stress and Aging 396
20. Wellness 418

Chapter 1. Introduction to Disease

Steady state	Steady state is a system in which a particular variable is not changing but energy must be continuously added to maintain this variable constant.
Homeostasis	Homeostasis is the property of an open system, especially living organisms, to regulate its internal environment to maintain a stable, constant condition, by means of multiple dynamic equilibrium adjustments, controlled by interrelated regulation mechanisms.
Common cold	An acute, self-limiting, and highly contagious virus infection of the upper respiratory tract that produces inflammation, profuse discharge, and other symptoms is referred to as the common cold.
Virus	Obligate intracellular parasite of living cells consisting of an outer capsid and an inner core of nucleic acid is referred to as virus. The term virus usually refers to those particles that infect eukaryotes whilst the term bacteriophage or phage is used to describe those infecting prokaryotes.
Antibiotic	Antibiotic refers to substance such as penicillin or streptomycin that is toxic to microorganisms. Usually a product of a particular microorvanism or plant.
Pain	Pain is an unpleasant sensation which may be associated with actual or potential tissue damage and which may have physical and emotional components.
Syndrome	Syndrome is the association of several clinically recognizable features, signs, symptoms, phenomena or characteristics which often occur together, so that the presence of one feature alerts the physician to the presence of the others
Eye	An eye is an organ that detects light. Different kinds of light-sensitive organs are found in a variety of creatures. The simplest eyes do nothing but detect whether the surroundings are light or dark, while more complex eyes can distinguish shapes and colors.
Hypothermia	Hypothermia is a low core body temperature, defined clinically as a temperature of less than 35 degrees celsius.
Freezing	Freezing is the process in which blood is frozen and all of the plasma and 99% of the WBCs are eliminated when thawing takes place and the nontransferable cryoprotectant is removed.
Blood	Blood is a circulating tissue composed of fluid plasma and cells. The main function of blood is to supply nutrients (oxygen, glucose) and constitutional elements to tissues and to remove waste products.
Blood vessel	A blood vessel is a part of the circulatory system and function to transport blood throughout the body. The most important types, arteries and veins, are so termed because they carry blood away from or towards the heart, respectively.
Muscle	Muscle is a contractile form of tissue. It is one of the four major tissue types, the other three being epithelium, connective tissue and nervous tissue. Muscle contraction is used to move parts of the body, as well as to move substances within the body.
Muscle contraction	A muscle contraction occurs when a muscle cell (called a muscle fiber) shortens. There are three general types: skeletal, heart, and smooth.
Etiology	The apparent causation and developmental history of an illness is an etiology.
Heredity	Heredity refers to the transmission of genetic information from parent to offspring.
Cancer	Cancer is a class of diseases or disorders characterized by uncontrolled division of cells and the ability of these cells to invade other tissues, either by direct growth into adjacent tissue through invasion or by implantation into distant sites by metastasis.
Bacteria	The domain that contains procaryotic cells with primarily diacyl glycerol diesters in their membranes and with bacterial rRNA. Bacteria also is a general term for organisms that are composed of procaryotic cells and are not multicellular.
Fungi	Fungi refers to simple parasitic life forms, including molds, mildews, yeasts, and mushrooms. They live on dead or decaying organic matter. Fungi can grow as single cells, like yeast, or as multicellular

Chapter 1. Introduction to Disease

	colonies, as seen with molds.
Agent	Agent refers to an epidemiological term referring to the organism or object that transmits a disease from the environment to the host.
Infection	The invasion and multiplication of microorganisms in body tissues is called an infection.
Malaria	Malaria refers to potentially fatal human disease caused by the protozoan parasite Plasmodium, which is transmitted by the bite of an infected mosquito.
Viral	Viral phenomena are objects or patterns able to replicate themselves or convert other objects into copies of themselves when these objects are exposed to them.
Skin	Skin is an organ of the integumentary system composed of a layer of tissues that protect underlying muscles and organs.
Microorganism	A microorganism or microbe is an organism that is so small that it is microscopic (invisible to the naked eye).
Misuse	Misuse refers to an unusual or illegal use of a prescription, usually for drug diversion purposes.
Resistance	Resistance refers to a nonspecific ability to ward off infection or disease regardless of whether the body has been previously exposed to it. A force that opposes the flow of a fluid such as air or blood. Compare with immunity.
Constant	A behavior or characteristic that does not vary from one observation to another is referred to as a constant.
Immunity	Resistance to the effects of specific disease-causing agents is called immunity.
Affect	Affect is the scientific term used to describe a subject's externally displayed mood. This can be assesed by the nurse by observing facial expression, tone of voice, and body language.
Idiopathic	Idiopathic is a medical adjective that indicates that a recognized cause has not yet been established.
Pathology	Pathology is the study of the processes underlying disease and other forms of illness, harmful abnormality, or dysfunction.
Medicine	Medicine is the branch of health science and the sector of public life concerned with maintaining or restoring human health through the study, diagnosis and treatment of disease and injury.
Measles	Measles refers to a highly contagious skin disease that is endemic throughout the world. It is caused by a morbilli virus in the family Paramyxoviridae, which enters the body through the respiratory tract or through the conjunctiva.
Rubella	An infectious disease that, if contracted by the mother during the first three months of pregnancy, has a high risk of causing mental retardation and physical deformity in the child is called rubella.
Alcohol	Alcohol is a general term, applied to any organic compound in which a hydroxyl group (-OH) is bound to a carbon atom, which in turn is bound to other hydrogen and/or carbon atoms. The general formula for a simple acyclic alcohol is $C_nH_{2n+1}OH$.
Oxygen	Oxygen is a chemical element in the periodic table. It has the symbol O and atomic number 8. Oxygen is the second most common element on Earth, composing around 46% of the mass of Earth's crust and 28% of the mass of Earth as a whole, and is the third most common element in the universe.
Leukemia	Leukemia refers to a type of cancer of the bloodforming tissues, characterized by an excessive production of white blood cells and an abnormally high number of them in the blood; cancer of the bone marrow cells that produce leukocytes.
Alcoholism	A disorder that involves long-term, repeated, uncontrolled, compulsive, and excessive use of alcoholic beverages and that impairs the drinker's health and work and social relationships is called alcoholism.

Chapter 1. Introduction to Disease

Chapter 1. Introduction to Disease

Stress	Stress refers to a condition that is a response to factors that change the human systems normal state.
Immune system	The immune system is the system of specialized cells and organs that protect an organism from outside biological influences. When the immune system is functioning properly, it protects the body against bacteria and viral infections, destroying cancer cells and foreign substances.
Asthma	Asthma is a complex disease characterized by bronchial hyperresponsiveness (BHR), inflammation, mucus production and intermittent airway obstruction.
Clubbing	In medicine, clubbing (or digital clubbing) is a deformity of the fingers and fingernails that is associated with a number of diseases, mostly of the heart and lungs.
Health	Health is a term that refers to a combination of the absence of illness, the ability to cope with everyday activities, physical fitness, and high quality of life.
Tissue	A collection of interconnected cells that perform a similar function within an organism is called tissue.
Connective tissue	Connective tissue is any type of biological tissue with an extensive extracellular matrix and often serves to support, bind together, and protect organs.
Compensation	Compensation refers to according to Adler, efforts to overcome imagined or real inferiorities by developing one's abilities.
Cirrhosis	Cirrhosis is a chronic disease of the liver in which liver tissue is replaced by connective tissue, resulting in the loss of liver function. Cirrhosis is caused by damage from toxins (including alcohol), metabolic problems, chronic viral hepatitis or other causes
Diabetes	Diabetes is a medical disorder characterized by varying or persistent elevated blood sugar levels, especially after eating. All types of diabetes share similar symptoms and complications at advanced stages: dehydration and ketoacidosis, cardiovascular disease, chronic renal failure, retinal damage which can lead to blindness, nerve damage which can lead to erectile dysfunction, gangrene with risk of amputation of toes, feet, and even legs.
Hypertrophy	Hypertrophy is the increase of the size of an organ. It should be distinguished from hyperplasia which occurs due to cell division; hypertrophy occurs due to an increase in cell size rather than division. It is most commonly seen in muscle that has been actively stimulated, the most well-known method being exercise.
Hyperplasia	Hyperplasia is a general term for an increase in the number of the cells of an organ or tissue causing it to increase in size.
Diagnosis	In medicine, diagnosis is the process of identifying a medical condition or disease by its signs, symptoms, and from the results of various diagnostic procedures.
Dysplasia	Dysplasia refers to a change in cell growth and behavior in a tissue in which the structure becomes disordered.
Atrophy	Atrophy is the partial or complete wasting away of a part of the body. Causes of atrophy include poor nourishment, poor circulation, loss of hormonal support, loss of nerve supply to the target organ, disuse or lack of exercise, or disease intrinsic to the tissue itself.
Lesion	A lesion is a non-specific term referring to abnormal tissue in the body. It can be caused by any disease process including trauma (physical, chemical, electrical), infection, neoplasm, metabolic and autoimmune.
Organ	Organ refers to a structure consisting of several tissues adapted as a group to perform specific functions.
Blood pressure	Blood pressure is the pressure exerted by the blood on the walls of the blood vessels.
Kidney	The kidney is a bean-shaped excretory organ in vertebrates. Part of the urinary system, the kidneys

Chapter 1. Introduction to Disease

Chapter 1. Introduction to Disease

	filter wastes (especially urea) from the blood and excrete them, along with water, as urine.
Tumor	An abnormal mass of cells that forms within otherwise normal tissue is a tumor. This growth can be either malignant or benign
Lead	Lead is a chemical element in the periodic table that has the symbol Pb and atomic number 82. A soft, heavy, toxic and malleable poor metal, lead is bluish white when freshly cut but tarnishes to dull gray when exposed to air. Lead is used in building construction, lead-acid batteries, bullets and shot, and is part of solder, pewter, and fusible alloys.
Anemia	Anemia is a deficiency of red blood cells and/or hemoglobin. This results in a reduced ability of blood to transfer oxygen to the tissues, and this causes hypoxia; since all human cells depend on oxygen for survival, varying degrees of anemia can have a wide range of clinical consequences.
Aplastic anemia	Aplastic anemia is a condition where the bone marrow does not produce enough, or any, new cells to replenish the blood cells.
Conversion	Conversion syndrome describes a condition in which physical symptoms arise for which there is no clear explanation.
Wound	A wound is type of physical trauma wherein the skin is torn, cut or punctured, or where blunt force trauma causes a contusion.
Radiography	Radiography is the creation of images by exposing a photographic film or other image receptor to X-rays. Since X-rays penetrate solid objects, but are weakened by them depending on the object's composition, the resulting picture reveals the internal structure of the object.
Urinalysis	A urinalysis (or "UA") is an array of tests performed on urine and one of the most common methods of medical diagnosis. A part of a urinalysis can be performed by using urine dipsticks, in which the test results can be read as color changes.
Ultrasound	Ultrasound is sound with a frequency greater than the upper limit of human hearing, approximately 20 kilohertz. Medical use can visualise muscle and soft tissue, making them useful for scanning the organs, and obstetric ultrasonography is commonly used during pregnancy.
Computed tomography	Computed tomography is an imaging method employing tomography where digital processing is used to generate a three-dimensional image of the internals of an object from a large series of two-dimensional X-ray images taken around a single axis of rotation.
Magnetic resonance imaging	Magnetic resonance imaging refers to imaging technology that uses magnetism and radio waves to induce hydrogen nuclei in water molecules to emit faint radio signals. A computer creates images of the body from the radio signals.
Prognosis	Prognosis refers to the prospects for the future or outcome of a disease.
Outcome	Outcome is the impact of care provided to a patient. They can be positive, such as the ability to walk freely as a result of rehabilitation, or negative, such as the occurrence of bedsores as a result of lack of mobility of a patient.
Course	Pattern of development and change of a disorder over time is a course.
Radiation	The emission of electromagnetic waves by all objects warmer than absolute zero is referred to as radiation.
Radiation therapy	Treatment for cancer in which parts of the body that have cancerous tumors are exposed to high-energy radiation to disrupt cell division of the cancer cells is called radiation therapy.
Acute	In medicine, an acute disease is a disease with either or both of: a rapid onset; and a short course (as opposed to a chronic course).
Acute Disease	An acute disease is defined as a short-term disease from which a person either dies or recovers.

Chapter 1. Introduction to Disease

Chapter 1. Introduction to Disease

Remission	Disappearance of the signs of a disease is called remission.
Chronic disease	Disease of long duration often not detected in its early stages and from which the patient will not recover is referred to as a chronic disease.
Exacerbation	Exacerbation is a period in an illness when the symptoms of the disease reappear.
Ulcerative colitis	Ulcerative colitis (UC) is a form of inflammatory bowel disease (IBD) featuring systemic inflammation specifically causing episodic mucosal inflammation of the colon (large bowel).
Pneumonia	Pneumonia is an illness of the lungs and respiratory system in which the microscopic, air-filled sacs (alveoli) responsible for absorbing oxygen from the atmosphere become inflamed and flooded with fluid.
Puberty	A time in the life of a developing individual characterized by the increasing production of sex hormones, which cause it to reach sexual maturity is called puberty.
Testes	The testes are the male generative glands in animals. Male mammals have two testes, which are often contained within an extension of the abdomen called the scrotum.
Mumps	Mumps is a viral disease of humans. Prior to the development of vaccination, it was a common childhood disease worldwide, and is still a significant threat to health in the third world.
Prostate	The prostate is a gland that is part of male mammalian sex organs. Its main function is to secrete and store a clear, slightly basic fluid that is part of semen. The prostate differs considerably between species anatomically, chemically and physiologically.
Gland	A gland is an organ in an animal's body that synthesizes a substance for release such as hormones, often into the bloodstream or into cavities inside the body or its outer surface.
Fever	Fever (also known as pyrexia, or a febrile response, and archaically known as ague) is a medical symptom that describes an increase in internal body temperature to levels that are above normal (37°C, 98.6°F).
Rheumatic fever	Rheumatic fever is an inflammatory disease which may develop after a Group A streptococcal infection (such as strep throat or scarlet fever) and can involve the heart, joints, skin, and brain.
Inflammation	Inflammation is the first response of the immune system to infection or irritation and may be referred to as the innate cascade.
Fallopian tube	The Fallopian tube is one of two very fine tubes leading from the ovaries of female mammals into the uterus. They deliver the ovum to the uterus.
Anxiety	Anxiety is a complex combination of the feeling of fear, apprehension and worry often accompanied by physical sensations such as palpitations, chest pain and/or shortness of breath.
Allergy	An allergy or Type I hypersensitivity is an immune malfunction whereby a person's body is hypersensitized to react immunologically to typically nonimmunogenic substances. When a person is hypersensitized, these substances are known as allergens.
Inflammatory response	Inflammatory response refers to a complex sequence of events involving chemicals and immune cells that results in the isolation and destruction of antigens and tissues near the antigens.

Chapter 1. Introduction to Disease

Chapter 2. Inflammation, Immunity, and Allergy

Tissue	A collection of interconnected cells that perform a similar function within an organism is called tissue.
Bacteria	The domain that contains procaryotic cells with primarily diacyl glycerol diesters in their membranes and with bacterial rRNA. Bacteria also is a general term for organisms that are composed of procaryotic cells and are not multicellular.
Fungi	Fungi refers to simple parasitic life forms, including molds, mildews, yeasts, and mushrooms. They live on dead or decaying organic matter. Fungi can grow as single cells, like yeast, or as multicellular colonies, as seen with molds.
Inflammation	Inflammation is the first response of the immune system to infection or irritation and may be referred to as the innate cascade.
Pain	Pain is an unpleasant sensation which may be associated with actual or potential tissue damage and which may have physical and emotional components.
Infection	The invasion and multiplication of microorganisms in body tissues is called an infection.
Toxin	Toxin refers to a microbial product or component that can injure another cell or organism at low concentrations. Often the term refers to a poisonous protein, but toxins may be lipids and other substances.
Virus	Obligate intracellular parasite of living cells consisting of an outer capsid and an inner core of nucleic acid is referred to as virus. The term virus usually refers to those particles that infect eukaryotes whilst the term bacteriophage or phage is used to describe those infecting prokaryotes.
DNA	Deoxyribonucleic acid (DNA) is a nucleic acid —usually in the form of a double helix— that contains the genetic instructions specifying the biological development of all cellular forms of life, and most viruses.
Capillaries	Capillaries refer to the smallest of the blood vessels and the sites of exchange between the blood and tissue cells.
Capillary	A capillary is the smallest of a body's blood vessels, measuring 5-10 micro meters. They connect arteries and veins, and most closely interact with tissues. Their walls are composed of a single layer of cells, the endothelium. This layer is so thin that molecules such as oxygen, water and lipids can pass through them by diffusion and enter the tissues.
Arteriole	An arteriole is a blood vessel that extends and branches out from an artery and leads to capillaries. They have thick muscular walls and are the primary site of vascular resistance.
Blood	Blood is a circulating tissue composed of fluid plasma and cells. The main function of blood is to supply nutrients (oxygen, glucose) and constitutional elements to tissues and to remove waste products.
Blood vessel	A blood vessel is a part of the circulatory system and function to transport blood throughout the body. The most important types, arteries and veins, are so termed because they carry blood away from or towards the heart, respectively.
Leukocyte	A white blood cell is a leukocyte. They help to defend the body against infectious disease and foreign materials as part of the immune system.
White blood cell	The white blood cell is a a component of blood. They help to defend the body against infectious disease and foreign materials as part of the immune system.
Neutrophil	Neutrophil refers to a type of phagocytic leukocyte.
Agent	Agent refers to an epidemiological term referring to the organism or object that transmits a disease from the environment to the host.

Go to **Cram101.com** for the Practice Tests for this Chapter.

Chapter 2. Inflammation, Immunity, and Allergy

Chapter 2. Inflammation, Immunity, and Allergy

Chemotaxis	Chemotaxis is the phenomenon in which bodily cells, bacteria, and other single-celled or multicellular organisms direct their movements according to certain chemicals in their environment.
Exudate	An exudate is any fluid that filters from the circulatory system into leisions or areas of inflamation. Its composition varies but generally includes water and the disolved solutes of the blood, some or all plasma proteins, white blood cells, platelets and red blood cells.
Plasma	Fluid portion of circulating blood is called plasma.
Nerve	A nerve is an enclosed, cable-like bundle of nerve fibers or axons, which includes the glia that ensheath the axons in myelin.
Radiation	The emission of electromagnetic waves by all objects warmer than absolute zero is referred to as radiation.
Allergen	An allergen is any substance (antigen), most often eaten or inhaled, that is recognized by the immune system and causes an allergic reaction.
Trauma	Trauma refers to a severe physical injury or wound to the body caused by an external force, or a psychological shock having a lasting effect on mental life.
Acid	An acid is a water-soluble, sour-tasting chemical compound that when dissolved in water, gives a solution with a pH of less than 7.
Inflammatory response	Inflammatory response refers to a complex sequence of events involving chemicals and immune cells that results in the isolation and destruction of antigens and tissues near the antigens.
Phagocytosis	Phagocytosis (literally, "cell eating") is a form of endocytosis where large particles are enveloped by the cell membrane of a (usually larger) cell and internalized to form a phagosome, or "food vacuole."
Bone marrow	Bone marrow is the tissue comprising the center of large bones. It is the place where new blood cells are produced. Bone marrow contains two types of stem cells: hemopoietic (which can produce blood cells) and stromal (which can produce fat, cartilage and bone).
Lymph node	A lymph node acts as a filter, with an internal honeycomb of connective tissue filled with lymphocytes that collect and destroy bacteria and viruses. When the body is fighting an infection, these lymphocytes multiply rapidly and produce a characteristic swelling of the lymph node.
Lymph	Lymph originates as blood plasma lost from the circulatory system, which leaks out into the surrounding tissues. The lymphatic system collects this fluid by diffusion into lymph capillaries, and returns it to the circulatory system.
Leukocytosis	Leukocytosis is an elevation of the white blood cell count above the normal range. The normal adult human leukocyte count in peripheral blood is 4.4-10.8 x 10^9/L. A white blood count of 11.0 or more suggests leukocytosis.
Protein	A protein is a complex, high-molecular-weight organic compound that consists of amino acids joined by peptide bonds. They are essential to the structure and function of all living cells and viruses. Many are enzymes or subunits of enzymes.
Fibrin	Fibrin is a protein involved in the clotting of blood. It is a fibrillar protein that is polymerized to form a "mesh" that forms a haemostatic plug or clot (in conjunction with platelets) over a wound site.
Wound	A wound is type of physical trauma wherein the skin is torn, cut or punctured, or where blunt force trauma causes a contusion.

Chapter 2. Inflammation, Immunity, and Allergy

Chapter 2. Inflammation, Immunity, and Allergy

Fiber	Fibers used by man come from a wide variety of sources: Natural fiber include those made out of plants, animal and mineral sources. Natural fibers can be classified according to their origin.
Connective tissue	Connective tissue is any type of biological tissue with an extensive extracellular matrix and often serves to support, bind together, and protect organs.
Scar	A scar results from the biologic process of wound repair in the skin and other tissues of the body. It is a connective tissue that fills the wound.
Immunity	Resistance to the effects of specific disease-causing agents is called immunity.
Cancer	Cancer is a class of diseases or disorders characterized by uncontrolled division of cells and the ability of these cells to invade other tissues, either by direct growth into adjacent tissue through invasion or by implantation into distant sites by metastasis.
Antigen	An antigen is a substance that stimulates an immune response, especially the production of antibodies. They are usually proteins or polysaccharides, but can be any type of molecule, including small molecules (haptens) coupled to a protein (carrier).
Immune response	The body's defensive reaction to invasion by bacteria, viral agents, or other foreign substances is called immune response.
Stomach	The stomach is an organ in the alimentary canal used to digest food. It's primary function is not the absorption of nutrients from digested food; rather, the main job of the stomach is to break down large food molecules into smaller ones, so that they can be absorbed into the blood more easily.
Skin	Skin is an organ of the integumentary system composed of a layer of tissues that protect underlying muscles and organs.
Lymphocyte	A lymphocyte is a type of white blood cell involved in the human body's immune system. There are two broad categories, namely T cells and B cells.
Antibody	An antibody is a protein used by the immune system to identify and neutralize foreign objects like bacteria and viruses. Each antibody recognizes a specific antigen unique to its target.
Humoral immunity	Humoral immunity is the aspect of immunity that is mediated by secreted antibodies, produced in the cells of the B lymphocyte lineage (B cell). Secreted antibodies bind to antigens on the surfaces of invading microbes, which flags them for destruction.
Lymphatic system	Lymph originates as blood plasma lost from the circulatory system, which leaks out into the surrounding tissues. The lymphatic system collects this fluid by diffusion into lymph capillaries, and returns it to the circulatory system.
Organ	Organ refers to a structure consisting of several tissues adapted as a group to perform specific functions.
Adenoids	Adenoids, or pharyngeal tonsils, are folds of lymphatic tissue covered by ciliated epithelium. They are found in the roof and posterior wall of the nasopharynx at the back of the throat behind the uvula.
Tonsils	The tonsils are areas of lymphoid tissue on either side of the throat. As with other organs of the lymphatic system, the tonsils act as part of the immune system to help protect against infection.
Adenoid	An adenoid is a fold of lymphatic tissue covered by ciliated epithelium. They are found in the roof and posterior wall of the nasopharynx at the back of the throat behind the uvula. They are part of the immune system, as they trap inhaled viruses and produce antibodies, particularly in children. This function decreases with age.

Chapter 2. Inflammation, Immunity, and Allergy

Chapter 2. Inflammation, Immunity, and Allergy

Tonsil	Tonsil refers to a patch of lymphatic tissue consisting of connective tissue that contains many lymphocytes; located in the pharynx and throat.
Spleen	The spleen is a ductless, vertebrate gland that is not necessary for life but is closely associated with the circulatory system, where it functions in the destruction of old red blood cells and removal of other debris from the bloodstream, and also in holding a reservoir of blood.
Salmonella	Salmonella is a genus of rod-shaped Gram-negative enterobacteria that causes typhoid fever, paratyphoid and foodborne illness. It is motile in nature and produces hydrogen sulfide.
Thymus	The thymus is a ductless gland located in the upper anterior portion of the chest cavity. It is most active during puberty, after which it shrinks in size and activity in most individuals and is replaced with fat. The thymus plays an important role in the development of the immune system.
Gland	A gland is an organ in an animal's body that synthesizes a substance for release such as hormones, often into the bloodstream or into cavities inside the body or its outer surface.
Intestine	The intestine is the portion of the alimentary canal extending from the stomach to the anus and, in humans and mammals, consists of two segments, the small intestine and the large intestine. The intestine is the part of the body responsible for extracting nutrition from food.
Globulin	Globulin is one of the two types of serum proteins, the other being albumin. This generic term encompasses a heterogenous series of families of proteins, with larger molecules and less soluble in pure water than albumin, which migrate less than albumin during serum electrophoresis.
Thoracic duct	The thoracic duct is an important part of the lymphatic system. It is the largest lymphatic vessel in the body. It collects most of the lymph in the body, neck and head, which is collected by the right lymphatic duct) and drains into the systemic (blood) circulation.
Immune system	The immune system is the system of specialized cells and organs that protect an organism from outside biological influences. When the immune system is functioning properly, it protects the body against bacteria and viral infections, destroying cancer cells and foreign substances.
Receptor	A receptor is a protein on the cell membrane or within the cytoplasm or cell nucleus that binds to a specific molecule (a ligand), such as a neurotransmitter, hormone, or other substance, and initiates the cellular response to the ligand. Receptor, in immunology, the region of an antibody which shows recognition of an antigen.
Lymphokine	Lymphokine refers to a biologically active glycoprotein secreted by activated lymphocytes, especially sensitized T cells. It acts as an intercellular mediator of the immune response and transmits growth, differentiation, and behavioral signals.
Autoimmunity	Autoimmunity is the failure of an organism to recognise its own constituent parts (down to the sub-molecular levels) as self, as a result of which it attempts to mount an immune response against its own cells and tissues.
Tolerance	Drug tolerance occurs when a subject's reaction to a drug decreases so that larger doses are required to achieve the same effect.
Autoimmune	Autoimmune refers to immune reactions against normal body cells; self against self.
Arthritis	Arthritis is a group of conditions that affect the health of the bone joints in the body. Arthritis can be caused from strains and injuries caused by repetitive motion, sports, overexertion, and falls. Unlike the autoimmune diseases, it largely affects older people and results from the degeneration of joint cartilage.

Chapter 2. Inflammation, Immunity, and Allergy

Fever	Fever (also known as pyrexia, or a febrile response, and archaically known as ague) is a medical symptom that describes an increase in internal body temperature to levels that are above normal (37°C, 98.6°F).
Rheumatoid arthritis	Rheumatoid arthritis is a chronic, inflammatory autoimmune disorder that causes the immune system to attack the joints. It is a disabling and painful inflammatory condition, which can lead to substantial loss of mobility due to pain and joint destruction.
Autoimmune disease	Disease that results when the immune system mistakenly attacks the body's own tissues is referred to as autoimmune disease.
Myasthenia gravis	Myasthenia gravis is a neuromuscular disease leading to fluctuating weakness and fatiguability.
Rheumatic fever	Rheumatic fever is an inflammatory disease which may develop after a Group A streptococcal infection (such as strep throat or scarlet fever) and can involve the heart, joints, skin, and brain.
Lupus erythematosus	Lupus erythematosus is a rheumatological autoimmune disorder in which antibodies are created against the patient's own DNA. It can cause various symptoms, but the main ones relate to the skin, kidney, joints, blood and immune system.
Systemic lupus erythematosus	An autoimmune, inflammatory disease that may affect every tissue of the body is called systemic lupus erythematosus.
Muscle	Muscle is a contractile form of tissue. It is one of the four major tissue types, the other three being epithelium, connective tissue and nervous tissue. Muscle contraction is used to move parts of the body, as well as to move substances within the body.
Joint	A joint (articulation) is the location at which two bones make contact (articulate). They are constructed to both allow movement and provide mechanical support.
Exacerbation	Exacerbation is a period in an illness when the symptoms of the disease reappear.
Remission	Disappearance of the signs of a disease is called remission.
Lesion	A lesion is a non-specific term referring to abnormal tissue in the body. It can be caused by any disease process including trauma (physical, chemical, electrical), infection, neoplasm, metabolic and autoimmune.
Affect	Affect is the scientific term used to describe a subject's externally displayed mood. This can be assesed by the nurse by observing facial expression, tone of voice, and body language.
Glomeruli	Glomeruli are important waystations in the pathway from the nose to the olfactory cortex. Each receives input from olfactory receptor neurons expressing only one type of olfactory receptor. There are tens of millions of olfactory receptor cells, but only about two thousand glomeruli. By combining so much input, the olfactory system is able to detect even very faint odors.
Excretion	Excretion is the biological process by which an organism chemically separates waste products from its body. The waste products are then usually expelled from the body by elimination.
Albumin	Albumin refers generally to any protein with water solubility, which is moderately soluble in concentrated salt solutions, and experiences heat coagulation (protein denaturation).
Kidney	The kidney is a bean-shaped excretory organ in vertebrates. Part of the urinary system, the kidneys filter wastes (especially urea) from the blood and excrete them, along with water, as urine.
Urine	Concentrated filtrate produced by the kidneys and excreted via the bladder is called urine.
Platelet	Cell fragment that is necessary to blood clotting is a platelet. They are the blood cell

Chapter 2. Inflammation, Immunity, and Allergy

Chapter 2. Inflammation, Immunity, and Allergy

	fragments that are involved in the cellular mechanisms that lead to the formation of blood clots.
Corticosteroid	Any steroid hormone secreted by the adrenal cortex, such as aldosterone, cortisol, and sex steroids is called a corticosteroid.
Resistance	Resistance refers to a nonspecific ability to ward off infection or disease regardless of whether the body has been previously exposed to it. A force that opposes the flow of a fluid such as air or blood. Compare with immunity.
Pneumonia	Pneumonia is an illness of the lungs and respiratory system in which the microscopic, air-filled sacs (alveoli) responsible for absorbing oxygen from the atmosphere become inflamed and flooded with fluid.
Population	Population refers to all members of a well-defined group of organisms, events, or things.
Syndrome	Syndrome is the association of several clinically recognizable features, signs, symptoms, phenomena or characteristics which often occur together, so that the presence of one feature alerts the physician to the presence of the others
Acquired immunodeficiency syndrome	Acquired Immunodeficiency Syndrome is defined as a collection of symptoms and infections resulting from the depletion of the immune system caused by infection with the human immunodeficiency virus, commonly called HIV.
Immunodeficiency	Immunodeficiency is a state in which the immune system's ability to fight infectious disease is compromised or entirely absent. Most cases of immunodeficiency are either congenital or acquired.
Homosexual	Homosexual refers to referring to people who are sexually aroused by and interested in forming romantic relationships with people of the same gender.
Hypodermic needle	A device for injecting a fluid into the body intramuscularly, intravenously, or subcutaneously is a hypodermic needle.
Heterosexual	Referring to people who are sexually aroused by and interested in forming romantic relationships with people of the other gender is referred to as heterosexual.
Incidence	In epidemiological studies of a particular disorder, the rate at which new cases occur in a given place at a given time is called incidence.
Retrovirus	A retrovirus is a virus which has a genome consisting of two RNA molecules, which may or may not be identical. It relies on the enzyme reverse transcriptase to perform the reverse transcription of its genome from RNA into DNA, which can then be integrated into the host's genome with an integrase enzyme.
HIV	The virus that causes AIDS is HIV (human immunodeficiency virus).
Human immunodeficiency virus	The human immunodeficiency virus is a retrovirus that primarily infects vital components of the human immune system. It is transmitted through penetrative and oral sex; blood transfusion; the sharing of contaminated needles in health care settings and through drug injection; and, between mother and infant, during pregnancy, childbirth and breastfeeding.
Causative agent	In the chain of infection, the organism capable of producing an infection is called a causative agent.
Tuberculosis	Tuberculosis is an infection caused by the bacterium Mycobacterium tuberculosis, which most commonly affects the lungs but can also affect the central nervous system, lymphatic system, circulatory system, genitourinary system, bones and joints.
Sarcoma	Cancer of the supportive tissues, such as bone, cartilage, and muscle is referred to as sarcoma.

Chapter 2. Inflammation, Immunity, and Allergy

Mycobacterium tuberculosis	Mycobacterium tuberculosis is the bacterium that causes most cases of tuberculosis. Its genome has been sequenced. It is an obligate aerobe mycobacterium (not gram positive/negative) that divides every 16 to 20 hours.
Mycobacterium	Mycobacterium is the a genus of actinobacteria, given its own family, the Mycobacteriaceae. It includes many pathogens known to cause serious diseases in mammals, including tuberculosis and leprosy.
Diarrhea	Diarrhea or diarrhoea is a condition in which the sufferer has frequent and watery, chunky, or loose bowel movements.
Lymphadenopathy	Lymphadenopathy is swelling of one or more lymph nodes.
Dementia	Dementia is progressive decline in cognitive function due to damage or disease in the brain beyond what might be expected from normal aging.
Brain	The part of the central nervous system involved in regulating and controlling body activity and interpreting information from the senses transmitted through the nervous system is referred to as the brain.
Encephalopathy	Encephalopathy is a nonspecific term describing a syndrome affecting the brain. Generally, it refers to involvement of large parts of the brain (or the whole organ), instead of identifiable changes confined to parts of the brain.
Semen	Semen is a fluid that contains spermatozoa. It is secreted by the gonads (sexual glands) of male or hermaphroditic animals including humans for fertilization of female ova. Semen discharged by an animal or human is known as ejaculate, and the process of discharge is called ejaculation.
Saliva	Saliva is the moist, clear, and usually somewhat frothy substance produced in the mouths of some animals, including humans.
Donor	Blood donation is a process by which a blood donor voluntarily has blood drawn for storage in a blood bank for subsequent use in a blood transfusion.
Asymptomatic	A disease is asymptomatic when it is at a stage where the patient does not experience symptoms. By their nature, asymptomatic diseases are not usually discovered until the patient undergoes medical tests (X-rays or other investigations). Some diseases remain asymptomatic for a remarkably long time, including some forms of cancer.
Health	Health is a term that refers to a combination of the absence of illness, the ability to cope with everyday activities, physical fitness, and high quality of life.
Variable	A characteristic or aspect in which people, objects, events, or conditions vary is called variable.
Latent	Hidden or concealed is a latent.
Epidemiology	Epidemiology is the study of the distribution and determinants of disease and disorders in human populations, and the use of its knowledge to control health problems. Epidemiology is considered the cornerstone methodology in all of public health research, and is highly regarded in evidence-based clinical medicine for identifying risk factors for disease and determining optimal treatment approaches to clinical practice.
Centers for Disease Control and Prevention	The Centers for Disease Control and Prevention in Atlanta, Georgia, is recognized as the lead United States agency for protecting the public health and safety of people by providing credible information to enhance health decisions, and promoting health through strong partnerships with state health departments and other organizations.
Pathogen	A pathogen or infectious agent is a biological agent that causes disease or illness to its host. The term is most often used for agents that disrupt the normal physiology of a

Chapter 2. Inflammation, Immunity, and Allergy

Chapter 2. Inflammation, Immunity, and Allergy

	multicellular animal or plant.
Eye	An eye is an organ that detects light. Different kinds of light-sensitive organs are found in a variety of creatures. The simplest eyes do nothing but detect whether the surroundings are light or dark, while more complex eyes can distinguish shapes and colors.
Hepatitis B	Hepatitis B is caused by a doublestranded DNA virus formerly called the 'Dane particle.' The virus is transmitted by body fluids.
Hepatitis	Hepatitis is a gastroenterological disease, featuring inflammation of the liver. The clinical signs and prognosis, as well as the therapy, depend on the cause.
Vaccine	A harmless variant or derivative of a pathogen used to stimulate a host organism's immune system to mount a long-term defense against the pathogen is referred to as vaccine.
Viral	Viral phenomena are objects or patterns able to replicate themselves or convert other objects into copies of themselves when these objects are exposed to them.
Nucleotide	A building block of a nucleic acid molecule, consisting of a sugar, a nitrogenous base, and a phosphate group is called a nucleotide.
Inhibitor	An inhibitor is a type of effector (biology) that decreases or prevents the rate of a chemical reaction. They are often called negative catalysts.
Protease	Protease refers to an enzyme that breaks peptide bonds between amino acids of proteins.
Protease inhibitor	A compound that interferes with the ability of certain enzymes to break down proteins is a protease inhibitor. They can keep a virus from making copies of itself (for example, AIDS virus protease inhibitors), and some can prevent cancer cells from spreading.
Chronic fatigue syndrome	Chronic fatigue syndrome is incapacitating exhaustion following only minimal exertion, accompanied by fever, headaches, muscle and joint pain, depression, and anxiety.
Depression	In everyday language depression refers to any downturn in mood, which may be relatively transitory and perhaps due to something trivial. This is differentiated from Clinical depression which is marked by symptoms that last two weeks or more and are so severe that they interfere with daily living.
Psychosomatic	A psychosomatic illness is one with physical manifestations and perhaps a supposed psychological cause. It is often diagnosed when any known or identifiable physical cause was excluded by medical examination.
Passive immunity	Passive immunity refers to temporary immunity obtained by acquiring ready-made antibodies or immune cells; lasts only a few weeks or months because the immune system has not been stimulated by antigens.
Toxoid	A bacterial exotoxmn that has been modified so that it is no longer toxic but will still stimulate antitoxin formation when injected into a person or animal is a toxoid.
Active immunity	Active immunity is produced when an animal's own immune system reacts to a stimulus e.g., a virus or bacteria, and produces antibodies and cells, which will protect it from the disease caused by the bacteria or virus.
Meningitis	Meningitis is inflammation of the membranes covering the brain and the spinal cord. Although the most common causes are infection (bacterial, viral, fungal or parasitic), chemical agents and even tumor cells may cause meningitis.
Measles	Measles refers to a highly contagious skin disease that is endemic throughout the world. It is caused by a morbilli virus in the family Paramyxoviridae, which enters the body through the respiratory tract or through the conjunctiva.
Immunization	Use of a vaccine to protect the body against specific disease-causing agents is called

Chapter 2. Inflammation, Immunity, and Allergy

Chapter 2. Inflammation, Immunity, and Allergy

	immunization.
Allergy	An allergy or Type I hypersensitivity is an immune malfunction whereby a person's body is hypersensitized to react immunologically to typically nonimmunogenic substances. When a person is hypersensitized, these substances are known as allergens.
Concept	A mental category used to class together objects, relations, events, abstractions, or qualities that have common properties is called concept.
Hypersensitivity	Hypersensitivity is an immune response that damages the body's own tissues. Four or five types of hypersensitivity are often described; immediate, antibody-dependent, immune complex, cell-mediated, and stimulatory.
Affinity	Chemical affinity results from electronic properties by which dissimilar substances are capable of forming chemical compounds. Specifically, the term refers to the tendency of an atom or compound to combine by chemical reaction with atoms or compounds of unlike composition.
Serotonin	Serotonin is a monoamine neurotransmitter synthesized in serotonergic neurons in the central nervous system and enterochromaffin cells in the gastrointestinal tract. It is believed to play an important part of the biochemistry of depression, migraine, bipolar disorder and anxiety.
Heparin	Heparin as a drug is used as an injectable anticoagulant. Heparin is a highly sulfated glycosaminoglycan widely used as an injectable anticoagulant. It is also used to form an inner anticoagulant surface on various experimental and medical devices such as test tubes and renal dialysis machines.
Congestion	In medicine and pathology the term congestion is used to describe excessive accumulation of blood or other fluid in a particular part of the body.
Hay fever	Hay fever is a collection of symptoms, predominantly in the nose and eyes, that occur after exposure to airborne particles of dust, dander, or the pollens of certain seasonal plants in people who are allergic to these substances.
Edema	Edema is swelling of any organ or tissue due to accumulation of excess fluid. Edema has many root causes, but its common mechanism is accumulation of fluid into the tissues.
Antihistamine	An antihistamine is a drug which serves to reduce or eliminate effects mediated by histamine, an endogenous chemical mediator released during allergic reactions, through action at the histamine receptor.
Shock	Circulatory shock, a state of cardiac output that is insufficient to meet the body's physiological needs, with consequences ranging from fainting to death is referred to as shock. Insulin shock, a state of severe hypoglycemia caused by administration of insulin.
Anaphylactic shock	A precipitous drop in blood pressure caused by loss of fluid from capillaries because of an increase in their permeability stimulated by an allergic reaction is called anaphylactic shock.
Anaphylaxis	Anaphylaxis refers to an immediate hypersensitivity reaction following exposure of a sensitized individual to the appropriate antigen.
Activation	As reflected by facial expressions, the degree of arousal a person is experiencing is referred to as activation.
Anaphylactic reaction	A severe overreaction or even fatal shock due to the effects of a drug is referred to as anaphylactic reaction.
Hypotension	In physiology and medicine, hypotension refers to an abnormally low blood pressure. It is often associated with shock, though not necessarily indicative of it.

Chapter 2. Inflammation, Immunity, and Allergy

Asthma	Asthma is a complex disease characterized by bronchial hyperresponsiveness (BHR), inflammation, mucus production and intermittent airway obstruction.
Muscle contraction	A muscle contraction occurs when a muscle cell (called a muscle fiber) shortens. There are three general types: skeletal, heart, and smooth.
Respiratory tract	In humans the respiratory tract is the part of the anatomy that has to do with the process of respiration or breathing.
Smooth muscle	Smooth muscle is a type of non-striated muscle, found within the "walls" of hollow organs; such as blood vessels, the bladder, the uterus, and the gastrointestinal tract. Smooth muscle is used to move matter within the body, via contraction; it generally operates "involuntarily", without nerve stimulation.
Tracheotomy	A tracheotomy is a surgical procedure performed on the neck to open a direct airway through an incision in the trachea
Trachea	Trachea is an airway through which respiratory gas transport takes place in organisms. In terrestrial vertebrates, such as birds and humans, the trachea lets air move from the throat to the lungs. In terrestrial invertebrates, such as onychophorans and beetles, they conduct air from outside the organism directly to all of its internal tissues.
Larynx	The larynx is an organ in the neck of mammals involved in protection of the trachea and sound production. The larynx houses the vocal cords, and is situated at the point where the upper tract splits into the trachea and the esophagus.
Cramp	A cramp is an unpleasant sensation caused by contraction, usually of a muscle. It can be caused by cold or overexertion.
Seizure	A seizure is a temporary alteration in brain function expressed as a changed mental state, tonic or clonic movements and various other symptoms. They are due to temporary abnormal electrical activity of a group of brain cells.
Blood pressure	Blood pressure is the pressure exerted by the blood on the walls of the blood vessels.
Epinephrine	Epinephrine is a hormone and a neurotransmitter. Epinephrine plays a central role in the short-term stress reaction—the physiological response to threatening or exciting conditions (fight-or-flight response). It is secreted by the adrenal medulla.
Injection	A method of rapid drug delivery that puts the substance directly in the bloodstream, in a muscle, or under the skin is called injection.
Intramuscular Injection	You have intramuscular injection when a needle is inserted in a muscle, usually a large muscle, and the drug is injected into that muscle.
Penicillin	Penicillin refers to a group of β-lactam antibiotics used in the treatment of bacterial infections caused by susceptible, usually Gram-positive, organisms.
Insulin	Insulin is a polypeptide hormone that regulates carbohydrate metabolism. Apart from being the primary effector in carbohydrate homeostasis, it also has a substantial effect on small vessel muscle tone, controls storage and release of fat (triglycerides) and cellular uptake of both amino acids and some electrolytes.
Serum	Serum is the same as blood plasma except that clotting factors (such as fibrin) have been removed. Blood plasma contains fibrinogen.
Hemolysis	The rupture of red blood cells accompanied by the release of hemoglobin is called hemolysis.
Red blood cells	Red blood cells are the most common type of blood cell and are the vertebrate body's principal means of delivering oxygen from the lungs or gills to body tissues via the blood.
Red blood cell	The red blood cell is the most common type of blood cell and is the vertebrate body's

Chapter 2. Inflammation, Immunity, and Allergy

Chapter 2. Inflammation, Immunity, and Allergy

	principal means of delivering oxygen from the lungs or gills to body tissues via the blood.
Fetus	Fetus refers to a developing human from the ninth week of gestation until birth; has all the major structures of an adult.
Inhalation	Inhalation is the movement of air from the external environment, through the airways, into the alveoli during breathing.
Glomerulonep-ritis	Glomerulonephritis is a primary or secondary autoimmune renal disease characterized by inflammation of the glomeruli. It may be asymptomatic, or present with hematuria and/or proteinuria (blood resp. protein in the urine).
Cytokine	A type of protein secreted by a T lymphocyte that attacks viruses, virally infected cells, and cancer cells is referred to as cytokine.
Acquired immune deficiency syndrome	Acquired Immune Deficiency Syndrome is defined as a collection of symptoms and infections resulting from the depletion of the immune system caused by infection with the human immunodeficiency virus, commonly called HIV.
Tetanus	Tetanus is a serious and often fatal disease caused by the neurotoxin tetanospasmin which is produced by the Gram-positive, obligate anaerobic bacterium Clostridium tetani. Tetanus also refers to a state of muscle tension.
Critical thinking	Critical thinking consists of a mental process of analyzing or evaluating information, particularly statements or propositions that people have offered as true. It forms a process of reflecting upon the meaning of statements, examining the offered evidence and reasoning, and forming judgments about the facts.
Antiserum	Serum containing induced antibodies is an antiserum.
Infectious disease	In medicine, infectious disease or communicable disease is disease caused by a biological agent such as by a virus, bacterium or parasite. This is contrasted to physical causes, such as burns or chemical ones such as through intoxication.
World Health Organization	The World Health Organization (WHO) is a specialized agency of the United Nations, acting as a coordinating authority on international public health, headquartered in Geneva, Switzerland.
Elderly	Old age consists of ages nearing the average life span of human beings, and thus the end of the human life cycle. Euphemisms for older people include advanced adult, elderly, and senior or senior citizen.

Chapter 2. Inflammation, Immunity, and Allergy

Chapter 3. Infectious Diseases

Infectious disease	In medicine, infectious disease or communicable disease is disease caused by a biological agent such as by a virus, bacterium or parasite. This is contrasted to physical causes, such as burns or chemical ones such as through intoxication.
Tuberculosis	Tuberculosis is an infection caused by the bacterium Mycobacterium tuberculosis, which most commonly affects the lungs but can also affect the central nervous system, lymphatic system, circulatory system, genitourinary system, bones and joints.
Microorganism	A microorganism or microbe is an organism that is so small that it is microscopic (invisible to the naked eye).
Influenza	Influenza or flu refers to an acute viral infection of the respiratory tract, occurring in isolated cases, epidemics, and pandemics. Influenza is caused by three strains of influenza virus, labeled types A, B, and C, based on the antigens of their protein coats.
Measles	Measles refers to a highly contagious skin disease that is endemic throughout the world. It is caused by a morbilli virus in the family Paramyxoviridae, which enters the body through the respiratory tract or through the conjunctiva.
Pathogen	A pathogen or infectious agent is a biological agent that causes disease or illness to its host. The term is most often used for agents that disrupt the normal physiology of a multicellular animal or plant.
Bacteria	The domain that contains procaryotic cells with primarily diacyl glycerol diesters in their membranes and with bacterial rRNA. Bacteria also is a general term for organisms that are composed of procaryotic cells and are not multicellular.
Organelle	Organelle refers to any structure within a cell that carries out one of its metabolic roles, such as mitochondria, centrioles, endoplasmic reticulum, and the nucleus.
Cell wall	A cell wall is a more or less solid layer surrounding a cell. They are found in bacteria, archaea, fungi, plants, and algae.
Diagnosis	In medicine, diagnosis is the process of identifying a medical condition or disease by its signs, symptoms, and from the results of various diagnostic procedures.
Mutation	A change in the structure of a gene is called a mutation.
Radiation	The emission of electromagnetic waves by all objects warmer than absolute zero is referred to as radiation.
Acid	An acid is a water-soluble, sour-tasting chemical compound that when dissolved in water, gives a solution with a pH of less than 7.
Botulism	Botulism is a rare but serious paralytic illness caused by a nerve toxin, botulin, that is produced by the bacterium Clostridium botulinum.
Tetanus	Tetanus is a serious and often fatal disease caused by the neurotoxin tetanospasmin which is produced by the Gram-positive, obligate anaerobic bacterium Clostridium tetani. Tetanus also refers to a state of muscle tension.
Wound	A wound is type of physical trauma wherein the skin is torn, cut or punctured, or where blunt force trauma causes a contusion.
Physiology	The study of the function of cells, tissues, and organs is referred to as physiology.
Toxin	Toxin refers to a microbial product or component that can injure another cell or organism at low concentrations. Often the term refers to a poisonous protein, but toxins may be lipids and other substances.
Muscle	Muscle is a contractile form of tissue. It is one of the four major tissue types, the other three being epithelium, connective tissue and nervous tissue. Muscle contraction is used to

Chapter 3. Infectious Diseases

Chapter 3. Infectious Diseases

	move parts of the body, as well as to move substances within the body.
Shock	Circulatory shock, a state of cardiac output that is insufficient to meet the body's physiological needs, with consequences ranging from fainting to death is referred to as shock. Insulin shock, a state of severe hypoglycemia caused by administration of insulin.
Infection	The invasion and multiplication of microorganisms in body tissues is called an infection.
Immune response	The body's defensive reaction to invasion by bacteria, viral agents, or other foreign substances is called immune response.
Fever	Fever (also known as pyrexia, or a febrile response, and archaically known as ague) is a medical symptom that describes an increase in internal body temperature to levels that are above normal (37°C, 98.6°F).
Pain	Pain is an unpleasant sensation which may be associated with actual or potential tissue damage and which may have physical and emotional components.
Peptic ulcer	Peptic ulcer is an ulcer of one of those areas of the gastrointestinal tract that are usually acidic.
Salmonella	Salmonella is a genus of rod-shaped Gram-negative enterobacteria that causes typhoid fever, paratyphoid and foodborne illness. It is motile in nature and produces hydrogen sulfide.
Pneumonia	Pneumonia is an illness of the lungs and respiratory system in which the microscopic, air-filled sacs (alveoli) responsible for absorbing oxygen from the atmosphere become inflamed and flooded with fluid.
Chlamydia	A sexually transmitted disease, caused by a bacterium, that causes inflammation of the urethra in males and of the urethra and cervix in females is referred to as chlamydia.
Bacillus	Bacillus is a genus of rod-shaped bacteria.
Diarrhea	Diarrhea or diarrhoea is a condition in which the sufferer has frequent and watery, chunky, or loose bowel movements.
Protein	A protein is a complex, high-molecular-weight organic compound that consists of amino acids joined by peptide bonds. They are essential to the structure and function of all living cells and viruses. Many are enzymes or subunits of enzymes.
Lipid	Lipid is one class of aliphatic hydrocarbon-containing organic compounds essential for the structure and function of living cells. They are characterized by being water-insoluble but soluble in nonpolar organic solvents.
Ulcer	An ulcer is an open sore of the skin, eyes or mucous membrane, often caused by an initial abrasion and generally maintained by an inflammation and/or an infection.
DNA	Deoxyribonucleic acid (DNA) is a nucleic acid —usually in the form of a double helix— that contains the genetic instructions specifying the biological development of all cellular forms of life, and most viruses.
Staphylococcus	Staphylococcus is a genus of gram-positive bacteria. Under the microscope they appear round (cocci), and form in grape-like clusters.
Epithelium	Epithelium is a tissue composed of a layer of cells. Epithelium can be found lining internal (e.g. endothelium, which lines the inside of blood vessels) or external (e.g. skin) free surfaces of the body. Functions include secretion, absorption and protection.
Immune system	The immune system is the system of specialized cells and organs that protect an organism from outside biological influences. When the immune system is functioning properly, it protects the body against bacteria and viral infections, destroying cancer cells and foreign substances.

Go to Cram101.com for the Practice Tests for this Chapter.

Chapter 3. Infectious Diseases

Chapter 3. Infectious Diseases

Latent	Hidden or concealed is a latent.
Immunodeficiency	Immunodeficiency is a state in which the immune system's ability to fight infectious disease is compromised or entirely absent. Most cases of immunodeficiency are either congenital or acquired.
Cancer	Cancer is a class of diseases or disorders characterized by uncontrolled division of cells and the ability of these cells to invade other tissues, either by direct growth into adjacent tissue through invasion or by implantation into distant sites by metastasis.
Human papillomavirus	Human papillomavirus is a member of a group of viruses in the genus Papillomavirus that can infect humans and cause changes in cells leading to abnormal tissue growth.
Cervical cancer	Cervical cancer is a malignancy of the cervix. Worldwide, it is the second most common cancer of women.
Eukaryotic	Eukaryotic cells are generally much larger than prokaryotes, typically a thousand times by volume. They have a variety of internal membranes and structures, called organelles, and a cytoskeleton composed of microtubules and microfilaments, which play an important role in defining the cell's organization.
Extension	Movement increasing the angle between parts at a joint is referred to as extension.
Dysentery	Dysentery is an illness involving severe diarrhea that is often associated with blood in the feces. It is caused by ingestion of food containing bacteria, causing a disease in which inflammation of the intestines affect the body significantly.
Health	Health is a term that refers to a combination of the absence of illness, the ability to cope with everyday activities, physical fitness, and high quality of life.
Giardiasis	Giardiasis is a disease caused by the flagellate protozoan Giardia lamblia. The giardia organism inhabits the digestinal tract of a wide variety of domestic and wild animal species as well as humans. It is a common cause of gastroenteritis in humans, infecting approximately 200 million people worldwide.
Sleeping sickness	Sleeping sickness or African trypanosomiasis is a parasitic disease in people and in animals. Caused by protozoa of genus Trypanosoma and transmitted by the tsetse fly, the disease is endemic in certain regions of Sub-Saharan Africa, covering about 36 countries and 60 million people.
Projection	Attributing one's own undesirable thoughts, impulses, traits, or behaviors to others is referred to as projection.
Cilia	Microscopic, hairlike processes on the exposed surfaces of certain epithelial cells are cilia.
Malaria	Malaria refers to potentially fatal human disease caused by the protozoan parasite Plasmodium, which is transmitted by the bite of an infected mosquito.
Tissue	A collection of interconnected cells that perform a similar function within an organism is called tissue.
Inflammatory response	Inflammatory response refers to a complex sequence of events involving chemicals and immune cells that results in the isolation and destruction of antigens and tissues near the antigens.
Fungi	Fungi refers to simple parasitic life forms, including molds, mildews, yeasts, and mushrooms. They live on dead or decaying organic matter. Fungi can grow as single cells, like yeast, or as multicellular colonies, as seen with molds.
Polysaccharide	A carbohydrate composed of many joined monosaccharides is called a polysaccharide.

Chapter 3. Infectious Diseases

Chapter 3. Infectious Diseases

Absorption	Absorption is a physical or chemical phenomenon or a process in which atoms, molecules, or ions enter some bulk phase - gas, liquid or solid material. In nutrition, amino acids are broken down through digestion, which begins in the stomach.
Inflammation	Inflammation is the first response of the immune system to infection or irritation and may be referred to as the innate cascade.
Allergy	An allergy or Type I hypersensitivity is an immune malfunction whereby a person's body is hypersensitized to react immunologically to typically nonimmunogenic substances. When a person is hypersensitized, these substances are known as allergens.
Organ	Organ refers to a structure consisting of several tissues adapted as a group to perform specific functions.
Candidiasis	Candidiasis, commonly called yeast infection, is a fungal infection of any of the Candida species. Yeast organisms are always present in all people, but are usually prevented from "overgrowth" by naturally occurring microorganisms.
Skin	Skin is an organ of the integumentary system composed of a layer of tissues that protect underlying muscles and organs.
Hepatitis A	Hepatitis A is an enterovirus transmitted by the orofecal route, such as contaminated food. It causes an acute form of hepatitis and does not have a chronic stage.
Hepatitis	Hepatitis is a gastroenterological disease, featuring inflammation of the liver. The clinical signs and prognosis, as well as the therapy, depend on the cause.
Shingles	A reactivated form of chickenpox caused by the varicella-zoster virus is shingles. It leads to a crop of painful blisters over the area of a dermatome.
Serum	Serum is the same as blood plasma except that clotting factors (such as fibrin) have been removed. Blood plasma contains fibrinogen.
Herpes simplex	Herpes simplex refers to two common types of viruses, herpes simplex virus 1 and herpes simplex virus 2. Herpes simplex virus 2 is responsible for the STD known as genital herpes.
Ringworm	Ringworm is a contagious fungal infection of the skin. Ringworm is very common, especially among children, and may be spread by skin-to-skin contact, as well as via contact with contaminated items such as hairbrushes.
Host	Host is an organism that harbors a parasite, mutual partner, or commensal partner; or a cell infected by a virus.
Intestine	The intestine is the portion of the alimentary canal extending from the stomach to the anus and, in humans and mammals, consists of two segments, the small intestine and the large intestine. The intestine is the part of the body responsible for extracting nutrition from food.
Large intestine	In anatomy of the digestive system, the colon, also called the large intestine or large bowel, is the part of the intestine from the cecum ('caecum' in British English) to the rectum. Its primary purpose is to extract water from feces.
Blood	Blood is a circulating tissue composed of fluid plasma and cells. The main function of blood is to supply nutrients (oxygen, glucose) and constitutional elements to tissues and to remove waste products.
Blood vessel	A blood vessel is a part of the circulatory system and function to transport blood throughout the body. The most important types, arteries and veins, are so termed because they carry blood away from or towards the heart, respectively.
Egg	An egg is the zygote, resulting from fertilization of the ovum. It nourishes and protects the

Chapter 3. Infectious Diseases

Chapter 3. Infectious Diseases

	embryo.
Urine	Concentrated filtrate produced by the kidneys and excreted via the bladder is called urine.
Exoskeleton	An exoskeleton is an external anatomical feature that supports and protects an animal's body. Many invertebrate animals such as insects, crustaceans and shellfish have an exoskeleton.
Vector	A vector is an organism that does not cause disease itself but which spreads infection by conveying pathogens from one host to another.
Reservoir	Reservoir is the source of infection. It is the environment in which microorganisms are able to live and grow.
Lyme disease	Lyme disease refers to a debilitating human disease caused by the bacterium Borrelia burgdorferi; characterized at first by a red rash at the site of a tick bite and, if not treated, by heart disease, arthritis, and nervous disorders.
Rabies	Rabies refers to an acute infectious disease of the central nervous system, which affects all warmblooded animals, It is caused by an ssRNA virus belonging to the genus Lv.ssaviru.s in the family Rhabdoviridae.
Epidemiology	Epidemiology is the study of the distribution and determinants of disease and disorders in human populations, and the use of its knowledge to control health problems. Epidemiology is considered the cornerstone methodology in all of public health research, and is highly regarded in evidence-based clinical medicine for identifying risk factors for disease and determining optimal treatment approaches to clinical practice.
Distribution	Distribution in pharmacology is a branch of pharmacokinetics describing reversible transfer of drug from one location to another within the body.
Semen	Semen is a fluid that contains spermatozoa. It is secreted by the gonads (sexual glands) of male or hermaphroditic animals including humans for fertilization of female ova. Semen discharged by an animal or human is known as ejaculate, and the process of discharge is called ejaculation.
Hepatitis B	Hepatitis B is caused by a doublestranded DNA virus formerly called the 'Dane particle.' The virus is transmitted by body fluids.
HIV	The virus that causes AIDS is HIV (human immunodeficiency virus).
Gonorrhea	Gonorrhea refers to an acute infectious sexually transmitted disease of the mucous membranes of the genitourinary tract, eye, rectum, and throat. It is caused by Neisseria gonorrhoeae.
Sexually transmitted disease	Infection transmitted from one individual to another by direct contact during sexual activity is referred to as a sexually transmitted disease.
Population	Population refers to all members of a well-defined group of organisms, events, or things.
Incidence	In epidemiological studies of a particular disorder, the rate at which new cases occur in a given place at a given time is called incidence.
Epidemic	An epidemic is a disease that appears as new cases in a given human population, during a given period, at a rate that substantially exceeds what is "expected", based on recent experience.
Pandemic	Pandemic refers to an increase in the occurrence of a disease within a large and geographically widespread population.
Constant	A behavior or characteristic that does not vary from one observation to another is referred to as a constant.

Go to Cram101.com for the Practice Tests for this Chapter.

Chapter 3. Infectious Diseases

Chapter 3. Infectious Diseases

Centers for Disease Control and Prevention	The Centers for Disease Control and Prevention in Atlanta, Georgia, is recognized as the lead United States agency for protecting the public health and safety of people by providing credible information to enhance health decisions, and promoting health through strong partnerships with state health departments and other organizations.
Isolation	Isolation refers to the degree to which groups do not live in the same communities.
Disinfection	Disinfection is the destruction of pathogenic and other kinds of microorganisms by physical or chemical means.
Standard precaution	Standard precaution refers to the recommended work practice for protection against transmission of bloodborne pathogens and other infectious diseases in the workplace
Cholera	Cholera is a water-borne disease caused by the bacterium Vibrio cholerae, which are typically ingested by drinking contaminated water, or by eating improperly cooked fish, especially shellfish.
Antibiotic	Antibiotic refers to substance such as penicillin or streptomycin that is toxic to microorganisms. Usually a product of a particular microorvanism or plant.
Penicillin	Penicillin refers to a group of β-lactam antibiotics used in the treatment of bacterial infections caused by susceptible, usually Gram-positive, organisms.
Resistance	Resistance refers to a nonspecific ability to ward off infection or disease regardless of whether the body has been previously exposed to it. A force that opposes the flow of a fluid such as air or blood. Compare with immunity.
Antibiotic resistance	Antibiotic resistance is the ability of a microorganism to withstand the effects of an antibiotic. Antibiotic resistance naturally develops via natural selection through random mutation and plasmid exchange between bacteria of the same species.
Adaptation	A biological adaptation is an anatomical structure, physiological process or behavioral trait of an organism that has evolved over a period of time by the process of natural selection such that it increases the expected long-term reproductive success of the organism.
Common cold	An acute, self-limiting, and highly contagious virus infection of the upper respiratory tract that produces inflammation, profuse discharge, and other symptoms is referred to as the common cold.
Viral	Viral phenomena are objects or patterns able to replicate themselves or convert other objects into copies of themselves when these objects are exposed to them.
Exudate	An exudate is any fluid that filters from the circulatory system into leisions or areas of inflamation. Its composition varies but generally includes water and the disolved solutes of the blood, some or all plasma proteins, white blood cells, platelets and red blood cells.
Antigen	An antigen is a substance that stimulates an immune response, especially the production of antibodies. They are usually proteins or polysaccharides, but can be any type of molecule, including small molecules (haptens) coupled to a protein (carrier).
Nucleic acid	A nucleic acid is a complex, high-molecular-weight biochemical macromolecule composed of nucleotide chains that convey genetic information.
Base	The common definition of a base is a chemical compound that absorbs hydronium ions when dissolved in water (a proton acceptor). An alkali is a special example of a base, where in an aqueous environment, hydroxide ions are donated.
Affect	Affect is the scientific term used to describe a subject's externally displayed mood. This can be assesed by the nurse by observing facial expression, tone of voice, and body language.
Metabolism	Metabolism is the biochemical modification of chemical compounds in living organisms and

Chapter 3. Infectious Diseases

Chapter 3. Infectious Diseases

	cells. This includes the biosynthesis of complex organic molecules (anabolism) and their breakdown (catabolism).
Carbohydrate	Carbohydrate is a chemical compound that contains oxygen, hydrogen, and carbon atoms. They consist of monosaccharide sugars of varying chain lengths and that have the general chemical formula $C_n(H_2O)_n$ or are derivatives of such.
Immunity	Resistance to the effects of specific disease-causing agents is called immunity.
Vaccine	A harmless variant or derivative of a pathogen used to stimulate a host organism's immune system to mount a long-term defense against the pathogen is referred to as vaccine.
Virus	Obligate intracellular parasite of living cells consisting of an outer capsid and an inner core of nucleic acid is referred to as virus. The term virus usually refers to those particles that infect eukaryotes whilst the term bacteriophage or phage is used to describe those infecting prokaryotes.
Smallpox	Once a highly contagious, often fatal disease caused by a poxvirus. Its most noticeable symptom was the appearance of blisters and pustules on the skin. Vaccination has eradicated smallpox throughout the world.
Diphtheria	Diphtheria refers to an acute, highly contagious childhood disease that generally affects the membranes of the throat and less frequently the nose. It is caused by Corynehacterium diphtheriae.
Morbidity	Morbidity refers to any condition that causes illness.
Mortality	The incidence of death in a population is mortality.
Pathology	Pathology is the study of the processes underlying disease and other forms of illness, harmful abnormality, or dysfunction.
Yellow fever	Yellow fever refers to an acute infectious disease caused by a flavivirus, which is transmitted to humans by mosquitoes. The liver is affected and the skin turns yellow in this disease.
Elevation	Elevation refers to upward movement of a part of the body.
World Health Organization	The World Health Organization (WHO) is a specialized agency of the United Nations, acting as a coordinating authority on international public health, headquartered in Geneva, Switzerland.
Malnutrition	Malnutrition is a general term for the medical condition in a person or animal caused by an unbalanced diet—either too little or too much food, or a diet missing one or more important nutrients.
Basic research	Basic research has as its primary objective the advancement of knowledge and the theoretical understanding of the relations among variables . It is exploratory and often driven by the researcher's curiosity, interest or hunch.
Critical thinking	Critical thinking consists of a mental process of analyzing or evaluating information, particularly statements or propositions that people have offered as true. It forms a process of reflecting upon the meaning of statements, examining the offered evidence and reasoning, and forming judgments about the facts.
Neoplasm	Neoplasm refers to abnormal growth of cells; often used to mean a tumor.

Chapter 3. Infectious Diseases

Chapter 4. Neoplasms

Cancer	Cancer is a class of diseases or disorders characterized by uncontrolled division of cells and the ability of these cells to invade other tissues, either by direct growth into adjacent tissue through invasion or by implantation into distant sites by metastasis.
Neoplasm	Neoplasm refers to abnormal growth of cells; often used to mean a tumor.
Tumor	An abnormal mass of cells that forms within otherwise normal tissue is a tumor. This growth can be either malignant or benign
Pain	Pain is an unpleasant sensation which may be associated with actual or potential tissue damage and which may have physical and emotional components.
Remission	Disappearance of the signs of a disease is called remission.
Epidemiology	Epidemiology is the study of the distribution and determinants of disease and disorders in human populations, and the use of its knowledge to control health problems. Epidemiology is considered the cornerstone methodology in all of public health research, and is highly regarded in evidence-based clinical medicine for identifying risk factors for disease and determining optimal treatment approaches to clinical practice.
Benzene	Benzene is an organic chemical compound that is a colorless and flammable liquid with a pleasant, sweet smell. Benzene is a known carcinogen. It is a minor, or additive, component of gasoline. It is an important industrial solvent and precursor in the production of drugs, plastics, gasoline, synthetic rubber, and dyes.
Arsenic	Arsenic is a chemical element in the periodic table that has the symbol As and atomic number 33. This is a notoriously poisonous metalloid that has many allotropic forms; yellow, black and grey are a few that are regularly seen. Arsenic and its compounds are used as pesticides, herbicides, insecticides and various alloys.
Risk factor	A risk factor is a variable associated with an increased risk of disease or infection but risk factors are not necessarily causal.
Skin	Skin is an organ of the integumentary system composed of a layer of tissues that protect underlying muscles and organs.
Radiation	The emission of electromagnetic waves by all objects warmer than absolute zero is referred to as radiation.
Leukemia	Leukemia refers to a type of cancer of the bloodforming tissues, characterized by an excessive production of white blood cells and an abnormally high number of them in the blood; cancer of the bone marrow cells that produce leukocytes.
Thyroid	The thyroid is one of the larger endocrine glands in the body. It is located in the neck and produces hormones, principally thyroxine and triiodothyronine, that regulate the rate of metabolism and affect the growth and rate of function of many other systems in the body.
Radon	Radon refers to a radioactive gas that is formed by the disintegration of radium, radon is one of the heaviest gases and is considered to be a health hazard.
Ionizing radiation	Ionizing radiation is a type of particle radiation in which an individual particle carries enough energy to ionize an atom or molecule. If the individual particles do not carry this amount of energy, it is essentially impossible for even a large flood of particles to cause ionization.
Lungs	Lungs are the essential organs of respiration in air-breathing vertebrates. Their principal function is to transport oxygen from the atmosphere into the bloodstream, and to excrete carbon dioxide from the bloodstream into the atmosphere.
Lung cancer	Lung cancer is a malignant tumour of the lungs. Most commonly it is bronchogenic carcinoma (about 90%).

Go to Cram101.com for the Practice Tests for this Chapter.

Chapter 4. Neoplasms

Chapter 4. Neoplasms

Genes	Genes are the units of heredity in living organisms. They are encoded in the organism's genetic material (usually DNA or RNA), and control the development and behavior of the organism.
Infection	The invasion and multiplication of microorganisms in body tissues is called an infection.
Viral	Viral phenomena are objects or patterns able to replicate themselves or convert other objects into copies of themselves when these objects are exposed to them.
Virus	Obligate intracellular parasite of living cells consisting of an outer capsid and an inner core of nucleic acid is referred to as virus. The term virus usually refers to those particles that infect eukaryotes whilst the term bacteriophage or phage is used to describe those infecting prokaryotes.
Colon	The colon is the part of the intestine from the cecum to the rectum. Its primary purpose is to extract water from feces.
Liver	The liver is an organ in vertebrates, including humans. It plays a major role in metabolism and has a number of functions in the body including drug detoxification, glycogen storage, and plasma protein synthesis. It also produces bile, which is important for digestion.
Lesion	A lesion is a non-specific term referring to abnormal tissue in the body. It can be caused by any disease process including trauma (physical, chemical, electrical), infection, neoplasm, metabolic and autoimmune.
Hormone	A hormone is a chemical messenger from one cell to another. All multicellular organisms produce hormones. The best known hormones are those produced by endocrine glands of vertebrate animals, but hormones are produced by nearly every organ system and tissue type in a human or animal body. Hormone molecules are secreted directly into the bloodstream, they move by circulation or diffusion to their target cells, which may be nearby cells in the same tissue or cells of a distant organ of the body.
Puberty	A time in the life of a developing individual characterized by the increasing production of sex hormones, which cause it to reach sexual maturity is called puberty.
Testosterone	Testosterone is a steroid hormone from the androgen group. Testosterone is secreted in the testes of men and the ovaries of women. It is the principal male sex hormone and the "original" anabolic steroid. In both males and females, it plays key roles in health and well-being.
Prostate	The prostate is a gland that is part of male mammalian sex organs. Its main function is to secrete and store a clear, slightly basic fluid that is part of semen. The prostate differs considerably between species anatomically, chemically and physiologically.
Gland	A gland is an organ in an animal's body that synthesizes a substance for release such as hormones, often into the bloodstream or into cavities inside the body or its outer surface.
Agent	Agent refers to an epidemiological term referring to the organism or object that transmits a disease from the environment to the host.
Predisposition	Predisposition refers to an inclination or diathesis to respond in a certain way, either inborn or acquired. In abnormal psychology, it is a factor that lowers the ability to withstand stress and inclines the individual toward pathology.
Estrogen	Estrogen is a steroid that functions as the primary female sex hormone. While present in both men and women, they are found in women in significantly higher quantities.
Ovaries	Ovaries are egg-producing reproductive organs found in female organisms.
Ovary	The primary reproductive organ of a female is called an ovary.

Chapter 4. Neoplasms

Chapter 4. Neoplasms

Chronic disease	Disease of long duration often not detected in its early stages and from which the patient will not recover is referred to as a chronic disease.
Carcinogen	A carcinogen is any substance or agent that promotes cancer. A carcinogen is often, but not necessarily, a mutagen or teratogen.
Carcinogenesis	Carcinogenesis is the process by which normal cells are transformed into cancer cells.
DNA	Deoxyribonucleic acid (DNA) is a nucleic acid —usually in the form of a double helix— that contains the genetic instructions specifying the biological development of all cellular forms of life, and most viruses.
Tissue	A collection of interconnected cells that perform a similar function within an organism is called tissue.
Immune system	The immune system is the system of specialized cells and organs that protect an organism from outside biological influences. When the immune system is functioning properly, it protects the body against bacteria and viral infections, destroying cancer cells and foreign substances.
Causative agent	In the chain of infection, the organism capable of producing an infection is called a causative agent.
Nerve	A nerve is an enclosed, cable-like bundle of nerve fibers or axons, which includes the glia that ensheath the axons in myelin.
Rectum	The rectum is the final straight portion of the large intestine in some mammals, and the gut in others, terminating in the anus.
Vagina	The vagina is the tubular tract leading from the uterus to the exterior of the body in female placental mammals and marsupials, or to the cloaca in female birds, monotremes, and some reptiles. Female insects and other invertebrates also have a vagina, which is the terminal part of the oviduct.
Sputum	The mucous secretion from the lungs, bronchi, and trachea that is ejected through the mouth is sputum.
Urine	Concentrated filtrate produced by the kidneys and excreted via the bladder is called urine.
Blood	Blood is a circulating tissue composed of fluid plasma and cells. The main function of blood is to supply nutrients (oxygen, glucose) and constitutional elements to tissues and to remove waste products.
Cyst	A cyst is a closed sac having a distinct membrane and developing abnormally in a cavity or structure of the body. They may occur as a result of a developmental error in the embryo during pregnancy or they may be caused by infections.
Mammography	Mammography is the process of using low-dose X-rays (usually around 0.7 mSv) to examine the human breast. It is used to look for different types of tumors and cysts.
Respiratory tract	In humans the respiratory tract is the part of the anatomy that has to do with the process of respiration or breathing.
Diarrhea	Diarrhea or diarrhoea is a condition in which the sufferer has frequent and watery, chunky, or loose bowel movements.
Constipation	Constipation is a condition of the digestive system where a person (or other animal) experiences hard feces that are difficult to eliminate; it may be extremely painful, and in severe cases (fecal impaction) lead to symptoms of bowel obstruction.
Urination	Urination is the process of disposing urine from the urinary bladder through the urethra to the outside of the body. The process of urination is usually under voluntary control.

Go to Cram101.com for the Practice Tests for this Chapter.

Chapter 4. Neoplasms

Urgency	Urgency is an intense and sudden desire to urinate.
Urinary system	The urinary system is the organ system that produces, stores, and carries urine. In humans it includes two kidneys, two ureters, the urinary bladder, two sphincter muscles, and the urethra.
Dysphagia	Dysphagia is the medical term for the symptom of difficulty in swallowing.
Anorexia	Anorexia nervosa is an eating disorder characterized by voluntary starvation and exercise stress.
Gastrointestnal tract	The gastrointestinal tract is the system of organs within multicellular animals which takes in food, digests it to extract energy and nutrients, and expels the remaining waste.
Bone marrow	Bone marrow is the tissue comprising the center of large bones. It is the place where new blood cells are produced. Bone marrow contains two types of stem cells: hemopoietic (which can produce blood cells) and stromal (which can produce fat, cartilage and bone).
Anemia	Anemia is a deficiency of red blood cells and/or hemoglobin. This results in a reduced ability of blood to transfer oxygen to the tissues, and this causes hypoxia; since all human cells depend on oxygen for survival, varying degrees of anemia can have a wide range of clinical consequences.
Affect	Affect is the scientific term used to describe a subject's externally displayed mood. This can be assesed by the nurse by observing facial expression, tone of voice, and body language.
Chemotherapy	Chemotherapy is the use of chemical substances to treat disease. In its modern-day use, it refers almost exclusively to cytostatic drugs used to treat cancer. In its non-oncological use, the term may also refer to antibiotics.
Endocrine gland	An endocrine gland is one of a set of internal organs involved in the secretion of hormones into the blood. These glands are known as ductless, which means they do not have tubes inside them.
Body cavity	A fluid-containing space between the digestive tract and the body wall is referred to as body cavity.
Carcinoma	Cancer that originates in the coverings of the body, such as the skin or the lining of the intestinal tract is a carcinoma.
Pancreas	The pancreas is a retroperitoneal organ that serves two functions: exocrine - it produces pancreatic juice containing digestive enzymes, and endocrine - it produces several important hormones, namely insulin.
Stomach	The stomach is an organ in the alimentary canal used to digest food. It's primary function is not the absorption of nutrients from digested food; rather, the main job of the stomach is to break down large food molecules into smaller ones, so that they can be absorbed into the blood more easily.
Sarcoma	Cancer of the supportive tissues, such as bone, cartilage, and muscle is referred to as sarcoma.
Cartilage	Cartilage is a type of dense connective tissue. Cartilage is composed of cells called chondrocytes which are dispersed in a firm gel-like ground substance, called the matrix. Cartilage is avascular (contains no blood vessels) and nutrients are diffused through the matrix.
Muscle	Muscle is a contractile form of tissue. It is one of the four major tissue types, the other three being epithelium, connective tissue and nervous tissue. Muscle contraction is used to move parts of the body, as well as to move substances within the body.

Chapter 4. Neoplasms

Chapter 4. Neoplasms

Connective tissue	Connective tissue is any type of biological tissue with an extensive extracellular matrix and often serves to support, bind together, and protect organs.
Lymph	Lymph originates as blood plasma lost from the circulatory system, which leaks out into the surrounding tissues. The lymphatic system collects this fluid by diffusion into lymph capillaries, and returns it to the circulatory system.
Benign tumor	A benign tumor does not invade neighboring tissues and do not seed metastases, but may locally grow to great size. They usually do not return after surgical removal.
Spinal cord	The spinal cord is a part of the vertebrate nervous system that is enclosed in and protected by the vertebral column (it passes through the spinal canal). It consists of nerve cells. The spinal cord carries sensory signals and motor innervation to most of the skeletal muscles in the body.
Brain	The part of the central nervous system involved in regulating and controlling body activity and interpreting information from the senses transmitted through the nervous system is referred to as the brain.
Nervous system	The nervous system of an animal coordinates the activity of the muscles, monitors the organs, constructs and processes input from the senses, and initiates actions.
Esophagus	The esophagus, or gullet is the muscular tube in vertebrates through which ingested food passes from the mouth area to the stomach. Food is passed through the esophagus by using the process of peristalsis.
Trachea	Trachea is an airway through which respiratory gas transport takes place in organisms. In terrestrial vertebrates, such as birds and humans, the trachea lets air move from the throat to the lungs. In terrestrial invertebrates, such as onychophorans and beetles, they conduct air from outside the organism directly to all of its internal tissues.
Lead	Lead is a chemical element in the periodic table that has the symbol Pb and atomic number 82. A soft, heavy, toxic and malleable poor metal, lead is bluish white when freshly cut but tarnishes to dull gray when exposed to air. Lead is used in building construction, lead-acid batteries, bullets and shot, and is part of solder, pewter, and fusible alloys.
Anterior pituitary	The anterior pituitary comprises the anterior lobe of the pituitary gland and is part of the endocrine system. Under the influence of the hypothalamus, the anterior pituitary produces and secretes several peptide hormones that regulate many physiological processes including stress, growth, and reproduction.
Pituitary gland	The pituitary gland or hypophysis is an endocrine gland about the size of a pea that sits in the small, bony cavity (sella turcica) at the base of the brain. Its posterior lobe is connected to a part of the brain called the hypothalamus via the infundibulum (or stalk), giving rise to the tuberoinfundibular pathway.
Growth hormone	Growth hormone is a polypeptide hormone synthesised and secreted by the anterior pituitary gland which stimulates growth and cell reproduction in humans and other vertebrate animals.
Androgen	Androgen is the generic term for any natural or synthetic compound, usually a steroid hormone, that stimulates or controls the development and maintenance of masculine characteristics in vertebrates by binding to androgen receptors.
Adrenal	In mammals, the adrenal glands are the triangle-shaped endocrine glands that sit atop the kidneys. They are chiefly responsible for regulating the stress response through the synthesis of corticosteroids and catecholamines, including cortisol and adrenaline.
Masculinization	Prenatal virilization, or masculinization, of a genetically female fetus can occur when an excessive amount of androgen is produced by the fetal adrenal glands or is present in maternal blood.

Go to Cram101.com for the Practice Tests for this Chapter.

Chapter 4. Neoplasms

Chapter 4. Neoplasms

Adrenal gland	In mammals, the adrenal gland (also known as suprarenal glands or colloquially as kidney hats) are the triangle-shaped endocrine glands that sit atop the kidneys; their name indicates that position.
Fibroids	Uterine fibroids are the most common neoplasm in females, and may affect about of 25 % of white and 50% of black women during the reproductive years. Fibroids may be removed simply by means of a hysterectomy, but much more favourably by a myomectomy or by uterine artery embolization, which preserve the uterus.
Uterus	The uterus is the major female reproductive organ of most mammals. One end, the cervix, opens into the vagina; the other is connected on both sides to the fallopian tubes. The main function is to accept a fertilized ovum which becomes implanted into the endometrium, and derives nourishment from blood vessels which develop exclusively for this purpose.
Smooth muscle	Smooth muscle is a type of non-striated muscle, found within the "walls" of hollow organs; such as blood vessels, the bladder, the uterus, and the gastrointestinal tract. Smooth muscle is used to move matter within the body, via contraction; it generally operates "involuntarily", without nerve stimulation.
Abortion	An abortion is the termination of a pregnancy associated with the death of an embryo or a fetus.
Spontaneous abortion	Spontaneous abortion is the natural or accidental termination of a pregnancy at a stage where the embryo or the fetus is incapable of surviving, generally defined at a gestation less than 20 weeks.
Port	A port is a central venous line that does not have an external connector; instead, it has a small reservoir implanted under the skin.
Blood vessel	A blood vessel is a part of the circulatory system and function to transport blood throughout the body. The most important types, arteries and veins, are so termed because they carry blood away from or towards the heart, respectively.
Lymph vessel	Lymph vessel refers to one of the system of vessels carrying lymph from the lymph capillaries to the veins.
Melanoma	Melanoma is a malignant tumor of melanocytes. Melanocytes predominantly occur in the skin but can be found elsewhere, especially the eye. The vast majority of melanomas originate in the skin.
Wart	A wart is a generally small, rough, cauliflower-like growth, of viral origin, typically on hands and feet.
Adenoma	Adenoma refers to a collection of growths of glandular origin. They can grow from many organs including the colon, adrenal, pituitary, thyroid, etc. These growths are benign, but some are known to have the potential, over time, to transform to malignancy
Sweat gland	Gland responsible for the loss of a watery fluid, consisting mainly of sodium chloride (commonly known as salt) and urea in solution, that is secreted through the skin is a sweat gland.
Epidermis	Epidermis is the outermost layer of the skin. It forms the waterproof, protective wrap over the body's surface and is made up of stratified squamous epithelium with an underlying basement membrane. It contains no blood vessels, and is nourished by diffusion from the dermis. In plants, the outermost layer of cells covering the leaves and young parts of a plant is the epidermis.
Sebaceous	The sebaceous glands are glands found in the skin of mammals. They secrete an oily substance called sebum that is made of fat (lipids) and the debris of dead fat-producing cells.

Chapter 4. Neoplasms

Chapter 4. Neoplasms

Acute	In medicine, an acute disease is a disease with either or both of: a rapid onset; and a short course (as opposed to a chronic course).
Amino acid	An amino acid is any molecule that contains both amino and carboxylic acid functional groups. They are the basic structural building units of proteins. They form short polymer chains called peptides or polypeptides which in turn form structures called proteins.
Glucose	Glucose, a simple monosaccharide sugar, is one of the most important carbohydrates and is used as a source of energy in animals and plants. Glucose is one of the main products of photosynthesis and starts respiration.
Acid	An acid is a water-soluble, sour-tasting chemical compound that when dissolved in water, gives a solution with a pH of less than 7.
Cachexia	Cachexia is loss of weight, muscle wasting, fatigue, weakness and anorexia (not anorexia nervosa) in someone who is not actively trying to lose weight.
Melanocyte	Melanocyte cells are located in the bottom layer of the skin's epidermis. With a process called melanogenesis, they produce melanin, a pigment in the skin, eyes, and hair.
Abdomen	The abdomen is a part of the body. In humans, and in many other vertebrates, it is the region between the thorax and the pelvis. In fully developed insects, the abdomen is the third (or posterior) segment, after the head and thorax.
Prognosis	Prognosis refers to the prospects for the future or outcome of a disease.
Metastasis	The spread of cancer cells beyond their original site are called metastasis.
Organ	Organ refers to a structure consisting of several tissues adapted as a group to perform specific functions.
Lymph node	A lymph node acts as a filter, with an internal honeycomb of connective tissue filled with lymphocytes that collect and destroy bacteria and viruses. When the body is fighting an infection, these lymphocytes multiply rapidly and produce a characteristic swelling of the lymph node.
Diagnosis	In medicine, diagnosis is the process of identifying a medical condition or disease by its signs, symptoms, and from the results of various diagnostic procedures.
Pathology	Pathology is the study of the processes underlying disease and other forms of illness, harmful abnormality, or dysfunction.
Cervix	The cervix is actually the lower, narrow portion of the uterus where it joins with the top end of the vagina. It is cylindrical or conical in shape and protrudes through the upper anterior vaginal wall.
Primary tumor	Primary tumor is the nomenclature used when the tumor has originated in the same organ, and has not metastasized to it.
Radiation therapy	Treatment for cancer in which parts of the body that have cancerous tumors are exposed to high-energy radiation to disrupt cell division of the cancer cells is called radiation therapy.
Inhibitor	An inhibitor is a type of effector (biology) that decreases or prevents the rate of a chemical reaction. They are often called negative catalysts.
Immunity	Resistance to the effects of specific disease-causing agents is called immunity.
Leukopenia	Too few leukocytes in the blood is called leukopenia.
White blood cell	The white blood cell is a a component of blood. They help to defend the body against infectious disease and foreign materials as part of the immune system.

Chapter 4. Neoplasms

Chapter 4. Neoplasms

Oral cavity	The mouth, also known as the buccal cavity or the oral cavity, is the opening through which an animal or human takes in food and water. It is usually located in the head, but not always; the mouth of a planarium is in the middle of its belly.
Testes	The testes are the male generative glands in animals. Male mammals have two testes, which are often contained within an extension of the abdomen called the scrotum.
Lifestyle	The culturally, socially, economically, and environmentally conditioned complex of actions characteristic of an individual, group, or community as a pattern of habituated behavior over time that is health related but not necessarily health directed is a lifestyle.
Bronchitis	Bronchitis is an obstructive pulmonary disease characterized by inflammation of the bronchi of the lungs.
Emphysema	Emphysema is a chronic lung disease. It is often caused by exposure to toxic chemicals or long-term exposure to tobacco smoke..
Chronic bronchitis	A persistent lung infection characterized by coughing, swelling of the lining of the respiratory tract, an increase in mucus production, a decrease in the number and activity of cilia, and produces sputum for at least three months in two consecutive years is called chronic bronchitis.
Fiber	Fibers used by man come from a wide variety of sources: Natural fiber include those made out of plants, animal and mineral sources. Natural fibers can be classified according to their origin.
Carotene	Carotene is an orange photosynthetic pigment important for photosynthesis. It is responsible for the orange color of the carrot and many other fruits and vegetables. It contributes to photosynthesis by transmitting the light energy it absorbs to chlorophyll.
Vitamin	An organic compound other than a carbohydrate, lipid, or protein that is needed for normal metabolism but that the body cannot synthesize in adequate amounts is called a vitamin.
Mortality	The incidence of death in a population is mortality.
Incidence	In epidemiological studies of a particular disorder, the rate at which new cases occur in a given place at a given time is called incidence.
Cervical cancer	Cervical cancer is a malignancy of the cervix. Worldwide, it is the second most common cancer of women.
Human papillomavirus	Human papillomavirus is a member of a group of viruses in the genus Papillomavirus that can infect humans and cause changes in cells leading to abnormal tissue growth.
Genital warts	A sexually transmitted disease, caused by a virus, that forms growths or bumps on the external genitalia, in or around the vagina or anus, or on the cervix in females or penis, scrotum, groin, or thigh in males are called genital warts.
Alcohol	Alcohol is a general term, applied to any organic compound in which a hydroxyl group (-OH) is bound to a carbon atom, which in turn is bound to other hydrogen and/or carbon atoms. The general formula for a simple acyclic alcohol is $C_nH_{2n+1}OH$.
Alcoholic	An alcoholic is dependent on alcohol as characterized by craving, loss of control, physical dependence and withdrawal symptoms, and tolerance.
Hip	In anatomy, the hip is the bony projection of the femur, known as the greater trochanter, and the overlying muscle and fat.
Palpation	Palpation is a method of examination in which the examiner feels the size or shape or firmness or location of something.
Areola	In anatomy, the term areola is used to describe any small circular area such as the colored

Chapter 4. Neoplasms

	skin surrounding the nipple.
Scrotum	In some male mammals the scrotum is an external bag of skin and muscle containing the testicles. It is an extension of the abdomen, and is located between the penis and anus.
Epididymis	The epididymis is part of the human male reproductive system and is present in all male mammals. It is a narrow, tightly-coiled tube connecting the efferent ducts from the rear of each testicle to its vas deferens.

Chapter 4. Neoplasms

Chapter 5. Hereditary Diseases

DNA	Deoxyribonucleic acid (DNA) is a nucleic acid —usually in the form of a double helix— that contains the genetic instructions specifying the biological development of all cellular forms of life, and most viruses.
Value	Value is worth in general, and it is thought to be connected to reasons for certain practices, policies, actions, beliefs or emotions. Value is "that which one acts to gain and/or keep."
Epidermis	Epidermis is the outermost layer of the skin. It forms the waterproof, protective wrap over the body's surface and is made up of stratified squamous epithelium with an underlying basement membrane. It contains no blood vessels, and is nourished by diffusion from the dermis. In plants, the outermost layer of cells covering the leaves and young parts of a plant is the epidermis.
Dermis	The dermis is the layer of skin beneath the epidermis that consists of connective tissue and cushions the body from stress and strain.
Skin	Skin is an organ of the integumentary system composed of a layer of tissues that protect underlying muscles and organs.
Protein	A protein is a complex, high-molecular-weight organic compound that consists of amino acids joined by peptide bonds. They are essential to the structure and function of all living cells and viruses. Many are enzymes or subunits of enzymes.
Acid	An acid is a water-soluble, sour-tasting chemical compound that when dissolved in water, gives a solution with a pH of less than 7.
Cell division	Cell division (or local doubling) is the process by which a cell, called the parent cell divides into two cells, called daughter cells. Cell division is usually a small segment of a larger cell cycle.
Chromosomes	Physical structures in the cell's nucleus that house the genes. Each human cell has 23 pairs of chromosomes.
Genes	Genes are the units of heredity in living organisms. They are encoded in the organism's genetic material (usually DNA or RNA), and control the development and behavior of the organism.
Autosomes	Autosomes refer to chromosomes number 1 to 22; do not include the sex chromosomes.
Karyotype	A set of chromosomes characteristic of a species arranged in homologous pairs is referred to as a karyotype. The human karyotype has 23 chromosome pairs.
Eye	An eye is an organ that detects light. Different kinds of light-sensitive organs are found in a variety of creatures. The simplest eyes do nothing but detect whether the surroundings are light or dark, while more complex eyes can distinguish shapes and colors.
Alleles	Genes coding for the same trait and found at the same locus on homologous chromosomes are called alleles.
Allele	Different forms of a gene are called an allele.
Homozygous	When an organism is referred to as being homozygous for a specific gene, it means that it carries two identical copies of that gene for a given trait on the two corresponding chromosomes (e.g., the genotype is AA or aa). Such a cell or such an organism is called a homozygote.
Heterozygous	When an organism is referred to as a heterozygote or as being heterozygous for a specific gene, it means that the organism carries a different version of that gene on each of the two corresponding chromosomes.

Chapter 5. Hereditary Diseases

Chapter 5. Hereditary Diseases

Blood type	A blood type is a description of an individual's characteristics of red blood cells due to substances (carbohydrates and proteins) on the cell membrane. The two most important classifications to describe blood types in humans are ABO and the Rhesus factor (Rh factor).
Blood	Blood is a circulating tissue composed of fluid plasma and cells. The main function of blood is to supply nutrients (oxygen, glucose) and constitutional elements to tissues and to remove waste products.
Autosomal dominant	An autosomal dominant gene is one that occurs on an autosomal (non-sex determining) chromosome. As it is dominant, the phenotype it gives will be expressed even if the gene is heterozygous. This contrasts with recessive genes, which need to be homozygous to be expressed.
Cartilage	Cartilage is a type of dense connective tissue. Cartilage is composed of cells called chondrocytes which are dispersed in a firm gel-like ground substance, called the matrix. Cartilage is avascular (contains no blood vessels) and nutrients are diffused through the matrix.
Achondroplasia	Achondroplasia refers to a form of human dwarfism caused by a single dominant allele. The homozygous condition is lethal.
Skeleton	In biology, the skeleton or skeletal system is the biological system providing physical support in living organisms.
Carrier	Person in apparent health whose chromosomes contain a pathologic mutant gene that may be transmitted to his or her children is a carrier.
Galactosemia	A rare genetic disease characterized by the buildup of the single sugar galactose in the bloodstream, resulting from the inability of the liver to metabolize it is called galactosemia.
Gamete	A gamete is a specialized germ cell that unites with another gamete during fertilization in organisms that reproduce sexually. They are haploid cells; that is, they contain one complete set of chromosomes. When they unite they form a zygote—a cell having two complete sets of chromosomes and therefore diploid.
Phenylketonuria	Phenylketonuria is a genetic disorder in which an individual cannot properly metabolize amino acids. The disorder is now easily detected but, if left untreated, results in mental retardation and hyperactivity.
Amino acid	An amino acid is any molecule that contains both amino and carboxylic acid functional groups. They are the basic structural building units of proteins. They form short polymer chains called peptides or polypeptides which in turn form structures called proteins.
Tyrosine	Tyrosine is one of the 20 amino acids that are used by cells to synthesize proteins. It plays a key role in signal transduction, since it can be tagged (phosphorylated) with a phosphate group by protein kinases to alter the functionality and activity of certain enzymes.
Enzyme	An enzyme is a protein that catalyzes, or speeds up, a chemical reaction. They are essential to sustain life because most chemical reactions in biological cells would occur too slowly, or would lead to different products, without them.
Phenylalanine	Phenylalanine is an essential amino acid. The genetic disorder phenylketonuria is an inability to metabolize phenylalanine.
Mental retardation	Mental retardation refers to having significantly below-average intellectual functioning and limitations in at least two areas of adaptive functioning. Many categorize retardation as mild, moderate, severe, or profound.
Severe mental	A limitation in mental development as measured on the Wechsler Adult Intelligence Scale with

Go to Cram101.com for the Practice Tests for this Chapter.

Chapter 5. Hereditary Diseases

retardation	scores between 20-34 is called severe mental retardation.
Melanin	Broadly, melanin is any of the polyacetylene, polyaniline, and polypyrrole "blacks" or their mixed copolymers. The most common form of biological melanin is a polymer of either or both of two monomer molecules: indolequinone, and dihydroxyindole carboxylic acid.
Convulsions	Involuntary muscle spasms, often severe, that can be caused by stimulant overdose or by depressant withdrawal are called convulsions.
Nervous system	The nervous system of an animal coordinates the activity of the muscles, monitors the organs, constructs and processes input from the senses, and initiates actions.
Metabolism	Metabolism is the biochemical modification of chemical compounds in living organisms and cells. This includes the biosynthesis of complex organic molecules (anabolism) and their breakdown (catabolism).
Inborn error of metabolism	An inborn error of metabolism comprises a large class of genetic diseases involving disorders of metabolism. The majority are due to defects of single genes that code for enzymes that facilitate conversion of various substances (substrates) into others (products).
Galactose	Galactose is a type of sugar found in dairy products, in sugar beets and other gums and mucilages. It is also synthesized by the body, where it forms part of glycolipids and glycoproteins in several tissues.
Liver	The liver is an organ in vertebrates, including humans. It plays a major role in metabolism and has a number of functions in the body including drug detoxification, glycogen storage, and plasma protein synthesis. It also produces bile, which is important for digestion.
Brain	The part of the central nervous system involved in regulating and controlling body activity and interpreting information from the senses transmitted through the nervous system is referred to as the brain.
Ascites	Serous fluid accumulation in the abdominal cavity is ascites.
Diarrhea	Diarrhea or diarrhoea is a condition in which the sufferer has frequent and watery, chunky, or loose bowel movements.
Diagnosis	In medicine, diagnosis is the process of identifying a medical condition or disease by its signs, symptoms, and from the results of various diagnostic procedures.
Lactose	Lactose is a disaccharide that makes up around 2-8% of the solids in milk. Lactose is a disaccharide consisting of two subunits, a galactose and a glucose linked together.
Anemia	Anemia is a deficiency of red blood cells and/or hemoglobin. This results in a reduced ability of blood to transfer oxygen to the tissues, and this causes hypoxia; since all human cells depend on oxygen for survival, varying degrees of anemia can have a wide range of clinical consequences.
Red blood cells	Red blood cells are the most common type of blood cell and are the vertebrate body's principal means of delivering oxygen from the lungs or gills to body tissues via the blood.
Red blood cell	The red blood cell is the most common type of blood cell and is the vertebrate body's principal means of delivering oxygen from the lungs or gills to body tissues via the blood.
Capillaries	Capillaries refer to the smallest of the blood vessels and the sites of exchange between the blood and tissue cells.
Capillary	A capillary is the smallest of a body's blood vessels, measuring 5-10 micro meters. They connect arteries and veins, and most closely interact with tissues. Their walls are composed of a single layer of cells, the endothelium. This layer is so thin that molecules such as oxygen, water and lipids can pass through them by diffusion and enter the tissues.

Chapter 5. Hereditary Diseases

Chapter 5. Hereditary Diseases

Necrosis	Necrosis is the name given to unprogrammed death of cells/living tissue. There are many causes of necrosis including injury, infection, cancer, infarction, and inflammation. Necrosis is caused by special enzymes that are released by lysosomes.
Tissue	A collection of interconnected cells that perform a similar function within an organism is called tissue.
Spleen	The spleen is a ductless, vertebrate gland that is not necessary for life but is closely associated with the circulatory system, where it functions in the destruction of old red blood cells and removal of other debris from the bloodstream, and also in holding a reservoir of blood.
Hemoglobin	Hemoglobin is the iron-containing oxygen-transport metalloprotein in the red cells of the blood in mammals and other animals. Hemoglobin transports oxygen from the lungs to the rest of the body, such as to the muscles, where it releases the oxygen load.
Sickle cell trait	Sickle cell trait describes the way a person can inherit some of the genes of sickle cell disease, but not develop symptoms.
Resistance	Resistance refers to a nonspecific ability to ward off infection or disease regardless of whether the body has been previously exposed to it. A force that opposes the flow of a fluid such as air or blood. Compare with immunity.
Malaria	Malaria refers to potentially fatal human disease caused by the protozoan parasite Plasmodium, which is transmitted by the bite of an infected mosquito.
Affect	Affect is the scientific term used to describe a subject's externally displayed mood. This can be assesed by the nurse by observing facial expression, tone of voice, and body language.
Lipid	Lipid is one class of aliphatic hydrocarbon-containing organic compounds essential for the structure and function of living cells. They are characterized by being water-insoluble but soluble in nonpolar organic solvents.
Y chromosome	Male sex chromosome that carries genes involved in sex determination is referred to as the Y chromosome. It contains the genes that cause testis development, thus determining maleness.
Recessive gene	Recessive gene refers to a gene that will not be expressed if paired with a dominant gene but will be expressed if paired with another recessive gene.
Receptor	A receptor is a protein on the cell membrane or within the cytoplasm or cell nucleus that binds to a specific molecule (a ligand), such as a neurotransmitter, hormone, or other substance, and initiates the cellular response to the ligand. Receptor, in immunology, the region of an antibody which shows recognition of an antigen.
Retina	The retina is a thin layer of cells at the back of the eyeball of vertebrates and some cephalopods; it is the part of the eye which converts light into nervous signals.
Hemophilia	Hemophilia is the name of any of several hereditary genetic illnesses that impair the body's ability to control bleeding. Genetic deficiencies cause lowered plasma clotting factor activity so as to compromise blood-clotting; when a blood vessel is injured, a scab will not form and the vessel can continue to bleed excessively for a very long period of time.
Epidemiology	Epidemiology is the study of the distribution and determinants of disease and disorders in human populations, and the use of its knowledge to control health problems. Epidemiology is considered the cornerstone methodology in all of public health research, and is highly regarded in evidence-based clinical medicine for identifying risk factors for disease and determining optimal treatment approaches to clinical practice.
Fragile X	The fragile X syndrome is a genetic disorder caused by mutation of the FMR1 gene on the X chromosome. Mutation at that site is found in 1 out of about every 2000 males and 1 out of

Go to Cram101.com for the Practice Tests for this Chapter.

Chapter 5. Hereditary Diseases

Chapter 5. Hereditary Diseases

	about every 4000 females.
Syndrome	Syndrome is the association of several clinically recognizable features, signs, symptoms, phenomena or characteristics which often occur together, so that the presence of one feature alerts the physician to the presence of the others
Fragile X syndrome	Fragile X Syndrome is the most common inherited cause of mental retardation, and the most common known cause of autism. Fragile X syndrome is a genetic disorder caused by mutation of the FMR1 gene on the X chromosome, a mutation found in 1 out of every 2000 males and 1 out of every 4000 females.
Population	Population refers to all members of a well-defined group of organisms, events, or things.
Joint	A joint (articulation) is the location at which two bones make contact (articulate). They are constructed to both allow movement and provide mechanical support.
Gametes	Gametes —also known as sex cells, or spores—are the specialized germ cells that come together during fertilization (conception) in organisms that reproduce sexually.
Intervention	Intervention refers to a planned attempt to break through addicts' or abusers' denial and get them into treatment. Interventions most often occur when legal, workplace, health, relationship, or financial problems have become intolerable.
Medical intervention	Medical intervention refers to the use of medications to treat a substance-related or mental disorder. This is usually done in combination with group/individual therapy or other treatment techniques.
Hyperactivity	Hyperactivity can be described as a state in which a individual is abnormally easily excitable and exuberant. Strong emotional reactions and a very short span of attention is also typical for the individual.
Physical therapy	Physical therapy is a health profession concerned with the assessment, diagnosis, and treatment of disease and disability through physical means. It is based upon principles of medical science, and is generally held to be within the sphere of conventional medicine.
Fetus	Fetus refers to a developing human from the ninth week of gestation until birth; has all the major structures of an adult.
Sperm	Sperm refers to the male sex cell with three distinct parts at maturity: head, middle piece, and tail.
Egg	An egg is the zygote, resulting from fertilization of the ovum. It nourishes and protects the embryo.
Nondisjunction	Nondisjunction is the failure of a chromosome to split correctly during meiosis. This results in the production of gametes which have either more or less of the usual amount of genetic material, and is a common mechanism for trisomy or monosomy. Nondisjunction can occur in the meiosis I or meiosis II phases of cellular reproduction.
Pneumonia	Pneumonia is an illness of the lungs and respiratory system in which the microscopic, air-filled sacs (alveoli) responsible for absorbing oxygen from the atmosphere become inflamed and flooded with fluid.
Infection	The invasion and multiplication of microorganisms in body tissues is called an infection.
Respiratory tract	In humans the respiratory tract is the part of the anatomy that has to do with the process of respiration or breathing.
Susceptibility	The degree of resistance of a host to a pathogen is susceptibility.
Incidence	In epidemiological studies of a particular disorder, the rate at which new cases occur in a given place at a given time is called incidence.

Go to **Cram101.com** for the Practice Tests for this Chapter.

Chapter 5. Hereditary Diseases

Leukemia	Leukemia refers to a type of cancer of the bloodforming tissues, characterized by an excessive production of white blood cells and an abnormally high number of them in the blood; cancer of the bone marrow cells that produce leukocytes.
Medial	In anatomical terms of location toward or near the midline is called medial.
Organ	Organ refers to a structure consisting of several tissues adapted as a group to perform specific functions.
Transverse	A transverse (also known as axial or horizontal) plane is an X-Y plane, parallel to the ground, which (in humans) separates the superior from the inferior, or put another way, the head from the feet.
Menstruation	Loss of blood and tissue from the uterine lining at the end of a female reproductive cycle are referred to as menstruation.
Ovulation	Ovulation is the process in the menstrual cycle by which a mature ovarian follicle ruptures and discharges an ovum (also known as an oocyte, female gamete, or casually, an egg) that participates in reproduction.
Ovaries	Ovaries are egg-producing reproductive organs found in female organisms.
Ovary	The primary reproductive organ of a female is called an ovary.
Puberty	A time in the life of a developing individual characterized by the increasing production of sex hormones, which cause it to reach sexual maturity is called puberty.
Secondary sex characteristics	Secondary sex characteristics are traits that distinguish the two sexes of a species, but that are not directly part of the reproductive system.
Distribution	Distribution in pharmacology is a branch of pharmacokinetics describing reversible transfer of drug from one location to another within the body.
Testes	The testes are the male generative glands in animals. Male mammals have two testes, which are often contained within an extension of the abdomen called the scrotum.
Hermaphrodite	Hermaphrodite refers to an organism of a species whose members possess both male and female sexual organs during their lives. In many species, hermaphroditism is a normal part of the life-cycle. Generally, hermaphroditism occurs in the invertebrates, although it occurs in a fair number of fish, and to a lesser degree in other vertebrates.
Anatomy	Anatomy is the branch of biology that deals with the structure and organization of living things. It can be divided into animal anatomy (zootomy) and plant anatomy (phytonomy).
Genitals	Genitals refers to the internal and external reproductive organs.
Conception	Conception is fusion of gametes to form a new organism. In animals, the process involves a sperm fusing with an ovum, which eventually leads to the development of an embryo.
Hormone	A hormone is a chemical messenger from one cell to another. All multicellular organisms produce hormones. The best known hormones are those produced by endocrine glands of vertebrate animals, but hormones are produced by nearly every organ system and tissue type in a human or animal body. Hormone molecules are secreted directly into the bloodstream, they move by circulation or diffusion to their target cells, which may be nearby cells in the same tissue or cells of a distant organ of the body.
Gland	A gland is an organ in an animal's body that synthesizes a substance for release such as hormones, often into the bloodstream or into cavities inside the body or its outer surface.
Gonad	Gonad refers to a sex organ in an animal; an ovary or a testis. It is the organ that makes gametes.

Go to Cram101.com for the Practice Tests for this Chapter.

Chapter 5. Hereditary Diseases

Chapter 5. Hereditary Diseases

Adrenal	In mammals, the adrenal glands are the triangle-shaped endocrine glands that sit atop the kidneys. They are chiefly responsible for regulating the stress response through the synthesis of corticosteroids and catecholamines, including cortisol and adrenaline.
Cortex	In anatomy and zoology the cortex is the outermost or superficial layer of an organ or the outer portion of the stem or root of a plant.
Adrenal cortex	Situated along the perimeter of the adrenal gland, the adrenal cortex mediates the stress response through the production of mineralocorticoids and glucocorticoids, including aldosterone and cortisol respectively. It is also a secondary site of androgen synthesis.
Genitalia	The Latin term genitalia is used to describe the sex organs, and in the English language this term and genital area are most often used to describe the externally visible sex organs or external genitalia: in males the penis and scrotum, in females the vulva.
Embryonic stage	The embryonic stage lasts from the third through the eighth week following conception. During this stage the major organ systems undergo rapid differentiation.
Malnutrition	Malnutrition is a general term for the medical condition in a person or animal caused by an unbalanced diet—either too little or too much food, or a diet missing one or more important nutrients.
Radiation	The emission of electromagnetic waves by all objects warmer than absolute zero is referred to as radiation.
Oxygen	Oxygen is a chemical element in the periodic table. It has the symbol O and atomic number 8. Oxygen is the second most common element on Earth, composing around 46% of the mass of Earth's crust and 28% of the mass of Earth as a whole, and is the third most common element in the universe.
Trimester	In human development, one of three 3-mnonth-long periods of pregnancy is called trimester.
First trimester	The first trimester is the period of time from the first day of the last menstrual period through 12 weeks of gestation. It is during this period that the embryo undergoes most of its early structural development. Most miscarriages occur during this period.
Rubella	An infectious disease that, if contracted by the mother during the first three months of pregnancy, has a high risk of causing mental retardation and physical deformity in the child is called rubella.
Embryo	A prenatal stage of development after germ layers form but before the rudiments of all organs are present is referred to as an embryo.
Virus	Obligate intracellular parasite of living cells consisting of an outer capsid and an inner core of nucleic acid is referred to as virus. The term virus usually refers to those particles that infect eukaryotes whilst the term bacteriophage or phage is used to describe those infecting prokaryotes.
Central nervous system	The central nervous system comprized of the brain and spinal cord, represents the largest part of the nervous system. Together with the peripheral nervous system, it has a fundamental role in the control of behavior.
Placental barrier	The placental barrier between the fetus and the wall of the mother's uterus allows for the transfer of materials from mother, and eliminates waste products of fetus.
Viral	Viral phenomena are objects or patterns able to replicate themselves or convert other objects into copies of themselves when these objects are exposed to them.
Cerebral palsy	Cerebral palsy is a group of permanent disorders associated with developmental brain injuries that occur during fetal development, birth, or shortly after birth. It is characterized by a disruption of motor skills, with symptoms such as spasticity, paralysis, or seizures.

Chapter 5. Hereditary Diseases

Chapter 5. Hereditary Diseases

Hydrocephalus	Hydrocephalus is an abnormal accumulation of cerebrospinal fluid in the ventricles of the brain. This increase in intracranial volume results in elevated intracranial pressure and compression of the brain.
Vaccine	A harmless variant or derivative of a pathogen used to stimulate a host organism's immune system to mount a long-term defense against the pathogen is referred to as vaccine.
Paralysis	Paralysis is the complete loss of muscle function for one or more muscle groups. Paralysis may be localized, or generalized, or it may follow a certain pattern.
Syphilis	Syphilis is a sexually transmitted disease that is caused by a spirochaete bacterium, Treponema pallidum. If not treated, syphilis can cause serious effects such as damage to the nervous system, heart, or brain. Untreated syphilis can be ultimately fatal.
Congenital syphilis	Syphilis that is acquired in utero from the mother is referred to as congenital syphilis.
Stillbirth	A stillbirth occurs when a fetus, of mid-second trimester to full term gestational age, which has died in the womb or during labour or delivery, exits the maternal body.
Penicillin	Penicillin refers to a group of β-lactam antibiotics used in the treatment of bacterial infections caused by susceptible, usually Gram-positive, organisms.
Atresia	Atresia is a condition in which a body orifice or passage in the body is abnormally closed or absent. Examples of atresia include biliary atresia.
Gastrointestinal tract	The gastrointestinal tract is the system of organs within multicellular animals which takes in food, digests it to extract energy and nutrients, and expels the remaining waste.
Esophagus	The esophagus, or gullet is the muscular tube in vertebrates through which ingested food passes from the mouth area to the stomach. Food is passed through the esophagus by using the process of peristalsis.
Trachea	Trachea is an airway through which respiratory gas transport takes place in organisms. In terrestrial vertebrates, such as birds and humans, the trachea lets air move from the throat to the lungs. In terrestrial invertebrates, such as onychophorans and beetles, they conduct air from outside the organism directly to all of its internal tissues.
Stomach	The stomach is an organ in the alimentary canal used to digest food. It's primary function is not the absorption of nutrients from digested food; rather, the main job of the stomach is to break down large food molecules into smaller ones, so that they can be absorbed into the blood more easily.
Esophageal atresia	Esophageal atresia is a congenital medical condition (birth defect) which affects the alimentary tract. It causes the esophagus to end in a blind-ended pouch rather than connecting normally to the stomach.
Dehydration	Dehydration is the removal of water from an object. Medically, dehydration is a serious and potentially life-threatening condition in which the body contains an insufficient volume of water for normal functioning.
Intestine	The intestine is the portion of the alimentary canal extending from the stomach to the anus and, in humans and mammals, consists of two segments, the small intestine and the large intestine. The intestine is the part of the body responsible for extracting nutrition from food.
Abdomen	The abdomen is a part of the body. In humans, and in many other vertebrates, it is the region between the thorax and the pelvis. In fully developed insects, the abdomen is the third (or posterior) segment, after the head and thorax.
Stool	Stool is the waste matter discharged in a bowel movement.

Chapter 5. Hereditary Diseases

Chapter 5. Hereditary Diseases

Bile duct	A bile duct is any of a number of long tube-like structures that carry bile. The top half of the common bile duct is associated with the liver, while the bottom half of the common bile duct is associated with the pancreas, through which it passes on its way to the intestine. It opens in the part of the intestine called the duodenum into a structure called the ampulla of Vater.
Duodenum	The duodenum is a hollow jointed tube connecting the stomach to the jejunum. It is the first part of the small intestine. Two very important ducts open into the duodenum, namely the bile duct and the pancreatic duct. The duodenum is largely responsible for the breakdown of food in the small intestine.
Jaundice	Jaundice is yellowing of the skin, sclera (the white of the eyes) and mucous membranes caused by increased levels of bilirubin in the human body.
Bile	Bile is a bitter, greenish-yellow alkaline fluid secreted by the liver of most vertebrates. In many species, it is stored in the gallbladder between meals and upon eating is discharged into the duodenum where it aids the process of digestion.
Sphincter	Muscle that surrounds a tube and closes or opens the tube by contracting and relaxing is referred to as sphincter.
Stenosis	A stenosis is an abnormal narrowing in a blood vessel or other tubular organ or structure. It is also sometimes called a "stricture" (as in urethral stricture).
Muscle	Muscle is a contractile form of tissue. It is one of the four major tissue types, the other three being epithelium, connective tissue and nervous tissue. Muscle contraction is used to move parts of the body, as well as to move substances within the body.
Pyloric stenosis	Infantile Pyloric stenosis is an uncommon paediatric condition where there is a congenital narrowing of the pylorus (the opening at the lower end of the stomach). Males are more commonly affected than females.
Constipation	Constipation is a condition of the digestive system where a person (or other animal) experiences hard feces that are difficult to eliminate; it may be extremely painful, and in severe cases (fecal impaction) lead to symptoms of bowel obstruction.
Diabetes	Diabetes is a medical disorder characterized by varying or persistent elevated blood sugar levels, especially after eating. All types of diabetes share similar symptoms and complications at advanced stages: dehydration and ketoacidosis, cardiovascular disease, chronic renal failure, retinal damage which can lead to blindness, nerve damage which can lead to erectile dysfunction, gangrene with risk of amputation of toes, feet, and even legs.
Epilepsy	Epilepsy is a chronic neurological condition characterized by recurrent unprovoked neural discharges. It is commonly controlled with medication, although surgical methods are used as well.
Allergy	An allergy or Type I hypersensitivity is an immune malfunction whereby a person's body is hypersensitized to react immunologically to typically nonimmunogenic substances. When a person is hypersensitized, these substances are known as allergens.
Lens	The lens or crystalline lens is a transparent, biconvex structure in the eye that, along with the cornea, helps to refract light to focus on the retina. Its function is thus similar to a man-made optical lens.
Alcoholism	A disorder that involves long-term, repeated, uncontrolled, compulsive, and excessive use of alcoholic beverages and that impairs the drinker's health and work and social relationships is called alcoholism.
Obesity	The state of being more than 20 percent above the average weight for a person of one's height is called obesity.

Chapter 5. Hereditary Diseases

Chapter 5. Hereditary Diseases

Go to **Cram101.com** for the Practice Tests for this Chapter.

Chapter 5. Hereditary Diseases

Chapter 6. Dietary Deficiencies and Excesses: Malnutrition, Obesity, and Alcoholism

Metabolism	Metabolism is the biochemical modification of chemical compounds in living organisms and cells. This includes the biosynthesis of complex organic molecules (anabolism) and their breakdown (catabolism).
Oxygen	Oxygen is a chemical element in the periodic table. It has the symbol O and atomic number 8. Oxygen is the second most common element on Earth, composing around 46% of the mass of Earth's crust and 28% of the mass of Earth as a whole, and is the third most common element in the universe.
Course	Pattern of development and change of a disorder over time is a course.
Glycogen	Glycogen refers to a complex, extensively branched polysaccharide of many glucose monomers; serves as an energy-storage molecule in liver and muscle cells.
Potassium	Potassium is a chemical element in the periodic table. It has the symbol K (L. kalium) and atomic number 19. Potassium is a soft silvery-white metallic alkali metal that occurs naturally bound to other elements in seawater and many minerals.
Minerals	Minerals refer to inorganic chemical compounds found in nature; salts.
Protein	A protein is a complex, high-molecular-weight organic compound that consists of amino acids joined by peptide bonds. They are essential to the structure and function of all living cells and viruses. Many are enzymes or subunits of enzymes.
Vitamin	An organic compound other than a carbohydrate, lipid, or protein that is needed for normal metabolism but that the body cannot synthesize in adequate amounts is called a vitamin.
Calcium	Calcium is the chemical element in the periodic table that has the symbol Ca and atomic number 20. Calcium is a soft grey alkaline earth metal that is used as a reducing agent in the extraction of thorium, zirconium and uranium. Calcium is also the fifth most abundant element in the Earth's crust.
Sugar	A sugar is the simplest molecule that can be identified as a carbohydrate. These include monosaccharides and disaccharides, trisaccharides and the oligosaccharides. The term "glyco-" indicates the presence of a sugar in an otherwise non-carbohydrate substance.
Carbohydrate	Carbohydrate is a chemical compound that contains oxygen, hydrogen, and carbon atoms. They consist of monosaccharide sugars of varying chain lengths and that have the general chemical formula $C_n(H_2O)_n$ or are derivatives of such.
Tissue	A collection of interconnected cells that perform a similar function within an organism is called tissue.
Value	Value is worth in general, and it is thought to be connected to reasons for certain practices, policies, actions, beliefs or emotions. Value is "that which one acts to gain and/or keep."
Homeostasis	Homeostasis is the property of an open system, especially living organisms, to regulate its internal environment to maintain a stable, constant condition, by means of multiple dynamic equilibrium adjustments, controlled by interrelated regulation mechanisms.
Malnutrition	Malnutrition is a general term for the medical condition in a person or animal caused by an unbalanced diet—either too little or too much food, or a diet missing one or more important nutrients.
Obesity	The state of being more than 20 percent above the average weight for a person of one's height is called obesity.
Alcoholism	A disorder that involves long-term, repeated, uncontrolled, compulsive, and excessive use of alcoholic beverages and that impairs the drinker's health and work and social relationships is called alcoholism.

Go to **Cram101.com** for the Practice Tests for this Chapter.

Chapter 6. Dietary Deficiencies and Excesses: Malnutrition, Obesity, and Alcoholism

Chapter 6. Dietary Deficiencies and Excesses: Malnutrition, Obesity, and Alcoholism

Concept	A mental category used to class together objects, relations, events, abstractions, or qualities that have common properties is called concept.
Gastrointestinal system	The gastrointestinal system is the system of organs within multicellular animals which takes in food, digests it to extract energy and nutrients, and expels the remaining waste.
Enzyme	An enzyme is a protein that catalyzes, or speeds up, a chemical reaction. They are essential to sustain life because most chemical reactions in biological cells would occur too slowly, or would lead to different products, without them.
Lipid	Lipid is one class of aliphatic hydrocarbon-containing organic compounds essential for the structure and function of living cells. They are characterized by being water-insoluble but soluble in nonpolar organic solvents.
Digestion	Digestion refers to the mechanical and chemical breakdown of food into molecules small enough for the body to absorb; the second main stage of food processing, following ingestion.
Pancreatitis	Pancreatitis is inflammation of the pancreas. The most common causes of pancreatitis are gallstones and frequent and excessive consumption of alcohol (80% of cases), and less common causes are drugs or medication.
Pancreas	The pancreas is a retroperitoneal organ that serves two functions: exocrine - it produces pancreatic juice containing digestive enzymes, and endocrine - it produces several important hormones, namely insulin.
Diarrhea	Diarrhea or diarrhoea is a condition in which the sufferer has frequent and watery, chunky, or loose bowel movements.
Hepatomegaly	Hepatomegaly is the condition of having an enlarged liver. It is a nonspecific medical sign having many causes, which can broadly be broken down into infection, direct toxicity, hepatic tumours, or metabolic disorder.
Steatorrhea	Steatorrhea is the formation of bulky, grey or light colored stools. There is increased fat excretion, which can be objectivated by determining the fecal fat levels. While definitions have not been standardised, fat excretion in feces in excess of 0.3 (g/kg)/day is considered indicative of steatorrhea.
Amenorrhea	Amenorrhea is the absence of a menstrual period in a woman of reproductive age. Physiologic states of amenorrhea are seen during pregnancy and lactation (breastfeeding).
Gingivitis	Gingivitis is the inflammation of the gums (gingiva) around the teeth.
Petechiae	A petechiae is a small red or purple spot on the body, caused by a minor hemorrhage
Cognition	The ability of an animal's nervous system to perceive, store, process, and use information obtained by its sensory receptors is referred to as cognition.
Estrogen	Estrogen is a steroid that functions as the primary female sex hormone. While present in both men and women, they are found in women in significantly higher quantities.
Syndrome	Syndrome is the association of several clinically recognizable features, signs, symptoms, phenomena or characteristics which often occur together, so that the presence of one feature alerts the physician to the presence of the others
Atrophy	Atrophy is the partial or complete wasting away of a part of the body. Causes of atrophy include poor nourishment, poor circulation, loss of hormonal support, loss of nerve supply to the target organ, disuse or lack of exercise, or disease intrinsic to the tissue itself.
Ascites	Serous fluid accumulation in the abdominal cavity is ascites.
Tremor	Tremor is the rhythmic, oscillating shaking movement of the whole body or just a certain part of it, caused by problems of the neurons responsible from muscle action.

Chapter 6. Dietary Deficiencies and Excesses: Malnutrition, Obesity, and Alcoholism

Chapter 6. Dietary Deficiencies and Excesses: Malnutrition, Obesity, and Alcoholism

Muscle	Muscle is a contractile form of tissue. It is one of the four major tissue types, the other three being epithelium, connective tissue and nervous tissue. Muscle contraction is used to move parts of the body, as well as to move substances within the body.
Wound	A wound is type of physical trauma wherein the skin is torn, cut or punctured, or where blunt force trauma causes a contusion.
Edema	Edema is swelling of any organ or tissue due to accumulation of excess fluid. Edema has many root causes, but its common mechanism is accumulation of fluid into the tissues.
Bile	Bile is a bitter, greenish-yellow alkaline fluid secreted by the liver of most vertebrates. In many species, it is stored in the gallbladder between meals and upon eating is discharged into the duodenum where it aids the process of digestion.
Congestive heart failure	Congestive heart failure is the inability of the heart to pump a sufficient amount of blood throughout the body, or requiring elevated filling pressures in order to pump effectively.
Vital capacity	Vital capacity is the total amount of air that a person can expire after a complete inspiration.
Consciousness	Consciousness refers to the ability to perceive, communicate, remember, understand, appreciate, and initiate voluntary movements; a functioning sensorium.
Constipation	Constipation is a condition of the digestive system where a person (or other animal) experiences hard feces that are difficult to eliminate; it may be extremely painful, and in severe cases (fecal impaction) lead to symptoms of bowel obstruction.
Gallbladder	The gallbladder is a pear-shaped organ that stores bile until the body needs it for digestion. It is connected to the liver and the duodenum by the biliary tract.
Absorption	Absorption is a physical or chemical phenomenon or a process in which atoms, molecules, or ions enter some bulk phase - gas, liquid or solid material. In nutrition, amino acids are broken down through digestion, which begins in the stomach.
Bile duct	A bile duct is any of a number of long tube-like structures that carry bile. The top half of the common bile duct is associated with the liver, while the bottom half of the common bile duct is associated with the pancreas, through which it passes on its way to the intestine. It opens in the part of the intestine called the duodenum into a structure called the ampulla of Vater.
Liver	The liver is an organ in vertebrates, including humans. It plays a major role in metabolism and has a number of functions in the body including drug detoxification, glycogen storage, and plasma protein synthesis. It also produces bile, which is important for digestion.
Stool	Stool is the waste matter discharged in a bowel movement.
Essential nutrient	An essential nutrient is a nutrient required for normal body functioning that can not be synthesized by the body. Categories of essential nutrient include vitamins, dietary minerals, essential fatty acids and essential amino acids.
Anemia	Anemia is a deficiency of red blood cells and/or hemoglobin. This results in a reduced ability of blood to transfer oxygen to the tissues, and this causes hypoxia; since all human cells depend on oxygen for survival, varying degrees of anemia can have a wide range of clinical consequences.
Intrinsic factor	A substance produced by the gastric glands that promotes absorption of vitamin is called an intrinsic factor.
Digestive tract	The digestive tract is the system of organs within multicellular animals which takes in food, digests it to extract energy and nutrients, and expels the remaining waste.

Go to **Cram101.com** for the Practice Tests for this Chapter.

Chapter 6. Dietary Deficiencies and Excesses: Malnutrition, Obesity, and Alcoholism

Chapter 6. Dietary Deficiencies and Excesses: Malnutrition, Obesity, and Alcoholism

Hepatitis	Hepatitis is a gastroenterological disease, featuring inflammation of the liver. The clinical signs and prognosis, as well as the therapy, depend on the cause.
Cirrhosis	Cirrhosis is a chronic disease of the liver in which liver tissue is replaced by connective tissue, resulting in the loss of liver function. Cirrhosis is caused by damage from toxins (including alcohol), metabolic problems, chronic viral hepatitis or other causes
Blood	Blood is a circulating tissue composed of fluid plasma and cells. The main function of blood is to supply nutrients (oxygen, glucose) and constitutional elements to tissues and to remove waste products.
Organ	Organ refers to a structure consisting of several tissues adapted as a group to perform specific functions.
Glucose	Glucose, a simple monosaccharide sugar, is one of the most important carbohydrates and is used as a source of energy in animals and plants. Glucose is one of the main products of photosynthesis and starts respiration.
Iron	Iron is essential to all organisms, except for a few bacteria. It is mostly stably incorporated in the inside of metalloproteins, because in exposed or in free form it causes production of free radicals that are generally toxic to cells.
Diabetes	Diabetes is a medical disorder characterized by varying or persistent elevated blood sugar levels, especially after eating. All types of diabetes share similar symptoms and complications at advanced stages: dehydration and ketoacidosis, cardiovascular disease, chronic renal failure, retinal damage which can lead to blindness, nerve damage which can lead to erectile dysfunction, gangrene with risk of amputation of toes, feet, and even legs.
Insulin	Insulin is a polypeptide hormone that regulates carbohydrate metabolism. Apart from being the primary effector in carbohydrate homeostasis, it also has a substantial effect on small vessel muscle tone, controls storage and release of fat (triglycerides) and cellular uptake of both amino acids and some electrolytes.
Diabetes mellitus	Diabetes mellitus is a medical disorder characterized by varying or persistent hyperglycemia (elevated blood sugar levels), especially after eating. All types of diabetes mellitus share similar symptoms and complications at advanced stages.
Urine	Concentrated filtrate produced by the kidneys and excreted via the bladder is called urine.
Lead	Lead is a chemical element in the periodic table that has the symbol Pb and atomic number 82. A soft, heavy, toxic and malleable poor metal, lead is bluish white when freshly cut but tarnishes to dull gray when exposed to air. Lead is used in building construction, lead-acid batteries, bullets and shot, and is part of solder, pewter, and fusible alloys.
Rhodopsin	Rhodopsin is expressed in vertebrate photoreceptor cells. It is a pigment of the retina that is responsible for both the formation of the photoreceptor cells and the first events in the perception of light. Rhodopsins belong to the class of G-protein coupled receptors. It is the chemical that allows night-vision, and is extremely sensitive to light.
Retina	The retina is a thin layer of cells at the back of the eyeball of vertebrates and some cephalopods; it is the part of the eye which converts light into nervous signals.
Rods	Rods, are photoreceptor cells in the retina of the eye that can function in less intense light than can the other type of photoreceptor, cone cells.
Conjunctiva	Conjunctiva refers to a mucous membrane that helps keep the eye moist; lines the inner surface of the eyelids and covers the front of the eyeball, except the cornea.
Carotene	Carotene is an orange photosynthetic pigment important for photosynthesis. It is responsible for the orange color of the carrot and many other fruits and vegetables. It contributes to

Go to **Cram101.com** for the Practice Tests for this Chapter.

Chapter 6. Dietary Deficiencies and Excesses: Malnutrition, Obesity, and Alcoholism

Chapter 6. Dietary Deficiencies and Excesses: Malnutrition, Obesity, and Alcoholism

	photosynthesis by transmitting the light energy it absorbs to chlorophyll.
Rickets	Rickets is a disorder which most commonly relates directly to Vitamin D deficiency, which causes a lack of calcium being absorbed. It can also arise, however, from other etiologies such as rare mesenchymal tumors or any phosphate-wasting disease. It is a disorder which most commonly relates directly to Vitamin D deficiency, which causes a lack of calcium being absorbed.
Yolk	Dense nutrient material that is present in the egg of a bird or reptile is referred to as yolk.
Egg	An egg is the zygote, resulting from fertilization of the ovum. It nourishes and protects the embryo.
Gastrointestinal tract	The gastrointestinal tract is the system of organs within multicellular animals which takes in food, digests it to extract energy and nutrients, and expels the remaining waste.
Osteomalacia	Osteomalacia is also referred to as bow-leggedness or rickets. It is a disorder which most commonly relates directly to Vitamin D deficiency, which causes a lack of calcium being absorbed. It can also arise, however, from other etiologies such as rare mesenchymal tumors or any phosphate-wasting disease.
Sterol	A sterol, or steroid alcohols are a subgroup of steroids with a hydroxyl group in the 3-position of the A-ring. They are amphipathic lipids synthetized from Acetyl coenzyme A.
Skin	Skin is an organ of the integumentary system composed of a layer of tissues that protect underlying muscles and organs.
Heart attack	A heart attack, is a serious, sudden heart condition usually characterized by varying degrees of chest pain or discomfort, weakness, sweating, nausea, vomiting, and arrhythmias, sometimes causing loss of consciousness. It occurs when the blood supply to a part of the heart is interrupted, causing death and scarring of the local heart tissue.
Folic acid	Folic acid and folate (the anion form) are forms of a water-soluble B vitamin. These occur naturally in food and can also be taken as supplements.
Acid	An acid is a water-soluble, sour-tasting chemical compound that when dissolved in water, gives a solution with a pH of less than 7.
Amino acid	An amino acid is any molecule that contains both amino and carboxylic acid functional groups. They are the basic structural building units of proteins. They form short polymer chains called peptides or polypeptides which in turn form structures called proteins.
Folate	Folic acid and folate (the anion form) are forms of a water-soluble B vitamin. These occur naturally in food and can also be taken as supplements.
Stroke	A stroke or cerebrovascular accident (CVA) occurs when the blood supply to a part of the brain is suddenly interrupted.
Intestine	The intestine is the portion of the alimentary canal extending from the stomach to the anus and, in humans and mammals, consists of two segments, the small intestine and the large intestine. The intestine is the part of the body responsible for extracting nutrition from food.
Prothrombin	Prothrombin refers to plasma protein that is converted to thrombin during the steps of blood clotting. Prothrombin is a blood plasma protein and is synthesized in the liver.
Coagulation	The coagulation of blood is a complex process during which blood forms solid clots. It is an important part of haemostasis (the cesztation of blood loss from a damaged vessel) whereby a damaged blood vessel wall is covered by a fibrin clot to stop hemorrhage and aid repair of the damaged vessel.

Go to Cram101.com for the Practice Tests for this Chapter.

Chapter 6. Dietary Deficiencies and Excesses: Malnutrition, Obesity, and Alcoholism

Chapter 6. Dietary Deficiencies and Excesses: Malnutrition, Obesity, and Alcoholism

Normal flora	The bacteria and fungi that live on animal body surfaces without causing disease is normal flora.
Antibiotic	Antibiotic refers to substance such as penicillin or streptomycin that is toxic to microorganisms. Usually a product of a particular microorvanism or plant.
Bacteria	The domain that contains procaryotic cells with primarily diacyl glycerol diesters in their membranes and with bacterial rRNA. Bacteria also is a general term for organisms that are composed of procaryotic cells and are not multicellular.
Ascorbic acid	Ascorbic acid is an organic acid with antioxidant properties. Its appearance is white to light yellow crystals or powder. It is water soluble. The L-enantiomer of ascorbic acid is commonly known as vitamin C.
Blood vessel	A blood vessel is a part of the circulatory system and function to transport blood throughout the body. The most important types, arteries and veins, are so termed because they carry blood away from or towards the heart, respectively.
Palpitation	A palpitation is an awareness of the beating of the heart, whether it is too slow, too fast, irregular, or at its normal frequency; brought on by overexertion, adrenaline, alcohol, disease or drugs, or as a symptom of panic disorder.
Lesion	A lesion is a non-specific term referring to abnormal tissue in the body. It can be caused by any disease process including trauma (physical, chemical, electrical), infection, neoplasm, metabolic and autoimmune.
Collagen	Collagen is the main protein of connective tissue in animals and the most abundant protein in mammals, making up about 1/4 of the total. It is one of the long, fibrous structural proteins whose functions are quite different from those of globular proteins such as enzymes.
Connective tissue	Connective tissue is any type of biological tissue with an extensive extracellular matrix and often serves to support, bind together, and protect organs.
Megadose	Generally an intake of a nutrient in excess of 10 times human need is called megadose.
Anticoagulant	A biochemical that inhibits blood clotting is referred to as an anticoagulant.
Cancer	Cancer is a class of diseases or disorders characterized by uncontrolled division of cells and the ability of these cells to invade other tissues, either by direct growth into adjacent tissue through invasion or by implantation into distant sites by metastasis.
Scurvy	Scurvy refers to the deficiency disease that results after a few weeks to months of consuming a diet that lacks vitamin C; pinpoint sites of bleeding on the skin are an early sign.
Trial	In classical conditioning, any presentation of a stimulus or pair of stimuli is called a trial.
Intracranial pressure	Intracranial pressure is the pressure of the brain, Cerebrospinal fluid (CSF), and the brain's blood supply within the intracranial space.
Stomach	The stomach is an organ in the alimentary canal used to digest food. It's primary function is not the absorption of nutrients from digested food; rather, the main job of the stomach is to break down large food molecules into smaller ones, so that they can be absorbed into the blood more easily.
Kidney	The kidney is a bean-shaped excretory organ in vertebrates. Part of the urinary system, the kidneys filter wastes (especially urea) from the blood and excrete them, along with water, as urine.
Lungs	Lungs are the essential organs of respiration in air-breathing vertebrates. Their principal function is to transport oxygen from the atmosphere into the bloodstream, and to excrete

Chapter 6. Dietary Deficiencies and Excesses: Malnutrition, Obesity, and Alcoholism

Chapter 6. Dietary Deficiencies and Excesses: Malnutrition, Obesity, and Alcoholism

	carbon dioxide from the bloodstream into the atmosphere.
Hypercalcemia	Hypercalcemia refers to an excess of calcium ions in the blood.
Polyuria	Excessive output of urine is called polyuria.
Digestive system	The organ system that ingests food, breaks it down into smaller chemical units, and absorbs the nutrient molecules is referred to as the digestive system.
Hemoglobin	Hemoglobin is the iron-containing oxygen-transport metalloprotein in the red cells of the blood in mammals and other animals. Hemoglobin transports oxygen from the lungs to the rest of the body, such as to the muscles, where it releases the oxygen load.
Goiter	Goiter refers to an enlargement of the thyroid gland resulting from a dietary iodine deficiency.
Iodine	Iodine is a chemical element in the periodic table that has the symbol I and atomic number 53. It is required as a trace element for most living organisms. Chemically, iodine is the least reactive of the halogens, and the most electropositive halogen. Iodine is primarily used in medicine, photography and in dyes.
Aldosterone	Aldosterone is a steroid hormone synthesized from cholesterol by the enzyme aldosterone synthase. It helps regulate the body's electrolyte balance by acting on the mineralocorticoid receptor. It diminishes the secretion of sodium ions and therefore, water and stimulates the secretion of potassium ions through the kidneys.
Adrenal	In mammals, the adrenal glands are the triangle-shaped endocrine glands that sit atop the kidneys. They are chiefly responsible for regulating the stress response through the synthesis of corticosteroids and catecholamines, including cortisol and adrenaline.
Cortex	In anatomy and zoology the cortex is the outermost or superficial layer of an organ or the outer portion of the stem or root of a plant.
Adrenal cortex	Situated along the perimeter of the adrenal gland, the adrenal cortex mediates the stress response through the production of mineralocorticoids and glucocorticoids, including aldosterone and cortisol respectively. It is also a secondary site of androgen synthesis.
Diuretic	A diuretic is any drug that elevates the rate of bodily urine excretion.
Sodium	Sodium is the chemical element in the periodic table that has the symbol Na (Natrium in Latin) and atomic number 11. Sodium is a soft, waxy, silvery reactive metal belonging to the alkali metals that is abundant in natural compounds (especially halite). It is highly reactive.
Nerve	A nerve is an enclosed, cable-like bundle of nerve fibers or axons, which includes the glia that ensheath the axons in myelin.
Muscle contraction	A muscle contraction occurs when a muscle cell (called a muscle fiber) shortens. There are three general types: skeletal, heart, and smooth.
Incidence	In epidemiological studies of a particular disorder, the rate at which new cases occur in a given place at a given time is called incidence.
Anorexia	Anorexia nervosa is an eating disorder characterized by voluntary starvation and exercise stress.
Obsession	An obsession is a thought or idea that the sufferer cannot stop thinking about. Common examples include fears of acquiring disease, getting hurt, or causing harm to someone. They are typically automatic, frequent, distressing, and difficult to control or put an end to by themselves.
Maladjustment	Maladjustment is the condition of being unable to adapt properly to your environment with

Go to **Cram101.com** for the Practice Tests for this Chapter.

Chapter 6. Dietary Deficiencies and Excesses: Malnutrition, Obesity, and Alcoholism

Chapter 6. Dietary Deficiencies and Excesses: Malnutrition, Obesity, and Alcoholism

	resulting emotional instability.
Blood clotting	A complex process by which platelets, the protein fibrin, and red blood cells block an irregular surface in or on the body, such as a damaged blood vessel, sealing the wound is referred to as blood clotting.
Anxiety	Anxiety is a complex combination of the feeling of fear, apprehension and worry often accompanied by physical sensations such as palpitations, chest pain and/or shortness of breath.
Calorie	Calorie refers to a unit used to measure heat energy and the energy contents of foods.
Laxatives	Medications used to soften stool and relieve constipation are referred to as laxatives.
Laxative	Laxative refers to a medication or other substance that stimulates evacuation of the intestinal tract.
Menstruation	Loss of blood and tissue from the uterine lining at the end of a female reproductive cycle are referred to as menstruation.
Gonadotropin	A hormone that stimulates the gonads is gonadotropin. They are protein hormones secreted by gonadotrope cells of the pituitary gland of vertebrates.
Ovaries	Ovaries are egg-producing reproductive organs found in female organisms.
Ovary	The primary reproductive organ of a female is called an ovary.
Anterior pituitary	The anterior pituitary comprises the anterior lobe of the pituitary gland and is part of the endocrine system. Under the influence of the hypothalamus, the anterior pituitary produces and secretes several peptide hormones that regulate many physiological processes including stress, growth, and reproduction.
Testosterone	Testosterone is a steroid hormone from the androgen group. Testosterone is secreted in the testes of men and the ovaries of women. It is the principal male sex hormone and the "original" anabolic steroid. In both males and females, it plays key roles in health and well-being.
Hormone	A hormone is a chemical messenger from one cell to another. All multicellular organisms produce hormones. The best known hormones are those produced by endocrine glands of vertebrate animals, but hormones are produced by nearly every organ system and tissue type in a human or animal body. Hormone molecules are secreted directly into the bloodstream, they move by circulation or diffusion to their target cells, which may be nearby cells in the same tissue or cells of a distant organ of the body.
Gonadotropic hormone	Substance secreted by anterior pituitary that regulates the activity of the ovaries and testes is referred to as gonadotropic hormone.
Dehydration	Dehydration is the removal of water from an object. Medically, dehydration is a serious and potentially life-threatening condition in which the body contains an insufficient volume of water for normal functioning.
Resistance	Resistance refers to a nonspecific ability to ward off infection or disease regardless of whether the body has been previously exposed to it. A force that opposes the flow of a fluid such as air or blood. Compare with immunity.
Infection	The invasion and multiplication of microorganisms in body tissues is called an infection.
Health	Health is a term that refers to a combination of the absence of illness, the ability to cope with everyday activities, physical fitness, and high quality of life.
Psychotherapy	Psychotherapy is a set of techniques based on psychological principles intended to improve mental health, emotional or behavioral issues.

Chapter 6. Dietary Deficiencies and Excesses: Malnutrition, Obesity, and Alcoholism

Chapter 6. Dietary Deficiencies and Excesses: Malnutrition, Obesity, and Alcoholism

Mortality	The incidence of death in a population is mortality.
Mortality rate	Mortality rate is the number of deaths (from a disease or in general) per 1000 people and typically reported on an annual basis.
Bulimia	Bulimia refers to a disorder in which a person binges on incredibly large quantities of food, then purges by vomiting or by using laxatives. Bulimia is often less about food, and more to do with deep psychological issues and profound feelings of lack of control.
Binge	Binge refers to relatively brief episode of uncontrolled, excessive consumption.
Constant	A behavior or characteristic that does not vary from one observation to another is referred to as a constant.
Gland	A gland is an organ in an animal's body that synthesizes a substance for release such as hormones, often into the bloodstream or into cavities inside the body or its outer surface.
Salivary gland	The salivary gland produces saliva, which keeps the mouth and other parts of the digestive system moist. It also helps break down carbohydrates and lubricates the passage of food down from the oro-pharynx to the esophagus to the stomach.
Electrolyte	An electrolyte is a substance that dissociates into free ions when dissolved (or molten), to produce an electrically conductive medium. Because they generally consist of ions in solution, they are also known as ionic solutions.
Depression	In everyday language depression refers to any downturn in mood, which may be relatively transitory and perhaps due to something trivial. This is differentiated from Clinical depression which is marked by symptoms that last two weeks or more and are so severe that they interfere with daily living.
Antidepressants	Antidepressants are medications used primarily in the treatment of clinical depression. Antidepressants create little if any immediate change in mood and require between several days and several weeks to take effect.
Antidepressant	An antidepressant is a medication used primarily in the treatment of clinical depression. They are not thought to produce tolerance, although sudden withdrawal may produce adverse effects. They create little if any immediate change in mood and require between several days and several weeks to take effect.
Affect	Affect is the scientific term used to describe a subject's externally displayed mood. This can be assesed by the nurse by observing facial expression, tone of voice, and body language.
Adipose tissue	Adipose tissue is an anatomical term for loose connective tissue composed of adipocytes. Its main role is to store energy in the form of fat, although it also cushions and insulates the body. It has an important endocrine function in producing recently-discovered hormones such as leptin, resistin and TNFalpha.
Mesentery	A mesentery is a part of the peritoneum that connects an internal organ, such as the small intestine, to the abdominal wall.
Omentum	Two notable sections of the peritoneum in humans are the omenta, the greater (gastrocolic) omentum and the lesser (gastrohepatic) omentum. They form a small cavity separate from the general cavity known as the lesser sac or omental bursa and lesser peritoneal cavity.
Subcutaneous	Subcutaneous injections are given by injecting a fluid into the subcutis. It is relatively painless and an effective way to administer particular types of medication.
Birth control pill	The birth control pill is a chemical taken by mouth to inhibit normal fertility. All act on the hormonal system.
Culture	Culture, generally refers to patterns of human activity and the symbolic structures that give

Chapter 6. Dietary Deficiencies and Excesses: Malnutrition, Obesity, and Alcoholism

Chapter 6. Dietary Deficiencies and Excesses: Malnutrition, Obesity, and Alcoholism

	such activity significance.
Central nervous system	The central nervous system comprized of the brain and spinal cord, represents the largest part of the nervous system. Together with the peripheral nervous system, it has a fundamental role in the control of behavior.
Nervous system	The nervous system of an animal coordinates the activity of the muscles, monitors the organs, constructs and processes input from the senses, and initiates actions.
Hypothalamus	Located below the thalamus, the hypothalamus links the nervous system to the endocrine system by synthesizing and secreting neurohormones often called releasing hormones because they function by stimulating the secretion of hormones from the anterior pituitary gland.
Satiety center	Satiety, or the feeling of fullness and disappearance of appetite after a meal, is a process mediated by the ventromedial nucleus in the hypothalamus. It is therefore the satiety center.
Thyroid	The thyroid is one of the larger endocrine glands in the body. It is located in the neck and produces hormones, principally thyroxine and triiodothyronine, that regulate the rate of metabolism and affect the growth and rate of function of many other systems in the body.
Stress	Stress refers to a condition that is a response to factors that change the human systems normal state.
Serum	Serum is the same as blood plasma except that clotting factors (such as fibrin) have been removed. Blood plasma contains fibrinogen.
Atherosclerosis	Process by which a fatty substance or plaque builds up inside arteries to form obstructions is called atherosclerosis.
Ventricle	In the heart, a ventricle is a heart chamber which collects blood from an atrium (another heart chamber) and pumps it out of the heart.
Left ventricle	The left ventricle is one of four chambers (two atria and two ventricles) in the human heart. It receives oxygenated blood from the left atrium via the mitral valve, and pumps it into the aorta via the aortic valve.
Hypertension	Hypertension is a medical condition where the blood pressure in the arteries is chronically elevated. Persistent hypertension is one of the risk factors for strokes, heart attacks, heart failure and arterial aneurysm, and is a leading cause of chronic renal failure.
Carbon	Carbon is a chemical element in the periodic table that has the symbol C and atomic number 6. An abundant nonmetallic, tetravalent element, carbon has several allotropic forms.
Hypoventilation	Hypoventilation occurs when ventilation is inadequate to perform gas exchange. It generally causes an increased concentration of carbon dioxide (hypercapnia) and respiratory acidosis. It can be caused by medical conditions, by holding one's breath, or by drugs. Hypoventilation may be dangerous for those with sleep apnea.
Carbon dioxide	Carbon dioxide is an atmospheric gas comprized of one carbon and two oxygen atoms. A very widely known chemical compound, it is frequently called by its formula CO_2. In its solid state, it is commonly known as dry ice.
Diaphragm	The diaphragm is a shelf of muscle extending across the bottom of the ribcage. It is critically important in respiration: in order to draw air into the lungs, the diaphragm contracts, thus enlarging the thoracic cavity and reducing intra-thoracic pressure.
Brain	The part of the central nervous system involved in regulating and controlling body activity and interpreting information from the senses transmitted through the nervous system is referred to as the brain.
Joint	A joint (articulation) is the location at which two bones make contact (articulate). They are

Chapter 6. Dietary Deficiencies and Excesses: Malnutrition, Obesity, and Alcoholism

Chapter 6. Dietary Deficiencies and Excesses: Malnutrition, Obesity, and Alcoholism

	constructed to both allow movement and provide mechanical support.
Osteoarthritis	Osteoarthritis is a condition in which low-grade inflammation results in pain in the joints, caused by wearing of the cartilage that covers and acts as a cushion inside joints.
Veins	Blood vessels that return blood toward the heart from the circulation are referred to as veins.
Vein	Vein in animals, is a vessel that returns blood to the heart. In plants, a vascular bundle in a leaf, composed of xylem and phloem.
Varicose veins	Varicose veins are veins on the leg which are large, twisted, and ropelike, and can cause pain, swelling, or itching. They are an extreme form of telangiectasia, or spider veins.
Hernia	Hernia refers to abnormal protrusion of an organ or a body part through the containing wall of its cavity. Commonly referred to as a rupture, a hernia often involves protrusion of the intestine through a break in the peritoneum.
Infiltration	Infiltration is the diffusion or accumulation (in a tissue or cells) of substances not normal to it or in amounts in excess of the normal. The material collected in those tissues or cells is also called infiltration.
Amphetamine	Amphetamine is a synthetic stimulant used to suppress the appetite, control weight, and treat disorders including narcolepsy and ADHD. It is also used recreationally and for performance enhancement.
Addiction	Addiction is an uncontrollable compulsion to repeat a behavior regardless of its consequences. Many drugs or behaviors can precipitate a pattern of conditions recognized as addiction, which include a craving for more of the drug or behavior, increased physiological tolerance to exposure, and withdrawal symptoms in the absence of the stimulus.
Unsaturated fat	An unsaturated fat is a fat or fatty acid in which there is one or more double bonds between carbon atoms of the fatty acid chain. Such fat molecules are monounsaturated if each contains one double bond, and polyunsaturated if each contain more than one.
Puberty	A time in the life of a developing individual characterized by the increasing production of sex hormones, which cause it to reach sexual maturity is called puberty.
Menopause	Menopause is the physiological cessation of menstrual cycles associated with advancing age in species that experience such cycles. Menopause is sometimes referred to as change of life or climacteric.
Alcohol	Alcohol is a general term, applied to any organic compound in which a hydroxyl group (-OH) is bound to a carbon atom, which in turn is bound to other hydrogen and/or carbon atoms. The general formula for a simple acyclic alcohol is $C_nH_{2n+1}OH$.
Blood pressure	Blood pressure is the pressure exerted by the blood on the walls of the blood vessels.
Epidemic	An epidemic is a disease that appears as new cases in a given human population, during a given period, at a rate that substantially exceeds what is "expected", based on recent experience.
Survey	A method of scientific investigation in which a large sample of people answer questions about their attitudes or behavior is referred to as a survey.
Centers for Disease Control and Prevention	The Centers for Disease Control and Prevention in Atlanta, Georgia, is recognized as the lead United States agency for protecting the public health and safety of people by providing credible information to enhance health decisions, and promoting health through strong partnerships with state health departments and other organizations.
Population	Population refers to all members of a well-defined group of organisms, events, or things.

Go to Cram101.com for the Practice Tests for this Chapter.

Chapter 6. Dietary Deficiencies and Excesses: Malnutrition, Obesity, and Alcoholism

Chapter 6. Dietary Deficiencies and Excesses: Malnutrition, Obesity, and Alcoholism

Marriage	A socially approved sexual and economic relationship between two or more individuals is a marriage.
Alcoholic	An alcoholic is dependent on alcohol as characterized by craving, loss of control, physical dependence and withdrawal symptoms, and tolerance.
Cardiovascular system	The circulatory system or cardiovascular system is the organ system which circulates blood around the body of most animals.
Etiology	The apparent causation and developmental history of an illness is an etiology.
Host	Host is an organism that harbors a parasite, mutual partner, or commensal partner; or a cell infected by a virus.
Intoxication	Condition in which a substance affecting the central nervous system has been ingested and certain maladaptive behaviors or psychological changes, such as belligerence and impaired function, are evident is called intoxication.
Amnesia	Amnesia is a condition in which memory is disturbed. The causes of amnesia are organic or functional. Organic causes include damage to the brain, through trauma or disease, or use of certain (generally sedative) drugs.
Shock	Circulatory shock, a state of cardiac output that is insufficient to meet the body's physiological needs, with consequences ranging from fainting to death is referred to as shock. Insulin shock, a state of severe hypoglycemia caused by administration of insulin.
Duodenum	The duodenum is a hollow jointed tube connecting the stomach to the jejunum. It is the first part of the small intestine. Two very important ducts open into the duodenum, namely the bile duct and the pancreatic duct. The duodenum is largely responsible for the breakdown of food in the small intestine.
Mucosa	The mucosa is a lining of ectodermic origin, covered in epithelium, and involved in absorption and secretion. They line various body cavities that are exposed to the external environment and internal organs.
Portal vein	The portal vein is the largest vein in the human body draining blood from the digestive system and its associated glands. It is formed by the union of the splenic vein and superior mesenteric vein and divides into a right and a left branch, before entering the liver.
Dependence	Dependence refers to a mental or physical craving for a drug and withdrawal symptoms when use of the drug is stopped.
Physical dependence	Physical dependence describes increased tolerance of a drug combined with a physical need of the drug to function. Abrupt cessation of the drug is typically associated with negative physical withdrawal symptoms. Physical dependence is distinguished from addiction. While addiction tends to describe psychological and behavioral attributes, physical dependence is defined primarily using physical and biological concepts.
Abstinence	Abstinence has diverse forms. In its oldest sense it is sexual, as in the practice of continence, chastity, and celibacy.
Thiamine	Thiamine, also known as vitamin B_1, is a colorless compound with chemical formula $C_{12}H_{17}ClN_4OS$. Systemic thiamine deficiency can lead to myriad problems including neurodegeneration, wasting, and death. Well-known syndromes caused by lack of thiamine due to malnutrition or a diet high in thiaminase-rich foods include Wernicke-Korsakoff syndrome and beriberi, diseases also common in chronic abusers of alcohol.
Encephalopathy	Encephalopathy is a nonspecific term describing a syndrome affecting the brain. Generally, it refers to involvement of large parts of the brain (or the whole organ), instead of identifiable changes confined to parts of the brain.

Chapter 6. Dietary Deficiencies and Excesses: Malnutrition, Obesity, and Alcoholism

Chapter 6. Dietary Deficiencies and Excesses: Malnutrition, Obesity, and Alcoholism

Delirium	Delirium is a medical term used to describe an acute decline in attention and cognition. Delirium is probably the single most common acute disorder affecting adults in general hospitals. It affects 10-20% of all adults in hospital, and 30-40% of older patients.
Eye	An eye is an organ that detects light. Different kinds of light-sensitive organs are found in a variety of creatures. The simplest eyes do nothing but detect whether the surroundings are light or dark, while more complex eyes can distinguish shapes and colors.
Delirium tremens	Delirium tremens refers to a condition characterized by sweating, restlessness, disorientation, and hallucinations. It occurs in some chronic alcohol users when there is a sudden decrease in usage.
Double vision	Diplopia, colloquially known as double vision, is the perception of two images from a single object. The images may be horizontal, vertical, or diagonal.
Fiber	Fibers used by man come from a wide variety of sources: Natural fiber include those made out of plants, animal and mineral sources. Natural fibers can be classified according to their origin.
Paralysis	Paralysis is the complete loss of muscle function for one or more muscle groups. Paralysis may be localized, or generalized, or it may follow a certain pattern.
Variable	A characteristic or aspect in which people, objects, events, or conditions vary is called variable.
Niacin	Niacin, also known as vitamin B3, is a water-soluble vitamin whose derivatives such as NADH play essential roles in energy metabolism in the living cell and DNA repair. The designation vitamin B3 also includes the amide form, nicotinamide or niacinamide.
Neuron	The neuron is a major class of cells in the nervous system. In vertebrates, they are found in the brain, the spinal cord and in the nerves and ganglia of the peripheral nervous system, and their primary role is to process and transmit neural information.
Addict	A person with an overpowering physical or psychological need to continue taking a particular substance or drug is referred to as an addict.
Hemorrhage	Loss of blood from the circulatory system is referred to as a hemorrhage.
Plasma	Fluid portion of circulating blood is called plasma.
Epistaxis	A nosebleed or nose bleed, medically known as epistaxis, is the relatively common occurrence of hemorrhage (bleeding) from the nose, usually noticed when it drains out through the nostrils.
Varices	Varices in general refers to distended veins. It derives from the latin word for twisted, "varix".
Esophageal varices	In medicine (gastroenterology), esophageal varices are extreme dilations of sub-mucosal veins in the mucosa of the esophagus in diseases featuring portal hypertension, secondary to cirrhosis primarily.
Gynecomastia	Gynecomastia is the development of abnormally large breasts on men. Gynecomastia is not simply a buildup of adipose tissue, but includes the development of glandular tissue as well.
Pain	Pain is an unpleasant sensation which may be associated with actual or potential tissue damage and which may have physical and emotional components.
Hallucination	Hallucination refers to a perception in the absence of sensory stimulation that is confused with reality.
Metabolic rate	Energy expended by the body per unit time is called metabolic rate.

Go to Cram101.com for the Practice Tests for this Chapter.

Chapter 6. Dietary Deficiencies and Excesses: Malnutrition, Obesity, and Alcoholism

Chapter 6. Dietary Deficiencies and Excesses: Malnutrition, Obesity, and Alcoholism

Pneumonia	Pneumonia is an illness of the lungs and respiratory system in which the microscopic, air-filled sacs (alveoli) responsible for absorbing oxygen from the atmosphere become inflamed and flooded with fluid.
Respiratory tract	In humans the respiratory tract is the part of the anatomy that has to do with the process of respiration or breathing.
Intravenous	Present or occurring within a vein, such as an intravenous blood clot is referred to as intravenous. Introduced directly into a vein, such as an intravenous injection or I.V. drip.
Ammonia	Ammonia is a compound of nitrogen and hydrogen with the formula NH_3. At standard temperature and pressure ammonia is a gas. It is toxic and corrosive to some materials, and has a characteristic pungent odor.
Urea	Urea is an organic compound of carbon, nitrogen, oxygen and hydrogen, CON_2H_4 or $(NH_2)_2CO$. Urea is essentially a waste product: it has no physiological function. It is dissolved in blood and excreted by the kidney.
Stimulus	Stimulus in a nervous system, a factor that triggers sensory transduction.
Respiratory center	The respiratory center regulates the rhythmic, alternating cycles of inspiration and expiration.
Dysrhythmia	Dysrhythmia is an abnormal cardiac rhythm.
Arrhythmia	Cardiac arrhythmia is a group of conditions in which muscle contraction of the heart is irregular for any reason.
Coronary	Referring to the heart or the blood vessels of the heart is referred to as coronary.
Artery	Vessel that takes blood away from the heart to the tissues and organs of the body is called an artery.
Coronary arteries	Arteries that directly supply the heart with blood are referred to as coronary arteries.
Coronary artery	An artery that supplies blood to the wall of the heart is called a coronary artery.
Congestion	In medicine and pathology the term congestion is used to describe excessive accumulation of blood or other fluid in a particular part of the body.
Placenta	The placenta is an organ present only in female placental mammals during gestation. It is composed of two parts, one genetically and biologically part of the fetus, the other part of the mother. It is implanted in the wall of the uterus, where it receives nutrients and oxygen from the mother's blood and passes out waste.
Fetus	Fetus refers to a developing human from the ninth week of gestation until birth; has all the major structures of an adult.
Fetal alcohol syndrome	A cluster of abnormalities that appears in the offspring of mothers who drink alcohol heavily during pregnancy is called fetal alcohol syndrome.
Mental retardation	Mental retardation refers to having significantly below-average intellectual functioning and limitations in at least two areas of adaptive functioning. Many categorize retardation as mild, moderate, severe, or profound.
Irritability	Irritability is an excessive response to stimuli. Irritability takes many forms, from the contraction of a unicellular organism when touched to complex reactions involving all the senses of higher animals.
Withdrawal symptoms	Withdrawal symptoms are physiological changes that occur when the use of a drug is stopped or dosage decreased.

Chapter 6. Dietary Deficiencies and Excesses: Malnutrition, Obesity, and Alcoholism

Chapter 6. Dietary Deficiencies and Excesses: Malnutrition, Obesity, and Alcoholism

Intervention	Intervention refers to a planned attempt to break through addicts' or abusers' denial and get them into treatment. Interventions most often occur when legal, workplace, health, relationship, or financial problems have become intolerable.
Alcoholics Anonymous	Alcoholics anonymous refers to the first 12-step, self-help, alcoholism recovery group; tens-of-thousands of chapters exist worldwide.
Community organization	The set of procedures and processes by which a population and its institutions mobilize and coordinate resources to solve a mutual problem or to pursue mutual goals is referred to as community organization.
Group therapy	Group therapy is a form of psychotherapy during which one or several therapists treat a small group of clients together as a group. This may be more cost effective than individual therapy, and possibly even more effective.
Rehabilitation	Rehabilitation is the restoration of lost capabilities, or the treatment aimed at producing it. Also refers to treatment for dependency on psychoactive substances such as alcohol, prescription drugs, and illicit drugs such as cocaine, heroin or amphetamines.
Halfway house	A home-like residence for people who are considered too disturbed to remain in their accustomed surroundings but who do not require the total care of a mental institution is a halfway house.
Chronic illness	A chronic illness is a persistent and lasting condition that generally involves progressive deteriation and an increase in symptoms and disability.
Respiratory system	The respiratory system is the biological system of any organism that engages in gas exchange. In humans and other mammals, the respiratory system consists of the airways, the lungs, and the respiratory muscles that mediate the movement of air into and out of the body.
Gastritis	Gastritis is a medical term for inflammation of the lining of the stomach. It means that white blood cells move into the wall of the stomach as a response to some type of injury.
Salt	Salt is a term used for ionic compounds composed of positively charged cations and negatively charged anions, so that the product is neutral and without a net charge.
Reproductive system	A reproductive system is the ensembles and interactions of organs and or substances within an organism that stricly pertain to reproduction. As an example, this would include in the case of female mammals, the hormone estrogen, the womb and eggs but not the breast.
Endocrine system	The endocrine system is a set of internal organs involved in the secretion of hormones into the blood. These glands are known as ductless, which means they do not have tubes inside them.
Antigen	An antigen is a substance that stimulates an immune response, especially the production of antibodies. They are usually proteins or polysaccharides, but can be any type of molecule, including small molecules (haptens) coupled to a protein (carrier).

Chapter 6. Dietary Deficiencies and Excesses: Malnutrition, Obesity, and Alcoholism

Chapter 7. Diseases of the Blood

Leukocyte	A white blood cell is a leukocyte. They help to defend the body against infectious disease and foreign materials as part of the immune system.
Platelet	Cell fragment that is necessary to blood clotting is a platelet. They are the blood cell fragments that are involved in the cellular mechanisms that lead to the formation of blood clots.
Plasma	Fluid portion of circulating blood is called plasma.
Blood	Blood is a circulating tissue composed of fluid plasma and cells. The main function of blood is to supply nutrients (oxygen, glucose) and constitutional elements to tissues and to remove waste products.
Erythrocyte	Red blood cells are the most common type of blood cell and are the vertebrate body's principal means of delivering oxygen from the lungs or gills to body tissues via the blood. Red blood cells are also known as erythrocyte.
Hemoglobin	Hemoglobin is the iron-containing oxygen-transport metalloprotein in the red cells of the blood in mammals and other animals. Hemoglobin transports oxygen from the lungs to the rest of the body, such as to the muscles, where it releases the oxygen load.
Oxygen	Oxygen is a chemical element in the periodic table. It has the symbol O and atomic number 8. Oxygen is the second most common element on Earth, composing around 46% of the mass of Earth's crust and 28% of the mass of Earth as a whole, and is the third most common element in the universe.
Lungs	Lungs are the essential organs of respiration in air-breathing vertebrates. Their principal function is to transport oxygen from the atmosphere into the bloodstream, and to excrete carbon dioxide from the bloodstream into the atmosphere.
Red blood cells	Red blood cells are the most common type of blood cell and are the vertebrate body's principal means of delivering oxygen from the lungs or gills to body tissues via the blood.
Red blood cell	The red blood cell is the most common type of blood cell and is the vertebrate body's principal means of delivering oxygen from the lungs or gills to body tissues via the blood.
White blood cell	The white blood cell is a a component of blood. They help to defend the body against infectious disease and foreign materials as part of the immune system.
Infection	The invasion and multiplication of microorganisms in body tissues is called an infection.
Neutrophil	Neutrophil refers to a type of phagocytic leukocyte.
Lymphocyte	A lymphocyte is a type of white blood cell involved in the human body's immune system. There are two broad categories, namely T cells and B cells.
Antibody	An antibody is a protein used by the immune system to identify and neutralize foreign objects like bacteria and viruses. Each antibody recognizes a specific antigen unique to its target.
Tissue	A collection of interconnected cells that perform a similar function within an organism is called tissue.
Tumor	An abnormal mass of cells that forms within otherwise normal tissue is a tumor. This growth can be either malignant or benign
Virus	Obligate intracellular parasite of living cells consisting of an outer capsid and an inner core of nucleic acid is referred to as virus. The term virus usually refers to those particles that infect eukaryotes whilst the term bacteriophage or phage is used to describe those infecting prokaryotes.
Monocyte	A monocyte is a leukocyte, part of the human body's immune system that protect against blood-borne pathogens and move quickly to sites of infection in the tissues.

Chapter 7. Diseases of the Blood

Chapter 7. Diseases of the Blood

Inflammation	Inflammation is the first response of the immune system to infection or irritation and may be referred to as the innate cascade.
Blood clotting	A complex process by which platelets, the protein fibrin, and red blood cells block an irregular surface in or on the body, such as a damaged blood vessel, sealing the wound is referred to as blood clotting.
Hemostasis	Hemostasis refers to a process whereby bleeding is halted in most animals with a closed circulatory system.
Hormone	A hormone is a chemical messenger from one cell to another. All multicellular organisms produce hormones. The best known hormones are those produced by endocrine glands of vertebrate animals, but hormones are produced by nearly every organ system and tissue type in a human or animal body. Hormone molecules are secreted directly into the bloodstream, they move by circulation or diffusion to their target cells, which may be nearby cells in the same tissue or cells of a distant organ of the body.
Kidney	The kidney is a bean-shaped excretory organ in vertebrates. Part of the urinary system, the kidneys filter wastes (especially urea) from the blood and excrete them, along with water, as urine.
Anemia	Anemia is a deficiency of red blood cells and/or hemoglobin. This results in a reduced ability of blood to transfer oxygen to the tissues, and this causes hypoxia; since all human cells depend on oxygen for survival, varying degrees of anemia can have a wide range of clinical consequences.
Denominator	To denominate means to "give a name" or "tell what kind"; thus the denominator tells us what kind of parts we have (halves, thirds, fourths, etc.).
Hemorrhage	Loss of blood from the circulatory system is referred to as a hemorrhage.
Hemolysis	The rupture of red blood cells accompanied by the release of hemoglobin is called hemolysis.
Bone marrow	Bone marrow is the tissue comprising the center of large bones. It is the place where new blood cells are produced. Bone marrow contains two types of stem cells: hemopoietic (which can produce blood cells) and stromal (which can produce fat, cartilage and bone).
Vitamin	An organic compound other than a carbohydrate, lipid, or protein that is needed for normal metabolism but that the body cannot synthesize in adequate amounts is called a vitamin.
Iron	Iron is essential to all organisms, except for a few bacteria. It is mostly stably incorporated in the inside of metalloproteins, because in exposed or in free form it causes production of free radicals that are generally toxic to cells.
Folic acid	Folic acid and folate (the anion form) are forms of a water-soluble B vitamin. These occur naturally in food and can also be taken as supplements.
Acid	An acid is a water-soluble, sour-tasting chemical compound that when dissolved in water, gives a solution with a pH of less than 7.
Life span	Life span refers to the upper boundary of life, the maximum number of years an individual can live. The maximum life span of human beings is about 120 years of age.
Pallor	Pallor is an abnormal loss of skin or mucous membrane color. It can develop suddenly or gradually, depending of the cause.
Dyspnea	Dyspnea or shortness of breath (SOB) is perceived difficulty breathing or pain on breathing. It is a common symptom of numerous medical disorders.
Intestine	The intestine is the portion of the alimentary canal extending from the stomach to the anus and, in humans and mammals, consists of two segments, the small intestine and the large

Chapter 7. Diseases of the Blood

Chapter 7. Diseases of the Blood

	intestine. The intestine is the part of the body responsible for extracting nutrition from food.
Intrinsic factor	A substance produced by the gastric glands that promotes absorption of vitamin is called an intrinsic factor.
Stomach	The stomach is an organ in the alimentary canal used to digest food. It's primary function is not the absorption of nutrients from digested food; rather, the main job of the stomach is to break down large food molecules into smaller ones, so that they can be absorbed into the blood more easily.
Small intestine	The small intestine is the part of the gastrointestinal tract between the stomach and the large intestine (colon). In humans over 5 years old it is about 7m long. It is divided into three structural parts: duodenum, jejunum and ileum.
Stool	Stool is the waste matter discharged in a bowel movement.
Egg	An egg is the zygote, resulting from fertilization of the ovum. It nourishes and protects the embryo.
Fak	FAK is a protein tyrosine kinase recruited at focal adhesions, which are sites at cell membranes where cytoskeletal elements interact with extracellular matrix proteins. Cell migration and differentiation are initiated at these sites.
Absorption	Absorption is a physical or chemical phenomenon or a process in which atoms, molecules, or ions enter some bulk phase - gas, liquid or solid material. In nutrition, amino acids are broken down through digestion, which begins in the stomach.
Nervous system	The nervous system of an animal coordinates the activity of the muscles, monitors the organs, constructs and processes input from the senses, and initiates actions.
Injection	A method of rapid drug delivery that puts the substance directly in the bloodstream, in a muscle, or under the skin is called injection.
Iron deficiency	Iron deficiency (or "sideropenia") is the most common known form of nutritional deficiency.
Lesion	A lesion is a non-specific term referring to abnormal tissue in the body. It can be caused by any disease process including trauma (physical, chemical, electrical), infection, neoplasm, metabolic and autoimmune.
Ulcer	An ulcer is an open sore of the skin, eyes or mucous membrane, often caused by an initial abrasion and generally maintained by an inflammation and/or an infection.
Protein	A protein is a complex, high-molecular-weight organic compound that consists of amino acids joined by peptide bonds. They are essential to the structure and function of all living cells and viruses. Many are enzymes or subunits of enzymes.
Bilirubin	A bile pigment produced from hemoglobin breakdown is bilirubin.
Liver	The liver is an organ in vertebrates, including humans. It plays a major role in metabolism and has a number of functions in the body including drug detoxification, glycogen storage, and plasma protein synthesis. It also produces bile, which is important for digestion.
Bile	Bile is a bitter, greenish-yellow alkaline fluid secreted by the liver of most vertebrates. In many species, it is stored in the gallbladder between meals and upon eating is discharged into the duodenum where it aids the process of digestion.
Spleen	The spleen is a ductless, vertebrate gland that is not necessary for life but is closely associated with the circulatory system, where it functions in the destruction of old red blood cells and removal of other debris from the bloodstream, and also in holding a reservoir of blood.

Chapter 7. Diseases of the Blood

Chapter 7. Diseases of the Blood

Autoimmune	Autoimmune refers to immune reactions against normal body cells; self against self.
Immune system	The immune system is the system of specialized cells and organs that protect an organism from outside biological influences. When the immune system is functioning properly, it protects the body against bacteria and viral infections, destroying cancer cells and foreign substances.
Fever	Fever (also known as pyrexia, or a febrile response, and archaically known as ague) is a medical symptom that describes an increase in internal body temperature to levels that are above normal (37°C, 98.6°F).
Blood pressure	Blood pressure is the pressure exerted by the blood on the walls of the blood vessels.
Jaundice	Jaundice is yellowing of the skin, sclera (the white of the eyes) and mucous membranes caused by increased levels of bilirubin in the human body.
Abdomen	The abdomen is a part of the body. In humans, and in many other vertebrates, it is the region between the thorax and the pelvis. In fully developed insects, the abdomen is the third (or posterior) segment, after the head and thorax.
Sclera	The sclera is the (usually) white outer coating of the eye made of tough fibrin connective tissue which gives the eye its shape and helps to protect the delicate inner parts.
Pain	Pain is an unpleasant sensation which may be associated with actual or potential tissue damage and which may have physical and emotional components.
Eye	An eye is an organ that detects light. Different kinds of light-sensitive organs are found in a variety of creatures. The simplest eyes do nothing but detect whether the surroundings are light or dark, while more complex eyes can distinguish shapes and colors.
Convulsions	Involuntary muscle spasms, often severe, that can be caused by stimulant overdose or by depressant withdrawal are called convulsions.
Blood clot	A blood clot is the final product of the blood coagulation step in hemostasis. It is achieved via the aggregation of platelets that form a platelet plug, and the activation of the humoral coagulation system
Paralysis	Paralysis is the complete loss of muscle function for one or more muscle groups. Paralysis may be localized, or generalized, or it may follow a certain pattern.
Crisis	A crisis is a temporary state of high anxiety where the persons usual coping mechanisims cease to work. This may have a result of disorganization or possibly personality growth.
Viral	Viral phenomena are objects or patterns able to replicate themselves or convert other objects into copies of themselves when these objects are exposed to them.
Hyperactivity	Hyperactivity can be described as a state in which a individual is abnormally easily excitable and exuberant. Strong emotional reactions and a very short span of attention is also typical for the individual.
Susceptibility	The degree of resistance of a host to a pathogen is susceptibility.
Aplastic anemia	Aplastic anemia is a condition where the bone marrow does not produce enough, or any, new cells to replenish the blood cells.
Radiation	The emission of electromagnetic waves by all objects warmer than absolute zero is referred to as radiation.
Polycythemia	Polycythemia is a condition in which there is a net increase in the total circulating red blood cell mass of the body.
Skin	Skin is an organ of the integumentary system composed of a layer of tissues that protect

Go to **Cram101.com** for the Practice Tests for this Chapter.

Chapter 7. Diseases of the Blood

Chapter 7. Diseases of the Blood

	underlying muscles and organs.
Reservoir	Reservoir is the source of infection. It is the environment in which microorganisms are able to live and grow.
Phlebotomy	Venipuncture or venepuncture (also known as phlebotomy, blood draw or simply bleeding) is the process of obtaining blood from someone, from one of their veins.
Hemophilia	Hemophilia is the name of any of several hereditary genetic illnesses that impair the body's ability to control bleeding. Genetic deficiencies cause lowered plasma clotting factor activity so as to compromise blood-clotting; when a blood vessel is injured, a scab will not form and the vessel can continue to bleed excessively for a very long period of time.
Affect	Affect is the scientific term used to describe a subject's externally displayed mood. This can be assesed by the nurse by observing facial expression, tone of voice, and body language.
Carrier	Person in apparent health whose chromosomes contain a pathologic mutant gene that may be transmitted to his or her children is a carrier.
Muscle	Muscle is a contractile form of tissue. It is one of the four major tissue types, the other three being epithelium, connective tissue and nervous tissue. Muscle contraction is used to move parts of the body, as well as to move substances within the body.
Joint	A joint (articulation) is the location at which two bones make contact (articulate). They are constructed to both allow movement and provide mechanical support.
Lead	Lead is a chemical element in the periodic table that has the symbol Pb and atomic number 82. A soft, heavy, toxic and malleable poor metal, lead is bluish white when freshly cut but tarnishes to dull gray when exposed to air. Lead is used in building construction, lead-acid batteries, bullets and shot, and is part of solder, pewter, and fusible alloys.
Organ	Organ refers to a structure consisting of several tissues adapted as a group to perform specific functions.
Petechiae	A petechiae is a small red or purple spot on the body, caused by a minor hemorrhage
Idiopathic	Idiopathic is a medical adjective that indicates that a recognized cause has not yet been established.
Leukemia	Leukemia refers to a type of cancer of the bloodforming tissues, characterized by an excessive production of white blood cells and an abnormally high number of them in the blood; cancer of the bone marrow cells that produce leukocytes.
Cancer	Cancer is a class of diseases or disorders characterized by uncontrolled division of cells and the ability of these cells to invade other tissues, either by direct growth into adjacent tissue through invasion or by implantation into distant sites by metastasis.
Lymph node	A lymph node acts as a filter, with an internal honeycomb of connective tissue filled with lymphocytes that collect and destroy bacteria and viruses. When the body is fighting an infection, these lymphocytes multiply rapidly and produce a characteristic swelling of the lymph node.
Medicine	Medicine is the branch of health science and the sector of public life concerned with maintaining or restoring human health through the study, diagnosis and treatment of disease and injury.
Lymph	Lymph originates as blood plasma lost from the circulatory system, which leaks out into the surrounding tissues. The lymphatic system collects this fluid by diffusion into lymph capillaries, and returns it to the circulatory system.
Lymphadenopathy	Lymphadenopathy is swelling of one or more lymph nodes.

Chapter 7. Diseases of the Blood

Chapter 7. Diseases of the Blood

Palpitation	A palpitation is an awareness of the beating of the heart, whether it is too slow, too fast, irregular, or at its normal frequency; brought on by overexertion, adrenaline, alcohol, disease or drugs, or as a symptom of panic disorder.
Infiltration	Infiltration is the diffusion or accumulation (in a tissue or cells) of substances not normal to it or in amounts in excess of the normal. The material collected in those tissues or cells is also called infiltration.
Hepatomegaly	Hepatomegaly is the condition of having an enlarged liver. It is a nonspecific medical sign having many causes, which can broadly be broken down into infection, direct toxicity, hepatic tumours, or metabolic disorder.
Bacteria	The domain that contains procaryotic cells with primarily diacyl glycerol diesters in their membranes and with bacterial rRNA. Bacteria also is a general term for organisms that are composed of procaryotic cells and are not multicellular.
Granulocytes	Granulocytes are a category of white blood cells, characterised by the fact that all types have differently staining granules in their cytoplasm on light microscopy. They are also called polymorphonuclear leukocytes (PMN or PML) because of the varying shapes of the nucleus, which is usually lobed into three segments.
Granulocyte	Granulocyte is a category of white blood cells, characterized by the fact that all types have differently staining granules in their cytoplasm on light microscopy.
Incidence	In epidemiological studies of a particular disorder, the rate at which new cases occur in a given place at a given time is called incidence.
Acute	In medicine, an acute disease is a disease with either or both of: a rapid onset; and a short course (as opposed to a chronic course).
Acute lymphocytic leukemia	Acute lymphocytic leukemia is a cancer of the white blood cells, characterized by the overproduction and continuous multiplication of malignant and immature white blood cells (referred to as lymphoblasts) in the bone marrow.
Course	Pattern of development and change of a disorder over time is a course.
Acute myelogenous leukemia	Acute myelogenous leukemia (AML), also known as acute myeloid leukemia, is a cancer of the myeloid line of blood cells. The median age of patients with AML is 70; it is rare among children.
Agent	Agent refers to an epidemiological term referring to the organism or object that transmits a disease from the environment to the host.
Chemotherapy	Chemotherapy is the use of chemical substances to treat disease. In its modern-day use, it refers almost exclusively to cytostatic drugs used to treat cancer. In its non-oncological use, the term may also refer to antibiotics.
Induction	A discipline technique in which a parent uses reason and explanation of the consequences for others of a child's actions is called induction.
Consolidation	A physiological change in the brain that must take place for encoded information to be stored in memory is a consolidation.
Remission	Disappearance of the signs of a disease is called remission.
Chemotherapeutic agent	Compound used in the treatment of disease that destroy pathogens or inhibit their growth at concentrations low enough to avoid doing undesirable damage to the host is referred to as a chemotherapeutic agent.
Serum	Serum is the same as blood plasma except that clotting factors (such as fibrin) have been removed. Blood plasma contains fibrinogen.

Chapter 7. Diseases of the Blood

Chapter 7. Diseases of the Blood

Lymphoma	Lymphoma is any of a variety of cancer that begins in the lymphatic system. In technical terms, lymphoma denotes malignancies of lymphocytes or, more rarely, of histiocytes.
Lymphatic system	Lymph originates as blood plasma lost from the circulatory system, which leaks out into the surrounding tissues. The lymphatic system collects this fluid by diffusion into lymph capillaries, and returns it to the circulatory system.
Lymph vessel	Lymph vessel refers to one of the system of vessels carrying lymph from the lymph capillaries to the veins.
Bone marrow transplant	Replacement of diseased bone marrow killed by radiation and chemicals with healthy bone marrow from a compatible donor is called bone marrow transplant.
Bone marrow transplantation	Bone marrow transplantation (BMT) or hematopoietic stem cell transplantation (HSCT) is a medical procedure in the field of hematology and oncology that involves transplantation of hematopoietic stem cells (HSC).
Autologous	In biology, autologous refers to cells, tissues or even proteins that are reimplanted in the same individual as they come from.
Donor	Blood donation is a process by which a blood donor voluntarily has blood drawn for storage in a blood bank for subsequent use in a blood transfusion.
Rejection	Rejection is a response by caregivers where they distance themselves emotionally from a chronically ill patient. Although they provide physical care they tend to scold and and correct the patient continuously.
Electrolyte	An electrolyte is a substance that dissociates into free ions when dissolved (or molten), to produce an electrically conductive medium. Because they generally consist of ions in solution, they are also known as ionic solutions.
Cholesterol	Cholesterol is a steroid, a lipid, and an alcohol, found in the cell membranes of all body tissues, and transported in the blood plasma of all animals. It is an important component of the membranes of cells, providing stability; it makes the membrane's fluidity stable over a bigger temperature interval.
Enzyme	An enzyme is a protein that catalyzes, or speeds up, a chemical reaction. They are essential to sustain life because most chemical reactions in biological cells would occur too slowly, or would lead to different products, without them.
Salt	Salt is a term used for ionic compounds composed of positively charged cations and negatively charged anions, so that the product is neutral and without a net charge.
Iliac	In human anatomy, iliac artery refers to several anatomical structures located in the pelvis.
Ratio	In number and more generally in algebra, a ratio is the linear relationship between two quantities.
Stress	Stress refers to a condition that is a response to factors that change the human systems normal state.
Venous blood	In the circulatory system, venous blood or peripheral blood is blood returning to the heart. With one exception (the pulmonary vein) this blood is deoxygenated and high in carbon dioxide, having released oxygen and absorbed CO_2 in the tissues.
Coagulation	The coagulation of blood is a complex process during which blood forms solid clots. It is an important part of haemostasis (the ceszation of blood loss from a damaged vessel) whereby a damaged blood vessel wall is covered by a fibrin clot to stop hemorrhage and aid repair of the damaged vessel.
Prothrombin	Prothrombin refers to plasma protein that is converted to thrombin during the steps of blood

Chapter 7. Diseases of the Blood

	clotting. Prothrombin is a blood plasma protein and is synthesized in the liver.
Prognosis	Prognosis refers to the prospects for the future or outcome of a disease.
Exacerbation	Exacerbation is a period in an illness when the symptoms of the disease reappear.
Ecchymosis	A bruise or contusion or ecchymosis is a kind of injury, usually caused by blunt impact, in which the capillaries are damaged, allowing blood to seep into the surrounding tissue.
Palpation	Palpation is a method of examination in which the examiner feels the size or shape or firmness or location of something.
Complaint	Complaint refers to report made by the police or some other agency to the court that initiates the intake process.
Biopsy	Removal of small tissue sample from the body for microscopic examination is called biopsy.
Intermittent fever	A intermittent fever is when the body temperature alternates between fever and normal or subnormal temperature.
Radiation therapy	Treatment for cancer in which parts of the body that have cancerous tumors are exposed to high-energy radiation to disrupt cell division of the cancer cells is called radiation therapy.
Critical thinking	Critical thinking consists of a mental process of analyzing or evaluating information, particularly statements or propositions that people have offered as true. It forms a process of reflecting upon the meaning of statements, examining the offered evidence and reasoning, and forming judgments about the facts.
Health	Health is a term that refers to a combination of the absence of illness, the ability to cope with everyday activities, physical fitness, and high quality of life.
Public health	Public health is concerned with threats to the overall health of a community based on population health analysis.

Chapter 7. Diseases of the Blood

Chapter 8. Diseases of the Heart

Mitral valve	The mitral valve, also known as the bicuspid valve, is a valve in the heart that lies between the left atrium (LA) and the left ventricle (LV). The mitral valve and the tricuspid valve are known as the atrioventricular valves because they lie between the atria and the ventricles of the heart.
Pericardium	The pericardium is a double-walled sac that contains the heart and the roots of the great vessels. There are two layers to this sac: the fibrous pericardium, serous pericardium.
Endocardium	In the heart, the endocardium is the innermost layer of cells, embryologically and biologically similar to the endothelium that lines blood vessels.
Myocardium	Myocardium is the muscular tissue of the heart. The myocardium is composed of specialized cardiac muscle cells with an ability not possessed by muscle tissue elsewhere in the body.
Organ	Organ refers to a structure consisting of several tissues adapted as a group to perform specific functions.
Tricuspid valve	The tricuspid valve is on the right side of the heart, between the right atrium and the right ventricle. Being the first valve after the venae cavae, and thus the whole venous system, it is the most common valve to be infected (endocarditis) in IV drug users.
Left atrium	The left atrium is one of four chambers (two atria and two ventricles) in the human heart. It receives oxygenated blood from the pulmonary veins, and pumps it into the left ventricle.
Ventricle	In the heart, a ventricle is a heart chamber which collects blood from an atrium (another heart chamber) and pumps it out of the heart.
Atrium	The atrium is the blood collection chamber of a heart. It has a thin-walled structure that allows blood to return to the heart. There is at least one atrium in an animal with a closed circulatory system
Left ventricle	The left ventricle is one of four chambers (two atria and two ventricles) in the human heart. It receives oxygenated blood from the left atrium via the mitral valve, and pumps it into the aorta via the aortic valve.
Muscle	Muscle is a contractile form of tissue. It is one of the four major tissue types, the other three being epithelium, connective tissue and nervous tissue. Muscle contraction is used to move parts of the body, as well as to move substances within the body.
Cardiac muscle	Cardiac muscle is a type of striated muscle found within the heart. Its function is to "pump" blood through the circulatory system. Unlike skeletal muscle, which contracts in response to nerve stimulation, and like smooth muscle, cardiac muscle is myogenic, meaning that it stimulates its own contraction without a requisite electrical impulse.
Blood	Blood is a circulating tissue composed of fluid plasma and cells. The main function of blood is to supply nutrients (oxygen, glucose) and constitutional elements to tissues and to remove waste products.
Blood vessel	A blood vessel is a part of the circulatory system and function to transport blood throughout the body. The most important types, arteries and veins, are so termed because they carry blood away from or towards the heart, respectively.
Septum	A septum, in general, is a wall separating two cavities or two spaces containing a less dense material. The muscle wall that divides the heart chambers.
AV valves	AV valves are large, multicusped valves that prevent backflow from the ventricles into the atria during systole. They are anchored to the wall of the ventricle by chordae tendinae, that prevent the valve from inverting.
Right ventricle	The right ventricle is one of four chambers (two atria and two ventricles) in the human heart. It receives de-oxygenated blood from the right atrium via the tricuspid valve, and

Go to Cram101.com for the Practice Tests for this Chapter.

Chapter 8. Diseases of the Heart

Chapter 8. Diseases of the Heart

	pumps it into the pulmonary artery via the pulmonary valve.
Artery	Vessel that takes blood away from the heart to the tissues and organs of the body is called an artery.
Aorta	The largest artery in the human body, the aorta originates from the left ventricle of the heart and brings oxygenated blood to all parts of the body in the systemic circulation.
Pulmonary artery	The pulmonary artery carrys blood from the heart to the lungs. They are the only arteries (other than umbilical arteries in the fetus) that carry deoxygenated blood.
Semilunar valve	Valve resembling a half moon located between the ventricles and their attached vessels is a semilunar valve. These are positioned on the pulmonary artery and the aorta. These valves do not have chordae tendinae, but are more similar to valves in veins.
Lungs	Lungs are the essential organs of respiration in air-breathing vertebrates. Their principal function is to transport oxygen from the atmosphere into the bloodstream, and to excrete carbon dioxide from the bloodstream into the atmosphere.
Tissue	A collection of interconnected cells that perform a similar function within an organism is called tissue.
Systole	The contraction stage of the heart cycle, when the heart chambers actively pump blood is systole.
Cardiac cycle	Cardiac cycle is the term used to describe the sequence of events that occur as a heart works to pump blood through the body. Every single 'beat' of the heart involves three major stages: atrial systole, ventricular systole and complete cardiac diastole.
Heart attack	A heart attack, is a serious, sudden heart condition usually characterized by varying degrees of chest pain or discomfort, weakness, sweating, nausea, vomiting, and arrhythmias, sometimes causing loss of consciousness. It occurs when the blood supply to a part of the heart is interrupted, causing death and scarring of the local heart tissue.
Coronary	Referring to the heart or the blood vessels of the heart is referred to as coronary.
Coronary arteries	Arteries that directly supply the heart with blood are referred to as coronary arteries.
Coronary artery	An artery that supplies blood to the wall of the heart is called a coronary artery.
Metabolism	Metabolism is the biochemical modification of chemical compounds in living organisms and cells. This includes the biosynthesis of complex organic molecules (anabolism) and their breakdown (catabolism).
Carbon	Carbon is a chemical element in the periodic table that has the symbol C and atomic number 6. An abundant nonmetallic, tetravalent element, carbon has several allotropic forms.
Oxygen	Oxygen is a chemical element in the periodic table. It has the symbol O and atomic number 8. Oxygen is the second most common element on Earth, composing around 46% of the mass of Earth's crust and 28% of the mass of Earth as a whole, and is the third most common element in the universe.
Carbon dioxide	Carbon dioxide is an atmospheric gas comprized of one carbon and two oxygen atoms. A very widely known chemical compound, it is frequently called by its formula CO_2. In its solid state, it is commonly known as dry ice.
Capillaries	Capillaries refer to the smallest of the blood vessels and the sites of exchange between the blood and tissue cells.
Capillary	A capillary is the smallest of a body's blood vessels, measuring 5-10 micro meters. They connect arteries and veins, and most closely interact with tissues. Their walls are composed

Go to **Cram101.com** for the Practice Tests for this Chapter.

Chapter 8. Diseases of the Heart

Chapter 8. Diseases of the Heart

	of a single layer of cells, the endothelium. This layer is so thin that molecules such as oxygen, water and lipids can pass through them by diffusion and enter the tissues.
Veins	Blood vessels that return blood toward the heart from the circulation are referred to as veins.
Vein	Vein in animals, is a vessel that returns blood to the heart. In plants, a vascular bundle in a leaf, composed of xylem and phloem.
Pulmonary vein	The pulmonary vein carries oxygen rich blood from the lungs to the left atrium of the heart. They are the only veins in the adult human body that carry oxygenated blood.
Diastole	The stage of the heart cycle in which the heart muscle is relaxed, allowing the chambers to fill with blood is called diastole.
Right coronary artery	The right coronary artery originates above the right cusp of the aortic valve. It travels down the right atrioventricular groove, towards the crux of the heart. At the origin of the RCA is the conus artery.
Aortic valve	The aortic valve lies between the left ventricle and the aorta. The most common congenital abnormality of the heart is the bicuspid aortic valve. In this condition, instead of three cusps, the aortic valve has two cusps.
Nerve	A nerve is an enclosed, cable-like bundle of nerve fibers or axons, which includes the glia that ensheath the axons in myelin.
Autonomic nervous system	The autonomic nervous system is the part of the nervous system that is not consciously controlled. It is commonly divided into two usually antagonistic subsystems: the sympathetic and parasympathetic nervous system.
Nervous system	The nervous system of an animal coordinates the activity of the muscles, monitors the organs, constructs and processes input from the senses, and initiates actions.
Sinoatrial node	Sinoatrial node refers to a small mass of specialized muscle in the wall of the right atrium; generates electrical signals rhythmically and spontaneously and serves as the heart's pacemaker.
Fiber	Fibers used by man come from a wide variety of sources: Natural fiber include those made out of plants, animal and mineral sources. Natural fibers can be classified according to their origin.
Purkinje fiber	A purkinje fiber is located in the inner ventricular walls of the heart, just beneath the endocardium. These fibers are specialized myocardial fibers that conduct an electrical stimulus or impulse that enables the heart to contract in a coordinated fashion.
Vagus nerve	The vagus nerve is tenth of twelve paired cranial nerves and is the only nerve that starts in the brainstem and extends all the way down past the head, right down to the abdomen. The vagus nerve is arguably the single most important nerve in the body.
Acetylcholine	The chemical compound acetylcholine was the first neurotransmitter to be identified. It is a chemical transmitter in both the peripheral nervous system (PNS) and central nervous system (CNS) in many organisms including humans.
Sympathetic	The sympathetic nervous system activates what is often termed the "fight or flight response". It is an automatic regulation system, that is, one that operates without the intervention of conscious thought.
Stress	Stress refers to a condition that is a response to factors that change the human systems normal state.
Epinephrine	Epinephrine is a hormone and a neurotransmitter. Epinephrine plays a central role in the

Chapter 8. Diseases of the Heart

Chapter 8. Diseases of the Heart

	short-term stress reaction—the physiological response to threatening or exciting conditions (fight-or-flight response). It is secreted by the adrenal medulla.
Coronary heart disease	Coronary heart disease is the end result of the accumulation of atheromatous plaques within the walls of the arteries that supply the myocardium (the muscle of the heart).
Coronary artery disease	Coronary artery disease (CAD) is the end result of the accumulation of atheromatous plaques within the walls of the arteries that supply the myocardium (the muscle of the heart).
Coronary circulation	The coronary circulation consists of the blood vessels that supply blood to, and remove blood from, the heart. The vessels that supply blood high in oxygen to the heart are known as coronary arteries.
Blood clot	A blood clot is the final product of the blood coagulation step in hemostasis. It is achieved via the aggregation of platelets that form a platelet plug, and the activation of the humoral coagulation system
Inhibitor	An inhibitor is a type of effector (biology) that decreases or prevents the rate of a chemical reaction. They are often called negative catalysts.
Occlusion	The term occlusion is often used to refer to blood vessels, arteries or veins which have become totally blocked to any blood flow.
Atherosclerosis	Process by which a fatty substance or plaque builds up inside arteries to form obstructions is called atherosclerosis.
Ischemia	Narrowing of arteries caused by plaque buildup within the arteries is called ischemia.
Cardiovascular disease	Cardiovascular disease refers to afflictions in the mechanisms, including the heart, blood vessels, and their controllers, that are responsible for transporting blood to the body's tissues and organs. Psychological factors may play important roles in such diseases and their treatments.
Scar	A scar results from the biologic process of wound repair in the skin and other tissues of the body. It is a connective tissue that fills the wound.
Pain	Pain is an unpleasant sensation which may be associated with actual or potential tissue damage and which may have physical and emotional components.
Infarction	The sudden death of tissue from a lack of blood perfusion is referred to as an infarction.
Prognosis	Prognosis refers to the prospects for the future or outcome of a disease.
Myocardial infarction	Acute myocardial infarction, commonly known as a heart attack, is a serious, sudden heart condition usually characterized by varying degrees of chest pain or discomfort, weakness, sweating, nausea, vomiting, and arrhythmias, sometimes causing loss of consciousness.
Congestive heart failure	Congestive heart failure is the inability of the heart to pump a sufficient amount of blood throughout the body, or requiring elevated filling pressures in order to pump effectively.
Sodium	Sodium is the chemical element in the periodic table that has the symbol Na (Natrium in Latin) and atomic number 11. Sodium is a soft, waxy, silvery reactive metal belonging to the alkali metals that is abundant in natural compounds (especially halite). It is highly reactive.
Salt	Salt is a term used for ionic compounds composed of positively charged cations and negatively charged anions, so that the product is neutral and without a net charge.
Atrioventricular node	The atrioventricular node is the tissue between the atria and the ventricles of the heart, which conducts the normal electrical impulse from the atria to the ventricles.
Enzyme	An enzyme is a protein that catalyzes, or speeds up, a chemical reaction. They are essential

Chapter 8. Diseases of the Heart

Chapter 8. Diseases of the Heart

	to sustain life because most chemical reactions in biological cells would occur too slowly, or would lead to different products, without them.
Channel	Channel, in communications (sometimes called communications channel), refers to the medium used to convey information from a sender (or transmitter) to a receiver.
Hypertension	Hypertension is a medical condition where the blood pressure in the arteries is chronically elevated. Persistent hypertension is one of the risk factors for strokes, heart attacks, heart failure and arterial aneurysm, and is a leading cause of chronic renal failure.
Lifestyle	The culturally, socially, economically, and environmentally conditioned complex of actions characteristic of an individual, group, or community as a pattern of habituated behavior over time that is health related but not necessarily health directed is a lifestyle.
Obesity	The state of being more than 20 percent above the average weight for a person of one's height is called obesity.
Bypass	In medicine, a bypass generally means an alternate or additional route for blood flow, which is created in bypass surgery, e.g. coronary artery bypass surgery by moving blood vessels or implanting synthetic tubing.
Angioplasty	Angioplasty is the mechanical, hydraulic dilation of a narrowed or totally obstructed arterial lumen, generally caused by atheroma (the lesion of atherosclerosis).
Angina	Angina pectoris is chest pain due to ischemia (a lack of blood and hence oxygen supply) to the heart muscle, generally due to obstruction or spasm of the coronary arteries (the heart's blood vessels). Coronary artery disease, the main cause of angina, is due to atherosclerosis of the cardiac arteries.
Unstable angina	Worsening angina attacks, sudden-onset angina at rest, and angina lasting more than 15 minutes are symptoms of unstable angina or acute coronary syndrome. As these may herald myocardial infarction (a heart attack), they require urgent medical attention and are generally treated quite similarly
Blood pressure	Blood pressure is the pressure exerted by the blood on the walls of the blood vessels.
Resistance	Resistance refers to a nonspecific ability to ward off infection or disease regardless of whether the body has been previously exposed to it. A force that opposes the flow of a fluid such as air or blood. Compare with immunity.
Pulmonary hypertension	Pulmonary hypertension (PH) is an increase in blood pressure in the pulmonary artery or lung vasculature.
Respiratory failure	Respiratory failure is a medical term for inadequate gas exchange by the respiratory system.
Ventilator	A medical ventilator is a device designed to provide mechanical ventilation to a patient. They are chiefly used in intensive care medicine, home care, and emergency medicine (as standalone units) and in anesthesia (as a component of an anesthesia machine).
Bronchodilator	A bronchodilator is a medication intended to improve bronchial airflow. Treatment of bronchial asthma is the most common application of these drugs.
Lead	Lead is a chemical element in the periodic table that has the symbol Pb and atomic number 82. A soft, heavy, toxic and malleable poor metal, lead is bluish white when freshly cut but tarnishes to dull gray when exposed to air. Lead is used in building construction, lead-acid batteries, bullets and shot, and is part of solder, pewter, and fusible alloys.
Infection	The invasion and multiplication of microorganisms in body tissues is called an infection.
Bacteria	The domain that contains procaryotic cells with primarily diacyl glycerol diesters in their

Chapter 8. Diseases of the Heart

Chapter 8. Diseases of the Heart

	membranes and with bacterial rRNA. Bacteria also is a general term for organisms that are composed of procaryotic cells and are not multicellular.
Mortality	The incidence of death in a population is mortality.
Mortality rate	Mortality rate is the number of deaths (from a disease or in general) per 1000 people and typically reported on an annual basis.
Foramen ovale	In the fetal heart, the foramen ovale is a shunt from the right to left atrium. At the base of the skull, the foramen ovale transmits the mandibular nerve, otic ganglion, accessory meningeal artery, and emissary veins.
Atrial septal defect	A atrial septal defect (ASD) is a group of congenital heart diseases that involve the interatrial septum of the heart.
Ventricular septal defect	A ventricular septal defect is a defect in the ventricular septum, the wall dividing the left and right ventricles of the heart.
Shunt	In medicine, a shunt is a hole or passage which moves, or allows movement of, fluid from one part of the body to another. The term may describe either congenital or acquired shunts; and acquired shunts may be either biological or mechanical.
Cyanosis	Bluish skin coloration due to decreased blood oxygen concentration is called cyanosis.
Hemoglobin	Hemoglobin is the iron-containing oxygen-transport metalloprotein in the red cells of the blood in mammals and other animals. Hemoglobin transports oxygen from the lungs to the rest of the body, such as to the muscles, where it releases the oxygen load.
Stenosis	A stenosis is an abnormal narrowing in a blood vessel or other tubular organ or structure. It is also sometimes called a "stricture" (as in urethral stricture).
Pulmonary stenosis	Pulmonary stenosis is the abnormal narrowing of the opening between the right ventricle and the pulmonary artery that slows blood flow to the lungs.
Hypertrophy	Hypertrophy is the increase of the size of an organ. It should be distinguished from hyperplasia which occurs due to cell division; hypertrophy occurs due to an increase in cell size rather than division. It is most commonly seen in muscle that has been actively stimulated, the most well-known method being exercise.
Red blood cells	Red blood cells are the most common type of blood cell and are the vertebrate body's principal means of delivering oxygen from the lungs or gills to body tissues via the blood.
Red blood cell	The red blood cell is the most common type of blood cell and is the vertebrate body's principal means of delivering oxygen from the lungs or gills to body tissues via the blood.
Dyspnea	Dyspnea or shortness of breath (SOB) is perceived difficulty breathing or pain on breathing. It is a common symptom of numerous medical disorders.
Lesion	A lesion is a non-specific term referring to abnormal tissue in the body. It can be caused by any disease process including trauma (physical, chemical, electrical), infection, neoplasm, metabolic and autoimmune.
Abdomen	The abdomen is a part of the body. In humans, and in many other vertebrates, it is the region between the thorax and the pelvis. In fully developed insects, the abdomen is the third (or posterior) segment, after the head and thorax.
Heart murmur	A heart murmur is produced as a result of turbulent flow of blood, turbulence sufficient to produce audible noise. This most commonly results from narrowing or leaking of valves or the presence of abnormal passages through which blood flows in or near the heart.
Murmurs	Murmurs are produced as a result of turbulent flow of blood, turbulence sufficient to produce audible noise.

Go to Cram101.com for the Practice Tests for this Chapter.

Chapter 8. Diseases of the Heart

Chapter 8. Diseases of the Heart

Mitral stenosis	Mitral stenosis is a narrowing of the orifice of the mitral valve of the heart.
Fever	Fever (also known as pyrexia, or a febrile response, and archaically known as ague) is a medical symptom that describes an increase in internal body temperature to levels that are above normal (37°C, 98.6°F).
Rheumatic fever	Rheumatic fever is an inflammatory disease which may develop after a Group A streptococcal infection (such as strep throat or scarlet fever) and can involve the heart, joints, skin, and brain.
Thrombus	Blood clot that remains in the blood vessel where it formed is called a thrombus.
Embolism	An embolism occurs when an object (the embolus) migrates from one part of the body and causes a blockage of a blood vessel in another part of the body.
Kidney	The kidney is a bean-shaped excretory organ in vertebrates. Part of the urinary system, the kidneys filter wastes (especially urea) from the blood and excrete them, along with water, as urine.
Brain	The part of the central nervous system involved in regulating and controlling body activity and interpreting information from the senses transmitted through the nervous system is referred to as the brain.
Congestion	In medicine and pathology the term congestion is used to describe excessive accumulation of blood or other fluid in a particular part of the body.
Edema	Edema is swelling of any organ or tissue due to accumulation of excess fluid. Edema has many root causes, but its common mechanism is accumulation of fluid into the tissues.
Papillary muscle	The papillary muscle of the heart serves to limit the movements of the mitral and tricuspid valves and prevent them from being reverted.
Aortic stenosis	Aortic stenosis is a heart condition caused by the incomplete opening of the aortic valve.
Syncope	Syncope is also the medical term for fainting.
Joint	A joint (articulation) is the location at which two bones make contact (articulate). They are constructed to both allow movement and provide mechanical support.
Young adult	An young adult is someone between the ages of 20 and 40 years old.
Autoimmune	Autoimmune refers to immune reactions against normal body cells; self against self.
Autoimmune disease	Disease that results when the immune system mistakenly attacks the body's own tissues is referred to as autoimmune disease.
Antibody	An antibody is a protein used by the immune system to identify and neutralize foreign objects like bacteria and viruses. Each antibody recognizes a specific antigen unique to its target.
Antigen	An antigen is a substance that stimulates an immune response, especially the production of antibodies. They are usually proteins or polysaccharides, but can be any type of molecule, including small molecules (haptens) coupled to a protein (carrier).
Antibiotic	Antibiotic refers to substance such as penicillin or streptomycin that is toxic to microorganisms. Usually a product of a particular microorvanism or plant.
Inflammation	Inflammation is the first response of the immune system to infection or irritation and may be referred to as the innate cascade.
Skin	Skin is an organ of the integumentary system composed of a layer of tissues that protect underlying muscles and organs.
Heart rate	Heart rate is a term used to describe the frequency of the cardiac cycle. It is considered

Chapter 8. Diseases of the Heart

Chapter 8. Diseases of the Heart

	one of the four vital signs. Usually it is calculated as the number of contractions of the heart in one minute and expressed as "beats per minute".
Physiology	The study of the function of cells, tissues, and organs is referred to as physiology.
Anatomy	Anatomy is the branch of biology that deals with the structure and organization of living things. It can be divided into animal anatomy (zootomy) and plant anatomy (phytonomy).
Fibrillation	Fibrillation is the rapid, irregular, and unsynchronized contraction of the muscle fibers of the heart. There are two major classes of fibrillation, atrial fibrillation and ventricular fibrillation.
Atrial fibrillation	Atrial fibrillation (AF or afib) is an abnormal heart rhythm (cardiac arrhythmia) which involves the two small, upper heart chambers (the atria).
Microorganism	A microorganism or microbe is an organism that is so small that it is microscopic (invisible to the naked eye).
Affect	Affect is the scientific term used to describe a subject's externally displayed mood. This can be assesed by the nurse by observing facial expression, tone of voice, and body language.
Ventricular fibrillation	Ventricular fibrillation is a cardiac condition that consists of a lack of coordination of the contraction of the muscle tissue of the large chambers of the heart that eventually leads to the heart stopping altogether.
Cardiac arrest	A cardiac arrest is the ceszation of normal circulation of the blood due to failure of the ventricles of the heart to contract effectively during systole.
Shock	Circulatory shock, a state of cardiac output that is insufficient to meet the body's physiological needs, with consequences ranging from fainting to death is referred to as shock. Insulin shock, a state of severe hypoglycemia caused by administration of insulin.
Arrhythmia	Cardiac arrhythmia is a group of conditions in which muscle contraction of the heart is irregular for any reason.
Cardiac arrhythmia	Cardiac arrhythmia is a group of conditions in which the muscle contraction of the heart is irregular or is faster or slower than normal.
Tachycardia	Tachycardia is an abnormally rapid beating of the heart, defined as a resting heart rate of over 100 beats per minute. Common causes are autonomic nervous system or endocrine system activity, hemodynamic responses, and various forms of cardiac arrhythmia.
Bradycardia	Bradycardia, as applied in adult medicine, is defined as a heart rate of under 60 beats per minute, though it is seldom symptomatic until the rate drops below 50 beat/min.
Medicine	Medicine is the branch of health science and the sector of public life concerned with maintaining or restoring human health through the study, diagnosis and treatment of disease and injury.
Electrocardigram	An electrocardiogram is a graphic produced by an electrocardiograph, which records the electrical voltage in the heart in the form of a continuous strip graph. It is the prime tool in cardiac electrophysiology, and has a prime function in screening and diagnosis of cardiovascular diseases..
Auscultation	Auscultation is the technical term for listening to the internal sounds of the body, usually using a stethoscope. Auscultation is normally performed for the purposes of examining the cardiovascular system and respiratory systems (heart and lung sounds), as well as the gastrointestinal system (bowel sounds).
Diagnosis	In medicine, diagnosis is the process of identifying a medical condition or disease by its signs, symptoms, and from the results of various diagnostic procedures.

Chapter 8. Diseases of the Heart

Chapter 8. Diseases of the Heart

Ultrasound	Ultrasound is sound with a frequency greater than the upper limit of human hearing, approximately 20 kilohertz. Medical use can visualise muscle and soft tissue, making them useful for scanning the organs, and obstetric ultrasonography is commonly used during pregnancy.
Catheter	A tubular surgical instrument for withdrawing fluids from a cavity of the body, especially one for introduction into the bladder through the urethra for the withdrawal of urine is referred to as a catheter.
Cardiac catheterization	Cardiac catheterization is the insertion of a catheter into a chamber or vessel of the heart. A small incision is made in a vessel in the groin, wrist or neck area (the femoral vessels or the carotid/jugular vessels), then a guidewire is inserted into the incision and threaded through the vessel into the area of the heart that requires treatment, visualized by fluoroscopy or echocardiogram, and a catheter is then threaded over the guidewire.
Basilic vein	In human anatomy, the basilic vein is a superficial vein of the upper limb. It communicates with the cephalic vein via the median cubital vein at the elbow and drains into the axillary vein.
Cardiovascular system	The circulatory system or cardiovascular system is the organ system which circulates blood around the body of most animals.
Cardiac output	Cardiac output is the volume of blood being pumped by the heart in a minute. It is equal to the heart rate multiplied by the stroke volume.
Injection	A method of rapid drug delivery that puts the substance directly in the bloodstream, in a muscle, or under the skin is called injection.
Tolerance	Drug tolerance occurs when a subject's reaction to a drug decreases so that larger doses are required to achieve the same effect.
Angina pectoris	Angina pectoris is chest pain due to ischemia (a lack of blood and hence oxygen supply) to the heart muscle, generally due to obstruction or spasm of the coronary arteries (the heart's blood vessels).
Referred pain	Referred pain is an unpleasant senzation localised to an area separate from the site of the causative injury or other painful stimulation. Often, referred pain arises when a nerve is compressed or damaged at or near its origin.
Consciousness	Consciousness refers to the ability to perceive, communicate, remember, understand, appreciate, and initiate voluntary movements; a functioning sensorium.
Implantation	Implantation refers to attachment and penetration of the embryo into the lining of the uterus.
Palpitation	A palpitation is an awareness of the beating of the heart, whether it is too slow, too fast, irregular, or at its normal frequency; brought on by overexertion, adrenaline, alcohol, disease or drugs, or as a symptom of panic disorder.
Right heart	Right heart is a term used to refer collectively to the right atrium and right ventricle of the heart; occasionally, this term is intended to reference the right atrium, right ventricle, and the pulmonary trunk collectively.
Angiography	Angiography is a medical imaging technique in which an X-Ray picture is taken to visualize the inner opening of blood filled structures, including arteries, veins and the heart chambers.
Petechiae	A petechiae is a small red or purple spot on the body, caused by a minor hemorrhage
Anorexia	Anorexia nervosa is an eating disorder characterized by voluntary starvation and exercise stress.

Chapter 8. Diseases of the Heart

Chapter 8. Diseases of the Heart

Diuretic	A diuretic is any drug that elevates the rate of bodily urine excretion.
Ligation	Ligation refers to enzymatically catalyzed formation of a phosphodiester bond that links two DNA molecules.
Steroid	A steroid is a lipid characterized by a carbon skeleton with four fused rings. Different steroids vary in the functional groups attached to these rings. Hundreds of distinct steroids have been identified in plants and animals. Their most important role in most living systems is as hormones.
Latent	Hidden or concealed is a latent.
Serum	Serum is the same as blood plasma except that clotting factors (such as fibrin) have been removed. Blood plasma contains fibrinogen.
Ductus arteriosus	In the developing fetus, the ductus arteriosus (DA) is a shunt connecting the pulmonary artery to the aortic arch that allows most of the blood from the right ventricle to bypass the fetus' fluid-filled lungs.
Critical thinking	Critical thinking consists of a mental process of analyzing or evaluating information, particularly statements or propositions that people have offered as true. It forms a process of reflecting upon the meaning of statements, examining the offered evidence and reasoning, and forming judgments about the facts.
Pulmonary edema	Pulmonary edema is swelling and/or fluid accumulation in the lungs. It leads to impaired gas exchange and may cause respiratory failure.
Asymptomatic	A disease is asymptomatic when it is at a stage where the patient does not experience symptoms. By their nature, asymptomatic diseases are not usually discovered until the patient undergoes medical tests (X-rays or other investigations). Some diseases remain asymptomatic for a remarkably long time, including some forms of cancer.
Productive cough	A cough in which phlegm or mucus is dislodged, enabling a person to clear mucus from the lungs is a productive cough.
Pulse	The rhythmic stretching of the arteries caused by the pressure of blood forced through the arteries by contractions of the ventricles during systole is a pulse.

Chapter 8. Diseases of the Heart

Chapter 9. Diseases of the Blood Vessels

Blood	Blood is a circulating tissue composed of fluid plasma and cells. The main function of blood is to supply nutrients (oxygen, glucose) and constitutional elements to tissues and to remove waste products.
Blood vessel	A blood vessel is a part of the circulatory system and function to transport blood throughout the body. The most important types, arteries and veins, are so termed because they carry blood away from or towards the heart, respectively.
Distribution	Distribution in pharmacology is a branch of pharmacokinetics describing reversible transfer of drug from one location to another within the body.
Cardiovascular system	The circulatory system or cardiovascular system is the organ system which circulates blood around the body of most animals.
Systemic circulation	Systemic circulation is a circuit of circulation in the cardiovascular system. Blood circulates from the left ventricle to the organs and tissues to the systemic veins to the right atrium.
Artery	Vessel that takes blood away from the heart to the tissues and organs of the body is called an artery.
Lungs	Lungs are the essential organs of respiration in air-breathing vertebrates. Their principal function is to transport oxygen from the atmosphere into the bloodstream, and to excrete carbon dioxide from the bloodstream into the atmosphere.
Aorta	The largest artery in the human body, the aorta originates from the left ventricle of the heart and brings oxygenated blood to all parts of the body in the systemic circulation.
Capillaries	Capillaries refer to the smallest of the blood vessels and the sites of exchange between the blood and tissue cells.
Capillary	A capillary is the smallest of a body's blood vessels, measuring 5-10 micro meters. They connect arteries and veins, and most closely interact with tissues. Their walls are composed of a single layer of cells, the endothelium. This layer is so thin that molecules such as oxygen, water and lipids can pass through them by diffusion and enter the tissues.
Arteriole	An arteriole is a blood vessel that extends and branches out from an artery and leads to capillaries. They have thick muscular walls and are the primary site of vascular resistance.
Veins	Blood vessels that return blood toward the heart from the circulation are referred to as veins.
Vein	Vein in animals, is a vessel that returns blood to the heart. In plants, a vascular bundle in a leaf, composed of xylem and phloem.
Lead	Lead is a chemical element in the periodic table that has the symbol Pb and atomic number 82. A soft, heavy, toxic and malleable poor metal, lead is bluish white when freshly cut but tarnishes to dull gray when exposed to air. Lead is used in building construction, lead-acid batteries, bullets and shot, and is part of solder, pewter, and fusible alloys.
Venule	A vessel that conveys blood between a capillary bed and a vein is a venule.
Pulmonary circulation	The pulmonary circulation is a circuit of blood circulation in the cardiovascular system, serving exclusively the lungs, where red blood cells pick up oxygen and release carbon dioxide during respiration.
Endothelium	The endothelium is the layer of thin, flat cells that lines the interior surface of blood vessels, forming an interface between circulating blood in the lumen and the rest of the vessel wall.
Intima	The tunica intima (or just intima) is the innermost layer of an artery. It is made up of one

Chapter 9. Diseases of the Blood Vessels

Chapter 9. Diseases of the Blood Vessels

	layer of endothelial cells and is supported by an internal elastic lamina. The endothelial cell are in direct contact with the blood flow.
Tissue	A collection of interconnected cells that perform a similar function within an organism is called tissue.
Muscle fiber	Cell with myofibrils containing actin and myosin filaments arranged within sarcomeres is a muscle fiber.
Muscle	Muscle is a contractile form of tissue. It is one of the four major tissue types, the other three being epithelium, connective tissue and nervous tissue. Muscle contraction is used to move parts of the body, as well as to move substances within the body.
Fiber	Fibers used by man come from a wide variety of sources: Natural fiber include those made out of plants, animal and mineral sources. Natural fibers can be classified according to their origin.
Smooth muscle	Smooth muscle is a type of non-striated muscle, found within the "walls" of hollow organs; such as blood vessels, the bladder, the uterus, and the gastrointestinal tract. Smooth muscle is used to move matter within the body, via contraction; it generally operates "involuntarily", without nerve stimulation.
Red blood cell	The red blood cell is the most common type of blood cell and is the vertebrate body's principal means of delivering oxygen from the lungs or gills to body tissues via the blood.
Oxygen	Oxygen is a chemical element in the periodic table. It has the symbol O and atomic number 8. Oxygen is the second most common element on Earth, composing around 46% of the mass of Earth's crust and 28% of the mass of Earth as a whole, and is the third most common element in the universe.
Metabolism	Metabolism is the biochemical modification of chemical compounds in living organisms and cells. This includes the biosynthesis of complex organic molecules (anabolism) and their breakdown (catabolism).
Diffusion	Random movement of molecules from a region of higher concentration toward one of lower concentration is referred to as diffusion.
Inferior vena cava	The inferior vena cava is a large vein that carries de-oxygenated blood from the lower half of the body into the heart. It is formed by the left and right common iliac veins and transports blood to the right atrium of the heart.
Superior vena cava	The superior vena cava is a large but short vein that carries de-oxygenated blood from the upper half of the body to the heart's right atrium. It is formed by the left and right brachiocephalic veins (also referred to as the innominate veins) which receive blood from the upper limbs and the head and neck.
Atherosclerosis	Process by which a fatty substance or plaque builds up inside arteries to form obstructions is called atherosclerosis.
Monocyte	A monocyte is a leukocyte, part of the human body's immune system that protect against blood-borne pathogens and move quickly to sites of infection in the tissues.
White blood cell	The white blood cell is a a component of blood. They help to defend the body against infectious disease and foreign materials as part of the immune system.
Calcium	Calcium is the chemical element in the periodic table that has the symbol Ca and atomic number 20. Calcium is a soft grey alkaline earth metal that is used as a reducing agent in the extraction of thorium, zirconium and uranium. Calcium is also the fifth most abundant element in the Earth's crust.
Carbohydrate	Carbohydrate is a chemical compound that contains oxygen, hydrogen, and carbon atoms. They

Go to **Cram101.com** for the Practice Tests for this Chapter.

Chapter 9. Diseases of the Blood Vessels

Chapter 9. Diseases of the Blood Vessels

	consist of monosaccharide sugars of varying chain lengths and that have the general chemical formula $C_n(H_2O)_n$ or are derivatives of such.
Infarction	The sudden death of tissue from a lack of blood perfusion is referred to as an infarction.
Occlusion	The term occlusion is often used to refer to blood vessels, arteries or veins which have become totally blocked to any blood flow.
Coronary	Referring to the heart or the blood vessels of the heart is referred to as coronary.
Ischemia	Narrowing of arteries caused by plaque buildup within the arteries is called ischemia.
Stroke	A stroke or cerebrovascular accident (CVA) occurs when the blood supply to a part of the brain is suddenly interrupted.
Organ	Organ refers to a structure consisting of several tissues adapted as a group to perform specific functions.
Brain	The part of the central nervous system involved in regulating and controlling body activity and interpreting information from the senses transmitted through the nervous system is referred to as the brain.
Myocardial infarction	Acute myocardial infarction, commonly known as a heart attack, is a serious, sudden heart condition usually characterized by varying degrees of chest pain or discomfort, weakness, sweating, nausea, vomiting, and arrhythmias, sometimes causing loss of consciousness.
Coronary arteries	Arteries that directly supply the heart with blood are referred to as coronary arteries.
Coronary artery	An artery that supplies blood to the wall of the heart is called a coronary artery.
Diabetes	Diabetes is a medical disorder characterized by varying or persistent elevated blood sugar levels, especially after eating. All types of diabetes share similar symptoms and complications at advanced stages: dehydration and ketoacidosis, cardiovascular disease, chronic renal failure, retinal damage which can lead to blindness, nerve damage which can lead to erectile dysfunction, gangrene with risk of amputation of toes, feet, and even legs.
Thrombosis	Thrombosis is the formation of a clot inside a blood vessel, obstructing the flow of blood through the circulatory system. A cerebral thrombosis can result in stroke.
Embolism	An embolism occurs when an object (the embolus) migrates from one part of the body and causes a blockage of a blood vessel in another part of the body.
Blood clot	A blood clot is the final product of the blood coagulation step in hemostasis. It is achieved via the aggregation of platelets that form a platelet plug, and the activation of the humoral coagulation system
Thrombus	Blood clot that remains in the blood vessel where it formed is called a thrombus.
Platelet	Cell fragment that is necessary to blood clotting is a platelet. They are the blood cell fragments that are involved in the cellular mechanisms that lead to the formation of blood clots.
Hypertension	Hypertension is a medical condition where the blood pressure in the arteries is chronically elevated. Persistent hypertension is one of the risk factors for strokes, heart attacks, heart failure and arterial aneurysm, and is a leading cause of chronic renal failure.
Hemorrhage	Loss of blood from the circulatory system is referred to as a hemorrhage.
Angina	Angina pectoris is chest pain due to ischemia (a lack of blood and hence oxygen supply) to the heart muscle, generally due to obstruction or spasm of the coronary arteries (the heart's blood vessels). Coronary artery disease, the main cause of angina, is due to atherosclerosis

Chapter 9. Diseases of the Blood Vessels

Chapter 9. Diseases of the Blood Vessels

	of the cardiac arteries.
Coronary artery disease	Coronary artery disease (CAD) is the end result of the accumulation of atheromatous plaques within the walls of the arteries that supply the myocardium (the muscle of the heart).
Cardiac arrest	A cardiac arrest is the ceszation of normal circulation of the blood due to failure of the ventricles of the heart to contract effectively during systole.
Anticoagulant	A biochemical that inhibits blood clotting is referred to as an anticoagulant.
Intravascular	Within the arteries, vessels, veins, or capillaries is intravascular.
Embolus	Embolus refers to any abnormal traveling object in the bloodstream, such as agglutinated bacteria or blood cells, a blood clot, or an air bubble.
Pulmonary artery	The pulmonary artery carrys blood from the heart to the lungs. They are the only arteries (other than umbilical arteries in the fetus) that carry deoxygenated blood.
Mitral valve	The mitral valve, also known as the bicuspid valve, is a valve in the heart that lies between the left atrium (LA) and the left ventricle (LV). The mitral valve and the tricuspid valve are known as the atrioventricular valves because they lie between the atria and the ventricles of the heart.
Kidney	The kidney is a bean-shaped excretory organ in vertebrates. Part of the urinary system, the kidneys filter wastes (especially urea) from the blood and excrete them, along with water, as urine.
Bacteria	The domain that contains procaryotic cells with primarily diacyl glycerol diesters in their membranes and with bacterial rRNA. Bacteria also is a general term for organisms that are composed of procaryotic cells and are not multicellular.
Cancer	Cancer is a class of diseases or disorders characterized by uncontrolled division of cells and the ability of these cells to invade other tissues, either by direct growth into adjacent tissue through invasion or by implantation into distant sites by metastasis.
Gangrene	Gangrene is necrosis and subsequent decay of body tissues caused by infection or thrombosis or lack of blood flow. It is usually the result of critically insufficient blood supply sometimes caused by injury and subsequent contamination with bacteria.
Necrosis	Necrosis is the name given to unprogrammed death of cells/living tissue. There are many causes of necrosis including injury, infection, cancer, infarction, and inflammation. Necrosis is caused by special enzymes that are released by lysosomes.
Coagulation	The coagulation of blood is a complex process during which blood forms solid clots. It is an important part of haemostasis (the ceszation of blood loss from a damaged vessel) whereby a damaged blood vessel wall is covered by a fibrin clot to stop hemorrhage and aid repair of the damaged vessel.
Aneurysm	An aneurysm is a localized dilation or ballooning of a blood vessel by more than 50% of the diameter of the vessel. Aneurysms most commonly occur in the arteries at the base of the brain and in the aorta (the main artery coming out of the heart) - this is an aortic aneurysm.
Abdomen	The abdomen is a part of the body. In humans, and in many other vertebrates, it is the region between the thorax and the pelvis. In fully developed insects, the abdomen is the third (or posterior) segment, after the head and thorax.
Ultrasound	Ultrasound is sound with a frequency greater than the upper limit of human hearing, approximately 20 kilohertz. Medical use can visualise muscle and soft tissue, making them useful for scanning the organs, and obstetric ultrasonography is commonly used during pregnancy.

Chapter 9. Diseases of the Blood Vessels

Chapter 9. Diseases of the Blood Vessels

Computed tomography	Computed tomography is an imaging method employing tomography where digital processing is used to generate a three-dimensional image of the internals of an object from a large series of two-dimensional X-ray images taken around a single axis of rotation.
Iliac	In human anatomy, iliac artery refers to several anatomical structures located in the pelvis.
Pulmonary embolism	A pulmonary embolism occurs when a blood clot, generally a venous thrombus, becomes dislodged from its site of formation and embolizes to the arterial blood supply of one of the lungs.
Petechiae	A petechiae is a small red or purple spot on the body, caused by a minor hemorrhage
Skin	Skin is an organ of the integumentary system composed of a layer of tissues that protect underlying muscles and organs.
Trauma	Trauma refers to a severe physical injury or wound to the body caused by an external force, or a psychological shock having a lasting effect on mental life.
Hemoglobin	Hemoglobin is the iron-containing oxygen-transport metalloprotein in the red cells of the blood in mammals and other animals. Hemoglobin transports oxygen from the lungs to the rest of the body, such as to the muscles, where it releases the oxygen load.
Stress	Stress refers to a condition that is a response to factors that change the human systems normal state.
Red blood cells	Red blood cells are the most common type of blood cell and are the vertebrate body's principal means of delivering oxygen from the lungs or gills to body tissues via the blood.
Phlebitis	Phlebitis is an inflammation of a vein, usually in the legs.
Inflammation	Inflammation is the first response of the immune system to infection or irritation and may be referred to as the innate cascade.
Infection	The invasion and multiplication of microorganisms in body tissues is called an infection.
Obesity	The state of being more than 20 percent above the average weight for a person of one's height is called obesity.
Edema	Edema is swelling of any organ or tissue due to accumulation of excess fluid. Edema has many root causes, but its common mechanism is accumulation of fluid into the tissues.
Thrombophlebitis	Thrombophlebitis is phlebitis (vein inflammation) related to a blood clot or thrombus. When this occurs repeatedly in different locations, it is known as Thrombophlebitis migrans.
Antibiotic	Antibiotic refers to substance such as penicillin or streptomycin that is toxic to microorganisms. Usually a product of a particular microorvanism or plant.
Medial	In anatomical terms of location toward or near the midline is called medial.
Varicose veins	Varicose veins are veins on the leg which are large, twisted, and ropelike, and can cause pain, swelling, or itching. They are an extreme form of telangiectasia, or spider veins.
Uterus	The uterus is the major female reproductive organ of most mammals. One end, the cervix, opens into the vagina; the other is connected on both sides to the fallopian tubes. The main function is to accept a fertilized ovum which becomes implanted into the endometrium, and derives nourishment from blood vessels which develop exclusively for this purpose.
Tumor	An abnormal mass of cells that forms within otherwise normal tissue is a tumor. This growth can be either malignant or benign
Resistance	Resistance refers to a nonspecific ability to ward off infection or disease regardless of whether the body has been previously exposed to it. A force that opposes the flow of a fluid such as air or blood. Compare with immunity.

Chapter 9. Diseases of the Blood Vessels

Chapter 9. Diseases of the Blood Vessels

Heredity	Heredity refers to the transmission of genetic information from parent to offspring.
Ulcer	An ulcer is an open sore of the skin, eyes or mucous membrane, often caused by an initial abrasion and generally maintained by an inflammation and/or an infection.
Scar	A scar results from the biologic process of wound repair in the skin and other tissues of the body. It is a connective tissue that fills the wound.
Solution	Solution refers to homogenous mixture formed when a solute is dissolved in a solvent.
Rectum	The rectum is the final straight portion of the large intestine in some mammals, and the gut in others, terminating in the anus.
Pain	Pain is an unpleasant sensation which may be associated with actual or potential tissue damage and which may have physical and emotional components.
Hemorrhoids	Hemorrhoids are varicosities or swelling and inflammation of veins in the rectum and anus.
Hemorrhoid	A pronounced swelling in a large vein, particularly veins found in the anal region is referred to as hemorrhoid.
Congestion	In medicine and pathology the term congestion is used to describe excessive accumulation of blood or other fluid in a particular part of the body.
Liver	The liver is an organ in vertebrates, including humans. It plays a major role in metabolism and has a number of functions in the body including drug detoxification, glycogen storage, and plasma protein synthesis. It also produces bile, which is important for digestion.
Varices	Varices in general refers to distended veins. It derives from the latin word for twisted, "varix".
Esophageal varices	In medicine (gastroenterology), esophageal varices are extreme dilations of sub-mucosal veins in the mucosa of the esophagus in diseases featuring portal hypertension, secondary to cirrhosis primarily.
Varicosity	Varicosity refers to a twisted, swollen vein.
Blood pressure	Blood pressure is the pressure exerted by the blood on the walls of the blood vessels.
Brain tumor	A brain tumor is any intracranial mass created by an abnormal and uncontrolled growth of cells either normally found in the brain itself: neurons, glial cells (astrocytes, oligodendrocytes, ependymal cells), lymphatic tissue, blood vessels), in the cranial nerves, in the brain envelopes (meninges), skull, pituitary and pineal gland, or spread from cancers primarily located in other organs.
Alcohol	Alcohol is a general term, applied to any organic compound in which a hydroxyl group (-OH) is bound to a carbon atom, which in turn is bound to other hydrogen and/or carbon atoms. The general formula for a simple acyclic alcohol is $C_nH_{2n+1}OH$.
Salt	Salt is a term used for ionic compounds composed of positively charged cations and negatively charged anions, so that the product is neutral and without a net charge.
Diastolic pressure	Diastolic pressure refers to arterial blood pressure during the diastolic phase of the cardiac cycle.
Ventricle	In the heart, a ventricle is a heart chamber which collects blood from an atrium (another heart chamber) and pumps it out of the heart.
Systolic pressure	The force of blood against the walls of the arteries when the heart contracts to pump blood to the rest of the body is systolic pressure.
Adjustment	Adjustment is an attempt to cope with a given situation.

Chapter 9. Diseases of the Blood Vessels

Chapter 9. Diseases of the Blood Vessels

Nervous system	The nervous system of an animal coordinates the activity of the muscles, monitors the organs, constructs and processes input from the senses, and initiates actions.
Sympathetic	The sympathetic nervous system activates what is often termed the "fight or flight response". It is an automatic regulation system, that is, one that operates without the intervention of conscious thought.
Parasympathetic nervous system	The parasympathetic nervous system is one of two divisions of the autonomic nervous system. It conserves energy as it slows the heart rate, increases intestinal and gland activity, and relaxes sphincter muscles in the gastro-intestinal tract. In other words, it acts to reverse the effects of the sympathetic nervous system.
Autonomic nervous system	The autonomic nervous system is the part of the nervous system that is not consciously controlled. It is commonly divided into two usually antagonistic subsystems: the sympathetic and parasympathetic nervous system.
Fight or flight response	The fight or flight response theory states that animals react to threats with a general discharge of the sympathetic nervous system.
Sympathetic nervous system	The sympathetic nervous system activates what is often termed the "fight or flight response". Messages travel through in a bidirectional flow. Efferent messages can trigger changes in different parts of the body simultaneously.
Renin	Renin is a circulating enzyme released mainly by juxtaglomerular cells of the kidneys in response to low blood volume or low body NaCl content.
Angiotensin	Angiotensin is a polypeptide in the blood that causes vasoconstriction, increased blood pressure, and aldosterone release from the adrenal cortex. Angiotensin is produced in the liver from precursor angiotensinogen, a serum globulin. It plays an important role in the renin-angiotensin system.
Hormone	A hormone is a chemical messenger from one cell to another. All multicellular organisms produce hormones. The best known hormones are those produced by endocrine glands of vertebrate animals, but hormones are produced by nearly every organ system and tissue type in a human or animal body. Hormone molecules are secreted directly into the bloodstream, they move by circulation or diffusion to their target cells, which may be nearby cells in the same tissue or cells of a distant organ of the body.
Aldosterone	Aldosterone is a steroid hormone synthesized from cholesterol by the enzyme aldosterone synthase. It helps regulate the body's electrolyte balance by acting on the mineralocorticoid receptor. It diminishes the secretion of sodium ions and therefore, water and stimulates the secretion of potassium ions through the kidneys.
Sodium	Sodium is the chemical element in the periodic table that has the symbol Na (Natrium in Latin) and atomic number 11. Sodium is a soft, waxy, silvery reactive metal belonging to the alkali metals that is abundant in natural compounds (especially halite). It is highly reactive.
Vasoconstriction	Vasoconstriction refers to a decrease in the diameter of a blood vessel.
Renal artery	The renal artery normally arise off the abdominal aorta and supply the kidneys with blood. The arterial supply of the kidneys is variable and there may be one or more supplying each kidney.
Renal	Pertaining to the kidney is referred to as renal.
Hypertrophy	Hypertrophy is the increase of the size of an organ. It should be distinguished from hyperplasia which occurs due to cell division; hypertrophy occurs due to an increase in cell size rather than division. It is most commonly seen in muscle that has been actively stimulated, the most well-known method being exercise.

Chapter 9. Diseases of the Blood Vessels

Chapter 9. Diseases of the Blood Vessels

Left ventricle	The left ventricle is one of four chambers (two atria and two ventricles) in the human heart. It receives oxygenated blood from the left atrium via the mitral valve, and pumps it into the aorta via the aortic valve.
Vitamin	An organic compound other than a carbohydrate, lipid, or protein that is needed for normal metabolism but that the body cannot synthesize in adequate amounts is called a vitamin.
Heart attack	A heart attack, is a serious, sudden heart condition usually characterized by varying degrees of chest pain or discomfort, weakness, sweating, nausea, vomiting, and arrhythmias, sometimes causing loss of consciousness. It occurs when the blood supply to a part of the heart is interrupted, causing death and scarring of the local heart tissue.
Angina pectoris	Angina pectoris is chest pain due to ischemia (a lack of blood and hence oxygen supply) to the heart muscle, generally due to obstruction or spasm of the coronary arteries (the heart's blood vessels).
Lifestyle	The culturally, socially, economically, and environmentally conditioned complex of actions characteristic of an individual, group, or community as a pattern of habituated behavior over time that is health related but not necessarily health directed is a lifestyle.
Cholesterol	Cholesterol is a steroid, a lipid, and an alcohol, found in the cell membranes of all body tissues, and transported in the blood plasma of all animals. It is an important component of the membranes of cells, providing stability; it makes the membrane's fluidity stable over a bigger temperature interval.
Health	Health is a term that refers to a combination of the absence of illness, the ability to cope with everyday activities, physical fitness, and high quality of life.
Catheter	A tubular surgical instrument for withdrawing fluids from a cavity of the body, especially one for introduction into the bladder through the urethra for the withdrawal of urine is referred to as a catheter.
Shock	Circulatory shock, a state of cardiac output that is insufficient to meet the body's physiological needs, with consequences ranging from fainting to death is referred to as shock. Insulin shock, a state of severe hypoglycemia caused by administration of insulin.
Plasma	Fluid portion of circulating blood is called plasma.
Hypovolemic shock	Hypovolemic shock refers to insufficient cardiac output resulting from a drop in blood volume.
Vasodilation	An increase in the diameter of superficial blood vessels triggered by nerve signals that relax the smooth muscles of the vessel walls is referred to as vasodilation.
Cardiac output	Cardiac output is the volume of blood being pumped by the heart in a minute. It is equal to the heart rate multiplied by the stroke volume.
Spinal cord	The spinal cord is a part of the vertebrate nervous system that is enclosed in and protected by the vertebral column (it passes through the spinal canal). It consists of nerve cells. The spinal cord carries sensory signals and motor innervation to most of the skeletal muscles in the body.
Anesthesia	Anesthesia is the process of blocking the perception of pain and other sensations. This allows patients to undergo surgery and other procedures without the distress and pain they would otherwise experience.
Antigen	An antigen is a substance that stimulates an immune response, especially the production of antibodies. They are usually proteins or polysaccharides, but can be any type of molecule, including small molecules (haptens) coupled to a protein (carrier).
Anaphylactic	A precipitous drop in blood pressure caused by loss of fluid from capillaries because of an

Chapter 9. Diseases of the Blood Vessels

Chapter 9. Diseases of the Blood Vessels

shock	increase in their permeability stimulated by an allergic reaction is called anaphylactic shock.
Extension	Movement increasing the angle between parts at a joint is referred to as extension.
Auscultation	Auscultation is the technical term for listening to the internal sounds of the body, usually using a stethoscope. Auscultation is normally performed for the purposes of examining the cardiovascular system and respiratory systems (heart and lung sounds), as well as the gastrointestinal system (bowel sounds).
Oscilloscope	An oscilloscope is a piece of electronic test equipment that allows signal voltages to be viewed, usually as a two-dimensional graph of one or more electrical potential differences (vertical axis) plotted as a function of time or of some other voltage (horizontal axis).
Stenosis	A stenosis is an abnormal narrowing in a blood vessel or other tubular organ or structure. It is also sometimes called a "stricture" (as in urethral stricture).
Anatomy	Anatomy is the branch of biology that deals with the structure and organization of living things. It can be divided into animal anatomy (zootomy) and plant anatomy (phytonomy).
Internal carotid artery	In human anatomy, the internal carotid artery is a major artery of the head and neck. It arises from the common carotid artery when it bifurcates into an internal and external branch. It has no branches in the neck. It ascends and enters the skull through the carotid canal. Inside the cranium, it gives off the ophthalmic artery.
Carotid artery	In human anatomy, the carotid artery refers to a number of major arteries in the head and neck.
Congestive heart failure	Congestive heart failure is the inability of the heart to pump a sufficient amount of blood throughout the body, or requiring elevated filling pressures in order to pump effectively.
Heart rate	Heart rate is a term used to describe the frequency of the cardiac cycle. It is considered one of the four vital signs. Usually it is calculated as the number of contractions of the heart in one minute and expressed as "beats per minute".
Wheezing	Wheezing is a continuous, coarse, whistling sound produced in the respiratory airways during breathing. For wheezing to occur, some part of the respiratory tree must be narrowed or obstructed, or airflow velocity within the respiratory tree must be heightened.
Angiography	Angiography is a medical imaging technique in which an X-Ray picture is taken to visualize the inner opening of blood filled structures, including arteries, veins and the heart chambers.
Activation	As reflected by facial expressions, the degree of arousal a person is experiencing is referred to as activation.
Steroid	A steroid is a lipid characterized by a carbon skeleton with four fused rings. Different steroids vary in the functional groups attached to these rings. Hundreds of distinct steroids have been identified in plants and animals. Their most important role in most living systems is as hormones.
Bypass	In medicine, a bypass generally means an alternate or additional route for blood flow, which is created in bypass surgery, e.g. coronary artery bypass surgery by moving blood vessels or implanting synthetic tubing.
Cramp	A cramp is an unpleasant sensation caused by contraction, usually of a muscle. It can be caused by cold or overexertion.
Protrusion	Protrusion is the anterior movement of an object. This term is often applied to the jaw.
Urinary system	The urinary system is the organ system that produces, stores, and carries urine. In humans it

Chapter 9. Diseases of the Blood Vessels

includes two kidneys, two ureters, the urinary bladder, two sphincter muscles, and the urethra.

Chapter 9. Diseases of the Blood Vessels

Chapter 10. Diseases of the Urinary System

Electrolyte	An electrolyte is a substance that dissociates into free ions when dissolved (or molten), to produce an electrically conductive medium. Because they generally consist of ions in solution, they are also known as ionic solutions.
Physiology	The study of the function of cells, tissues, and organs is referred to as physiology.
Muscle	Muscle is a contractile form of tissue. It is one of the four major tissue types, the other three being epithelium, connective tissue and nervous tissue. Muscle contraction is used to move parts of the body, as well as to move substances within the body.
Nerve	A nerve is an enclosed, cable-like bundle of nerve fibers or axons, which includes the glia that ensheath the axons in myelin.
Calcium	Calcium is the chemical element in the periodic table that has the symbol Ca and atomic number 20. Calcium is a soft grey alkaline earth metal that is used as a reducing agent in the extraction of thorium, zirconium and uranium. Calcium is also the fifth most abundant element in the Earth's crust.
Sodium	Sodium is the chemical element in the periodic table that has the symbol Na (Natrium in Latin) and atomic number 11. Sodium is a soft, waxy, silvery reactive metal belonging to the alkali metals that is abundant in natural compounds (especially halite). It is highly reactive.
Renal	Pertaining to the kidney is referred to as renal.
Salt	Salt is a term used for ionic compounds composed of positively charged cations and negatively charged anions, so that the product is neutral and without a net charge.
Kidney	The kidney is a bean-shaped excretory organ in vertebrates. Part of the urinary system, the kidneys filter wastes (especially urea) from the blood and excrete them, along with water, as urine.
Blood	Blood is a circulating tissue composed of fluid plasma and cells. The main function of blood is to supply nutrients (oxygen, glucose) and constitutional elements to tissues and to remove waste products.
Acid	An acid is a water-soluble, sour-tasting chemical compound that when dissolved in water, gives a solution with a pH of less than 7.
Acidosis	Acidosis is an increased acidity (i.e. hydrogen ion concentration) of blood plasma. Generally acidosis is said to occur when arterial pH falls below 7.35, while its counterpart (alkalosis) occurs at a pH over 7.45.
Diabetes	Diabetes is a medical disorder characterized by varying or persistent elevated blood sugar levels, especially after eating. All types of diabetes share similar symptoms and complications at advanced stages: dehydration and ketoacidosis, cardiovascular disease, chronic renal failure, retinal damage which can lead to blindness, nerve damage which can lead to erectile dysfunction, gangrene with risk of amputation of toes, feet, and even legs.
Diabetes mellitus	Diabetes mellitus is a medical disorder characterized by varying or persistent hyperglycemia (elevated blood sugar levels), especially after eating. All types of diabetes mellitus share similar symptoms and complications at advanced stages.
Alkalosis	Alkalosis refers to a condition reducing hydrogen ion concentration of arterial blood plasma (alkalemia). Generally alkalosis is said to occur when arterial pH exceeds 7.45.
Urine	Concentrated filtrate produced by the kidneys and excreted via the bladder is called urine.
Hormone	A hormone is a chemical messenger from one cell to another. All multicellular organisms produce hormones. The best known hormones are those produced by endocrine glands of vertebrate animals, but hormones are produced by nearly every organ system and tissue type in

Go to Cram101.com for the Practice Tests for this Chapter.

Chapter 10. Diseases of the Urinary System

Chapter 10. Diseases of the Urinary System

	a human or animal body. Hormone molecules are secreted directly into the bloodstream, they move by circulation or diffusion to their target cells, which may be nearby cells in the same tissue or cells of a distant organ of the body.
Erythropoietin	Erythropoietin is a glycoprotein hormone that is a growth factor for erythrocyte (red blood cell) precursors in the bone marrow. It increases the number of red blood cells in the blood.
Red blood cell	The red blood cell is the most common type of blood cell and is the vertebrate body's principal means of delivering oxygen from the lungs or gills to body tissues via the blood.
Arteriole	An arteriole is a blood vessel that extends and branches out from an artery and leads to capillaries. They have thick muscular walls and are the primary site of vascular resistance.
Juxtaglomerular apparatus	The juxtaglomerular apparatus is a renal structure consisting of the macula densa and juxtaglomerular cells. Juxtaglomerular cells (JG cells) are the site of renin secretion.
Nephron	A nephron is the basic structural and functional unit of the kidney. Its chief function is to regulate water and soluble substances by filtering the blood, reabsorbing what is needed and excreting the rest as urine. They eliminate wastes from the body, regulate blood volume and pressure, control levels of electrolytes and metabolites, and regulate blood pH.
Amino acid	An amino acid is any molecule that contains both amino and carboxylic acid functional groups. They are the basic structural building units of proteins. They form short polymer chains called peptides or polypeptides which in turn form structures called proteins.
Glucose	Glucose, a simple monosaccharide sugar, is one of the most important carbohydrates and is used as a source of energy in animals and plants. Glucose is one of the main products of photosynthesis and starts respiration.
Lead	Lead is a chemical element in the periodic table that has the symbol Pb and atomic number 82. A soft, heavy, toxic and malleable poor metal, lead is bluish white when freshly cut but tarnishes to dull gray when exposed to air. Lead is used in building construction, lead-acid batteries, bullets and shot, and is part of solder, pewter, and fusible alloys.
Proximal convoluted tubule	Highly coiled region of a nephron near the glomerular capsule, where tubular reabsorption takes place is called the proximal convoluted tubule.
Distal convoluted tubule	The distal convoluted tubule is a portion of kidney nephron between the loop of Henle and the collecting duct system. It is partly responsible for the regulation of potassium, sodium, calcium, and pH.
Capillaries	Capillaries refer to the smallest of the blood vessels and the sites of exchange between the blood and tissue cells.
Glomerulus	A glomerulus is a capillary tuft surrounded by Bowman's capsule in nephrons of the vertebrate kidney. It receives its blood supply from an afferent arteriole of the renal circulation, and empties into an efferent arteriole.
Capillary	A capillary is the smallest of a body's blood vessels, measuring 5-10 micro meters. They connect arteries and veins, and most closely interact with tissues. Their walls are composed of a single layer of cells, the endothelium. This layer is so thin that molecules such as oxygen, water and lipids can pass through them by diffusion and enter the tissues.
Plasma	Fluid portion of circulating blood is called plasma.
Protein	A protein is a complex, high-molecular-weight organic compound that consists of amino acids joined by peptide bonds. They are essential to the structure and function of all living cells and viruses. Many are enzymes or subunits of enzymes.
Red blood cells	Red blood cells are the most common type of blood cell and are the vertebrate body's

Chapter 10. Diseases of the Urinary System

Chapter 10. Diseases of the Urinary System

	principal means of delivering oxygen from the lungs or gills to body tissues via the blood.
Creatinine	Creatinine is a nitrogenous organic acid that helps supply energy to muscle cells. Creatinine is a breakdown product of creatine phosphate in muscle, and is usually produced at a fairly constant rate by the body.
Metabolism	Metabolism is the biochemical modification of chemical compounds in living organisms and cells. This includes the biosynthesis of complex organic molecules (anabolism) and their breakdown (catabolism).
Urea	Urea is an organic compound of carbon, nitrogen, oxygen and hydrogen, CON_2H_4 or $(NH_2)_2CO$. Urea is essentially a waste product: it has no physiological function. It is dissolved in blood and excreted by the kidney.
Hydrogen ion	A single proton with a charge of + 1. The dissociation of a water molecule leads to the generation of a hydroxide ion and a hydrogen ion. The hydrogen ion is hydrated in aqueous solutions and is usually written as H_2O^+.
Hydrogen	Hydrogen is a chemical element in the periodic table that has the symbol H and atomic number 1. At standard temperature and pressure it is a colorless, odorless, nonmetallic, univalent, tasteless, highly flammable diatomic gas.
Ion	Ion refers to an atom or molecule that has gained or lost one or more electrons, thus acquiring an electrical charge.
Renal artery	The renal artery normally arise off the abdominal aorta and supply the kidneys with blood. The arterial supply of the kidneys is variable and there may be one or more supplying each kidney.
Renal vein	The renal vein is the vein that drains the kidney. The filtered blood returns to circulation through the renal veins which join into the inferior vena cava.
Artery	Vessel that takes blood away from the heart to the tissues and organs of the body is called an artery.
Ureter	A ureter is a duct that carries urine from the kidneys to the urinary bladder. They are muscular tubes that can propel urine along by the motions of peristalsis.
Vein	Vein in animals, is a vessel that returns blood to the heart. In plants, a vascular bundle in a leaf, composed of xylem and phloem.
Afferent arteriole	The afferent arteriole is a blood vessel that supply the nephrons in many excretory systems. They branch from the renal artery which supplies blood to the kidneys, and later diverge into the capillaries of the glomerulus.
Urethra	In anatomy, the urethra is a tube which connects the urinary bladder to the outside of the body. The urethra has an excretory function in both sexes, to pass urine to the outside, and also a reproductive function in the male, as a passage for sperm.
Bladder	A hollow muscular storage organ for storing urine is a bladder.
Urinary system	The urinary system is the organ system that produces, stores, and carries urine. In humans it includes two kidneys, two ureters, the urinary bladder, two sphincter muscles, and the urethra.
Infection	The invasion and multiplication of microorganisms in body tissues is called an infection.
Prostate	The prostate is a gland that is part of male mammalian sex organs. Its main function is to secrete and store a clear, slightly basic fluid that is part of semen. The prostate differs considerably between species anatomically, chemically and physiologically.
Tumor	An abnormal mass of cells that forms within otherwise normal tissue is a tumor. This growth

Chapter 10. Diseases of the Urinary System

Chapter 10. Diseases of the Urinary System

	can be either malignant or benign
Gland	A gland is an organ in an animal's body that synthesizes a substance for release such as hormones, often into the bloodstream or into cavities inside the body or its outer surface.
Bacteria	The domain that contains procaryotic cells with primarily diacyl glycerol diesters in their membranes and with bacterial rRNA. Bacteria also is a general term for organisms that are composed of procaryotic cells and are not multicellular.
Young adult	An young adult is someone between the ages of 20 and 40 years old.
Glomerulonep-ritis	Glomerulonephritis is a primary or secondary autoimmune renal disease characterized by inflammation of the glomeruli. It may be asymptomatic, or present with hematuria and/or proteinuria (blood resp. protein in the urine).
Fever	Fever (also known as pyrexia, or a febrile response, and archaically known as ague) is a medical symptom that describes an increase in internal body temperature to levels that are above normal (37°C, 98.6°F).
Rheumatic fever	Rheumatic fever is an inflammatory disease which may develop after a Group A streptococcal infection (such as strep throat or scarlet fever) and can involve the heart, joints, skin, and brain.
Scarlet fever	Scarlet fever refers to a disease that results from infection with a strain of Streptococcus pyogenes that carries a lysogenic phage with the gene for erythrogenic toxin. The toxin causes shedding of the skin. This is a communicable disease spread by respiratory droplets.
Edema	Edema is swelling of any organ or tissue due to accumulation of excess fluid. Edema has many root causes, but its common mechanism is accumulation of fluid into the tissues.
Albuminuria	Albuminuria is a pathological condition where albumin is present in the urine. The kidneys normally filter out large molecules from the urine, so albuminuria can be an indicator of damage to the kidneys.
Urinalysis	A urinalysis (or "UA") is an array of tests performed on urine and one of the most common methods of medical diagnosis. A part of a urinalysis can be performed by using urine dipsticks, in which the test results can be read as color changes.
Albumin	Albumin refers generally to any protein with water solubility, which is moderately soluble in concentrated salt solutions, and experiences heat coagulation (protein denaturation).
Hematuria	In medicine, hematuria is the presence of blood in the urine. It is a sign of a large number of diseases of the kidneys and the urinary tract, ranging from trivial to lethal.
Glomeruli	Glomeruli are important waystations in the pathway from the nose to the olfactory cortex. Each receives input from olfactory receptor neurons expressing only one type of olfactory receptor. There are tens of millions of olfactory receptor cells, but only about two thousand glomeruli. By combining so much input, the olfactory system is able to detect even very faint odors.
Acute	In medicine, an acute disease is a disease with either or both of: a rapid onset; and a short course (as opposed to a chronic course).
Inflammation	Inflammation is the first response of the immune system to infection or irritation and may be referred to as the innate cascade.
Antigen	An antigen is a substance that stimulates an immune response, especially the production of antibodies. They are usually proteins or polysaccharides, but can be any type of molecule, including small molecules (haptens) coupled to a protein (carrier).
Antibody	An antibody is a protein used by the immune system to identify and neutralize foreign objects

Go to Cram101.com for the Practice Tests for this Chapter.

Chapter 10. Diseases of the Urinary System

Chapter 10. Diseases of the Urinary System

	like bacteria and viruses. Each antibody recognizes a specific antigen unique to its target.
Blocking	A sudden break or interuption in the flow of thinking or speech that is seen as an absence in thought is refered to as blocking.
Inflammatory response	Inflammatory response refers to a complex sequence of events involving chemicals and immune cells that results in the isolation and destruction of antigens and tissues near the antigens.
Neutrophil	Neutrophil refers to a type of phagocytic leukocyte.
Filtration	Filtration involved in passive transport is the movement of water and solute molecules across the cell membrane due to hydrostatic pressure by the cardiovascular system.
Prognosis	Prognosis refers to the prospects for the future or outcome of a disease.
Exacerbation	Exacerbation is a period in an illness when the symptoms of the disease reappear.
Remission	Disappearance of the signs of a disease is called remission.
Hypertension	Hypertension is a medical condition where the blood pressure in the arteries is chronically elevated. Persistent hypertension is one of the risk factors for strokes, heart attacks, heart failure and arterial aneurysm, and is a leading cause of chronic renal failure.
Uremia	Uremia is a toxic condition resulting from renal failure, when kidney function is compromised and urea, a waste product normally excreted in the urine, is retained in the blood. Uremia can lead to disturbances in the platelets, among other effects.
Fusion	Fusion refers to the combination of two atoms into a single atom as a result of a collision, usually accompanied by the release of energy.
Convulsions	Involuntary muscle spasms, often severe, that can be caused by stimulant overdose or by depressant withdrawal are called convulsions.
Dialysis	Dialysis refers to separation and disposal of metabolic wastes from the blood by mechanical means; an artificial method of performing the functions of the kidneys.
Renal failure	Renal failure is the condition where the kidneys fail to function properly. Physiologically, renal failure is described as a decrease in the glomerular filtration rate. Clinically, this manifests in an elevated serum creatinine.
Hemorrhage	Loss of blood from the circulatory system is referred to as a hemorrhage.
Excretion	Excretion is the biological process by which an organism chemically separates waste products from its body. The waste products are then usually expelled from the body by elimination.
Liver	The liver is an organ in vertebrates, including humans. It plays a major role in metabolism and has a number of functions in the body including drug detoxification, glycogen storage, and plasma protein synthesis. It also produces bile, which is important for digestion.
Azotemia	Azotemia is a medical condition characterized by abnormal levels of urea, creatinine, various body waste compounds, and other nitrogen-rich compounds in the blood as a result of insufficient filtering of the blood by the kidneys.
Assess	Assess is to systematically and continuously collect, validate, and communicate patient data.
Serum	Serum is the same as blood plasma except that clotting factors (such as fibrin) have been removed. Blood plasma contains fibrinogen.
Dehydration	Dehydration is the removal of water from an object. Medically, dehydration is a serious and potentially life-threatening condition in which the body contains an insufficient volume of water for normal functioning.

Go to Cram101.com for the Practice Tests for this Chapter.

Chapter 10. Diseases of the Urinary System

Chapter 10. Diseases of the Urinary System

Shock	Circulatory shock, a state of cardiac output that is insufficient to meet the body's physiological needs, with consequences ranging from fainting to death is referred to as shock. Insulin shock, a state of severe hypoglycemia caused by administration of insulin.
Trauma	Trauma refers to a severe physical injury or wound to the body caused by an external force, or a psychological shock having a lasting effect on mental life.
Oliguria	Oliguria is the decreased production of urine. The decreased production may be a sign of dehydration, renal failure or urinary obstruction/urinary retention.
Anuria	Oliguria and anuria are the decreased or absent production of urine, respectively. The decreased production of urine may be a sign of dehydration, renal failure or urinary obstruction/urinary retention.
Ammonia	Ammonia is a compound of nitrogen and hydrogen with the formula NH_3. At standard temperature and pressure ammonia is a gas. It is toxic and corrosive to some materials, and has a characteristic pungent odor.
Hyperkalemia	Hyperkalemia is an elevated blood level (above 5.0 mmol/L) of the electrolyte potassium.
Potassium	Potassium is a chemical element in the periodic table. It has the symbol K (L. kalium) and atomic number 19. Potassium is a soft silvery-white metallic alkali metal that occurs naturally bound to other elements in seawater and many minerals.
Cardiac arrest	A cardiac arrest is the cesztation of normal circulation of the blood due to failure of the ventricles of the heart to contract effectively during systole.
Chronic renal failure	Chronic renal failure is a slowly progressive loss of renal function over a period of months or years and defined as an abnormally low glomerular filtration rate, which is usually determined indirectly by the creatinine level in blood serum.
Acute renal failure	Acute renal failure is a rapid loss of function due to damage to the kidneys, resulting in retention of nitrogenous (urea and creatinine) and non-nitrogenous waste products that are normally excreted by the kidney.
Diabetic nephropathy	Diabetic nephropathy (nephropatia diabetica), also known as Kimmelstiel-Wilson syndrome and intercapillary glomerulonephritis, is a progressive kidney disease caused by angiopathy of capillaries in the kidney glomeruli.
Diarrhea	Diarrhea or diarrhoea is a condition in which the sufferer has frequent and watery, chunky, or loose bowel movements.
Gastrointestnal tract	The gastrointestinal tract is the system of organs within multicellular animals which takes in food, digests it to extract energy and nutrients, and expels the remaining waste.
Nervous system	The nervous system of an animal coordinates the activity of the muscles, monitors the organs, constructs and processes input from the senses, and initiates actions.
Hemodialysis	Hemodialysis is a method for removing waste products such as potassium and urea, as well as free water from the blood when the kidneys are incapable of this. It is a form of renal dialysis and is therefore a renal replacement therapy.
Peritoneum	In higher vertebrates, the peritoneum is the serous membrane that forms the lining of the abdominal cavity - it covers most of the intra-abdominal organs. The peritoneum both supports the abdominal organs and serves as a conduit for their blood and lymph vessels and nerves.
Pelvis	The pelvis is the bony structure located at the base of the spine (properly known as the caudal end). The pelvis incorporates the socket portion of the hip joint for each leg (in bipeds) or hind leg (in quadrupeds). It forms the lower limb (or hind-limb) girdle of the skeleton.

Go to Cram101.com for the Practice Tests for this Chapter.

Chapter 10. Diseases of the Urinary System

Chapter 10. Diseases of the Urinary System

Pyelonephritis	Pyelonephritis is an ascending urinary tract infection that has reached the pyelum of the kidney.
Tissue	A collection of interconnected cells that perform a similar function within an organism is called tissue.
Lymph	Lymph originates as blood plasma lost from the circulatory system, which leaks out into the surrounding tissues. The lymphatic system collects this fluid by diffusion into lymph capillaries, and returns it to the circulatory system.
Renal pelvis	The renal pelvis represents the funnel-like dilated proximal part of the ureter. The major function of the renal pelvis is to act as a funnel for urine flowing to the ureter.
Scar	A scar results from the biologic process of wound repair in the skin and other tissues of the body. It is a connective tissue that fills the wound.
Abdomen	The abdomen is a part of the body. In humans, and in many other vertebrates, it is the region between the thorax and the pelvis. In fully developed insects, the abdomen is the third (or posterior) segment, after the head and thorax.
Pain	Pain is an unpleasant sensation which may be associated with actual or potential tissue damage and which may have physical and emotional components.
Antibiotic	Antibiotic refers to substance such as penicillin or streptomycin that is toxic to microorganisms. Usually a product of a particular microorvanism or plant.
Microorganism	A microorganism or microbe is an organism that is so small that it is microscopic (invisible to the naked eye).
Urination	Urination is the process of disposing urine from the urinary bladder through the urethra to the outside of the body. The process of urination is usually under voluntary control.
Urgency	Urgency is an intense and sudden desire to urinate.
Diagnosis	In medicine, diagnosis is the process of identifying a medical condition or disease by its signs, symptoms, and from the results of various diagnostic procedures.
Carcinoma	Cancer that originates in the coverings of the body, such as the skin or the lining of the intestinal tract is a carcinoma.
Organ	Organ refers to a structure consisting of several tissues adapted as a group to perform specific functions.
Metastasis	The spread of cancer cells beyond their original site are called metastasis.
Lungs	Lungs are the essential organs of respiration in air-breathing vertebrates. Their principal function is to transport oxygen from the atmosphere into the bloodstream, and to excrete carbon dioxide from the bloodstream into the atmosphere.
Brain	The part of the central nervous system involved in regulating and controlling body activity and interpreting information from the senses transmitted through the nervous system is referred to as the brain.
Anemia	Anemia is a deficiency of red blood cells and/or hemoglobin. This results in a reduced ability of blood to transfer oxygen to the tissues, and this causes hypoxia; since all human cells depend on oxygen for survival, varying degrees of anemia can have a wide range of clinical consequences.
White blood cell	The white blood cell is a a component of blood. They help to defend the body against infectious disease and foreign materials as part of the immune system.
Lymph vessel	Lymph vessel refers to one of the system of vessels carrying lymph from the lymph capillaries

Go to **Cram101.com** for the Practice Tests for this Chapter.

Chapter 10. Diseases of the Urinary System

Chapter 10. Diseases of the Urinary System

	to the veins.
Cancer	Cancer is a class of diseases or disorders characterized by uncontrolled division of cells and the ability of these cells to invade other tissues, either by direct growth into adjacent tissue through invasion or by implantation into distant sites by metastasis.
Solution	Solution refers to homogenous mixture formed when a solute is dissolved in a solvent.
Parathyroid gland	One of four endocrine glands embedded in the surface of the thyroid gland that secrete parathyroid hormone is called a parathyroid gland.
Urinary tract infection	A urinary tract infection is an infection anywhere from the kidneys to the ureters to the bladder to the urethra.
Extracorporeal	Extracorporeal refers to out of the body.
Uric acid	An insoluble precipitate of nitrogenous waste excreted by land snails, insects, birds, and some reptiles is called uric acid.
Phosphate	A phosphate is a polyatomic ion or radical consisting of one phosphorus atom and four oxygen. In the ionic form, it carries a -3 formal charge, and is denoted PO_4^{3-}.
Magnesium	Magnesium is the chemical element in the periodic table that has the symbol Mg and atomic number 12 and an atomic mass of 24.31.
Ammonium	The ammonium cation is a positively charged polyatomic ion of the chemical formula NH_4^+ and a molecular mass of 18.04, resulting from protonation of ammonia (NH_3).
Incidence	In epidemiological studies of a particular disorder, the rate at which new cases occur in a given place at a given time is called incidence.
Bypass	In medicine, a bypass generally means an alternate or additional route for blood flow, which is created in bypass surgery, e.g. coronary artery bypass surgery by moving blood vessels or implanting synthetic tubing.
Pyuria	Pyuria refers to urine which contains white blood cells. It can be sign of a bacterial urinary tract infection. Pyuria may be present in the septic patient, or in an older patient with pneumonia.
Genes	Genes are the units of heredity in living organisms. They are encoded in the organism's genetic material (usually DNA or RNA), and control the development and behavior of the organism.
Autosomal dominant	An autosomal dominant gene is one that occurs on an autosomal (non-sex determining) chromosome. As it is dominant, the phenotype it gives will be expressed even if the gene is heterozygous. This contrasts with recessive genes, which need to be homozygous to be expressed.
Recessive gene	Recessive gene refers to a gene that will not be expressed if paired with a dominant gene but will be expressed if paired with another recessive gene.
Affect	Affect is the scientific term used to describe a subject's externally displayed mood. This can be assesed by the nurse by observing facial expression, tone of voice, and body language.
Cyst	A cyst is a closed sac having a distinct membrane and developing abnormally in a cavity or structure of the body. They may occur as a result of a developmental error in the embryo during pregnancy or they may be caused by infections.
Polyuria	Excessive output of urine is called polyuria.
Cystitis	Cystitis is the inflammation of the bladder. The condition primarily affects women, but can affect all age groups from either sex.

Chapter 10. Diseases of the Urinary System

Chapter 10. Diseases of the Urinary System

Urinary bladder	In the anatomy of mammals, the urinary bladder is the organ that collects urine excreted by the kidneys prior to disposal by urination. Urine enters the bladder via the ureters and exits via the urethra.
Agent	Agent refers to an epidemiological term referring to the organism or object that transmits a disease from the environment to the host.
Escherichia coli	Escherichia coli is one of the main species of bacteria that live in the lower intestines of warm-blooded animals, including birds and mammals. They are necessary for the proper digestion of food and are part of the intestinal flora. Its presence in groundwater is a common indicator of fecal contamination.
Causative agent	In the chain of infection, the organism capable of producing an infection is called a causative agent.
Projection	Attributing one's own undesirable thoughts, impulses, traits, or behaviors to others is referred to as projection.
Ileal conduit	An ileal conduit urinary diversion is a surgically-created urinary diversion used to create a way for the body to store and eliminate urine for patients who have had their urinary bladders removed as a result of bladder cancer or pelvic exenteration.
Dysuria	In medicine, specifically urology, dysuria refers to any difficulty in urination. It is sometimes accompanied by pain. It is most often a result of an infection of the urinary tract.
Hypoproteinemia	Hypoproteinemia refers to a low concentration of blood proteins.
Blood vessel	A blood vessel is a part of the circulatory system and function to transport blood throughout the body. The most important types, arteries and veins, are so termed because they carry blood away from or towards the heart, respectively.
Intestine	The intestine is the portion of the alimentary canal extending from the stomach to the anus and, in humans and mammals, consists of two segments, the small intestine and the large intestine. The intestine is the part of the body responsible for extracting nutrition from food.
Stoma	A stoma is an artificial opening for waste excretion located on the body.
Ileum	The ileum is the final section of the small intestine. Its function is to absorb vitamin B12 and bile salts. The wall itself made up of folds, each of which has many tiny finger-like projections known as villi, on its surface.
Skin	Skin is an organ of the integumentary system composed of a layer of tissues that protect underlying muscles and organs.
Small intestine	The small intestine is the part of the gastrointestinal tract between the stomach and the large intestine (colon). In humans over 5 years old it is about 7m long. It is divided into three structural parts: duodenum, jejunum and ileum.
Urinary incontinence	Urinary incontinence is the involuntary excretion of urine from one's body. It is often temporary, and it almost always results from an underlying medical condition.
Spinal nerve	The spinal nerve is usually a mixed nerve, formed from the dorsal and ventral roots that come out of the spinal cord.
Estrogen	Estrogen is a steroid that functions as the primary female sex hormone. While present in both men and women, they are found in women in significantly higher quantities.
Sphincter	Muscle that surrounds a tube and closes or opens the tube by contracting and relaxing is referred to as sphincter.

Go to **Cram101.com** for the Practice Tests for this Chapter.

Chapter 10. Diseases of the Urinary System

Chapter 10. Diseases of the Urinary System

Collagen	Collagen is the main protein of connective tissue in animals and the most abundant protein in mammals, making up about 1/4 of the total. It is one of the long, fibrous structural proteins whose functions are quite different from those of globular proteins such as enzymes.
Sugar	A sugar is the simplest molecule that can be identified as a carbohydrate. These include monosaccharides and disaccharides, trisaccharides and the oligosaccharides. The term "glyco-" indicates the presence of a sugar in an otherwise non-carbohydrate substance.
Eye	An eye is an organ that detects light. Different kinds of light-sensitive organs are found in a variety of creatures. The simplest eyes do nothing but detect whether the surroundings are light or dark, while more complex eyes can distinguish shapes and colors.
Tuberculosis	Tuberculosis is an infection caused by the bacterium Mycobacterium tuberculosis, which most commonly affects the lungs but can also affect the central nervous system, lymphatic system, circulatory system, genitourinary system, bones and joints.
Rods	Rods, are photoreceptor cells in the retina of the eye that can function in less intense light than can the other type of photoreceptor, cone cells.
Intravenous	Present or occurring within a vein, such as an intravenous blood clot is referred to as intravenous. Introduced directly into a vein, such as an intravenous injection or I.V. drip.
Veins	Blood vessels that return blood toward the heart from the circulation are referred to as veins.
Suppression	Suppression is the defense mechanism where a memory is deliberately forgotten.
Steroid	A steroid is a lipid characterized by a carbon skeleton with four fused rings. Different steroids vary in the functional groups attached to these rings. Hundreds of distinct steroids have been identified in plants and animals. Their most important role in most living systems is as hormones.
Critical thinking	Critical thinking consists of a mental process of analyzing or evaluating information, particularly statements or propositions that people have offered as true. It forms a process of reflecting upon the meaning of statements, examining the offered evidence and reasoning, and forming judgments about the facts.
Asymptomatic	A disease is asymptomatic when it is at a stage where the patient does not experience symptoms. By their nature, asymptomatic diseases are not usually discovered until the patient undergoes medical tests (X-rays or other investigations). Some diseases remain asymptomatic for a remarkably long time, including some forms of cancer.
Case study	A carefully drawn biography that may be obtained through interviews, questionnaires, and psychological tests is called a case study.
Menstrual cycle	The menstrual cycle is the set of recurring physiological changes in a female's body that are under the control of the reproductive hormone system and necessary for reproduction. Besides humans, only other great apes exhibit menstrual cycles, in contrast to the estrus cycle of most mammalian species.
Value	Value is worth in general, and it is thought to be connected to reasons for certain practices, policies, actions, beliefs or emotions. Value is "that which one acts to gain and/or keep."
Digestive tract	The digestive tract is the system of organs within multicellular animals which takes in food, digests it to extract energy and nutrients, and expels the remaining waste.
Fatty acid	A fatty acid is a carboxylic acid (or organic acid), often with a long aliphatic tail (long chains), either saturated or unsaturated.
Lipid	Lipid is one class of aliphatic hydrocarbon-containing organic compounds essential for the

	structure and function of living cells. They are characterized by being water-insoluble but soluble in nonpolar organic solvents.
Digestive system	The organ system that ingests food, breaks it down into smaller chemical units, and absorbs the nutrient molecules is referred to as the digestive system.
Carbohydrate	Carbohydrate is a chemical compound that contains oxygen, hydrogen, and carbon atoms. They consist of monosaccharide sugars of varying chain lengths and that have the general chemical formula $C_n(H_2O)_n$ or are derivatives of such.

Chapter 10. Diseases of the Urinary System

Chapter 11. Diseases of the Digestive Tract

Intestine	The intestine is the portion of the alimentary canal extending from the stomach to the anus and, in humans and mammals, consists of two segments, the small intestine and the large intestine. The intestine is the part of the body responsible for extracting nutrition from food.
Esophagus	The esophagus, or gullet is the muscular tube in vertebrates through which ingested food passes from the mouth area to the stomach. Food is passed through the esophagus by using the process of peristalsis.
Pharynx	The pharynx is the part of the digestive system and respiratory system of many animals immediately behind the mouth and in front of the esophagus.
Stomach	The stomach is an organ in the alimentary canal used to digest food. It's primary function is not the absorption of nutrients from digested food; rather, the main job of the stomach is to break down large food molecules into smaller ones, so that they can be absorbed into the blood more easily.
Ulcer	An ulcer is an open sore of the skin, eyes or mucous membrane, often caused by an initial abrasion and generally maintained by an inflammation and/or an infection.
Large intestine	In anatomy of the digestive system, the colon, also called the large intestine or large bowel, is the part of the intestine from the cecum ('caecum' in British English) to the rectum. Its primary purpose is to extract water from feces.
Small intestine	The small intestine is the part of the gastrointestinal tract between the stomach and the large intestine (colon). In humans over 5 years old it is about 7m long. It is divided into three structural parts: duodenum, jejunum and ileum.
Digestive tract	The digestive tract is the system of organs within multicellular animals which takes in food, digests it to extract energy and nutrients, and expels the remaining waste.
Gallbladder	The gallbladder is a pear-shaped organ that stores bile until the body needs it for digestion. It is connected to the liver and the duodenum by the biliary tract.
Pancreas	The pancreas is a retroperitoneal organ that serves two functions: exocrine - it produces pancreatic juice containing digestive enzymes, and endocrine - it produces several important hormones, namely insulin.
Organ	Organ refers to a structure consisting of several tissues adapted as a group to perform specific functions.
Liver	The liver is an organ in vertebrates, including humans. It plays a major role in metabolism and has a number of functions in the body including drug detoxification, glycogen storage, and plasma protein synthesis. It also produces bile, which is important for digestion.
Acid	An acid is a water-soluble, sour-tasting chemical compound that when dissolved in water, gives a solution with a pH of less than 7.
Digestion	Digestion refers to the mechanical and chemical breakdown of food into molecules small enough for the body to absorb; the second main stage of food processing, following ingestion.
Protein	A protein is a complex, high-molecular-weight organic compound that consists of amino acids joined by peptide bonds. They are essential to the structure and function of all living cells and viruses. Many are enzymes or subunits of enzymes.
Sphincter	Muscle that surrounds a tube and closes or opens the tube by contracting and relaxing is referred to as sphincter.
Muscle	Muscle is a contractile form of tissue. It is one of the four major tissue types, the other three being epithelium, connective tissue and nervous tissue. Muscle contraction is used to move parts of the body, as well as to move substances within the body.

Chapter 11. Diseases of the Digestive Tract

Chapter 11. Diseases of the Digestive Tract

Catalyst	A chemical that speeds up a reaction but is not used up in the reaction is a catalyst.
Enzyme	An enzyme is a protein that catalyzes, or speeds up, a chemical reaction. They are essential to sustain life because most chemical reactions in biological cells would occur too slowly, or would lead to different products, without them.
Gastric juice	Gastric juice is a strong acidic liquid, pH 1 to 3, which is close to being colorless. It is secreted by the glands in the lining of the stomach.
Hydrochloric acid	The chemical substance hydrochloric acid is the aqueous solution of hydrogen chloride gas. It is a strong acid, the major component of gastric acid.
Mucus	Mucus is a slippery secretion of the lining of various membranes in the body (mucous membranes). Mucus aids in the protection of the lungs by trapping foreign particles that enter the nose during normal breathing. Additionally, it prevents tissues from drying out.
Pyloric sphincter	Pyloric sphincter in the vertebrate digestive tract, a muscular ring that regulates the passage of food out of the stomach and into the small intestine.
Chyme	Chyme is the liquid substance found in the stomach before passing the pyloric valve and entering the duodenum. It consists of partially digested food, water, hydrochloric acid, and various digestive enzymes.
Peristalsis	Peristalsis is the process of involuntary wave-like successive muscular contractions by which food is moved through the digestive tract. The large, hollow organs of the digestive system contains muscles that enable their walls to move.
Course	Pattern of development and change of a disorder over time is a course.
Muscle contraction	A muscle contraction occurs when a muscle cell (called a muscle fiber) shortens. There are three general types: skeletal, heart, and smooth.
Smooth muscle	Smooth muscle is a type of non-striated muscle, found within the "walls" of hollow organs; such as blood vessels, the bladder, the uterus, and the gastrointestinal tract. Smooth muscle is used to move matter within the body, via contraction; it generally operates "involuntarily", without nerve stimulation.
Duodenum	The duodenum is a hollow jointed tube connecting the stomach to the jejunum. It is the first part of the small intestine. Two very important ducts open into the duodenum, namely the bile duct and the pancreatic duct. The duodenum is largely responsible for the breakdown of food in the small intestine.
Lipid	Lipid is one class of aliphatic hydrocarbon-containing organic compounds essential for the structure and function of living cells. They are characterized by being water-insoluble but soluble in nonpolar organic solvents.
Carbohydrate	Carbohydrate is a chemical compound that contains oxygen, hydrogen, and carbon atoms. They consist of monosaccharide sugars of varying chain lengths and that have the general chemical formula $C_n(H_2O)_n$ or are derivatives of such.
Solution	Solution refers to homogenous mixture formed when a solute is dissolved in a solvent.
Neutralization	A chemical reaction involved in mixing an acid with a base which produces a salt and water is referred to as neutralization.
Bile duct	A bile duct is any of a number of long tube-like structures that carry bile. The top half of the common bile duct is associated with the liver, while the bottom half of the common bile duct is associated with the pancreas, through which it passes on its way to the intestine. It opens in the part of the intestine called the duodenum into a structure called the ampulla of Vater.

Chapter 11. Diseases of the Digestive Tract

Chapter 11. Diseases of the Digestive Tract

Bile	Bile is a bitter, greenish-yellow alkaline fluid secreted by the liver of most vertebrates. In many species, it is stored in the gallbladder between meals and upon eating is discharged into the duodenum where it aids the process of digestion.
Common bile duct	The common bile duct begins at the junction of the common hepatic duct and the cystic duct and ends at the Ampulla of Vater which drains into the second part of the duodenum. It carries bile from the liver and gallbladder to the gastrointestinal tract.
Lymph vessel	Lymph vessel refers to one of the system of vessels carrying lymph from the lymph capillaries to the veins.
Capillaries	Capillaries refer to the smallest of the blood vessels and the sites of exchange between the blood and tissue cells.
Capillary	A capillary is the smallest of a body's blood vessels, measuring 5-10 micro meters. They connect arteries and veins, and most closely interact with tissues. Their walls are composed of a single layer of cells, the endothelium. This layer is so thin that molecules such as oxygen, water and lipids can pass through them by diffusion and enter the tissues.
Lymph	Lymph originates as blood plasma lost from the circulatory system, which leaks out into the surrounding tissues. The lymphatic system collects this fluid by diffusion into lymph capillaries, and returns it to the circulatory system.
Blood	Blood is a circulating tissue composed of fluid plasma and cells. The main function of blood is to supply nutrients (oxygen, glucose) and constitutional elements to tissues and to remove waste products.
Absorption	Absorption is a physical or chemical phenomenon or a process in which atoms, molecules, or ions enter some bulk phase - gas, liquid or solid material. In nutrition, amino acids are broken down through digestion, which begins in the stomach.
Minerals	Minerals refer to inorganic chemical compounds found in nature; salts.
Affect	Affect is the scientific term used to describe a subject's externally displayed mood. This can be assesed by the nurse by observing facial expression, tone of voice, and body language.
Neoplasm	Neoplasm refers to abnormal growth of cells; often used to mean a tumor.
Cancer	Cancer is a class of diseases or disorders characterized by uncontrolled division of cells and the ability of these cells to invade other tissues, either by direct growth into adjacent tissue through invasion or by implantation into distant sites by metastasis.
Risk factor	A risk factor is a variable associated with an increased risk of disease or infection but risk factors are not necessarily causal.
Alcohol	Alcohol is a general term, applied to any organic compound in which a hydroxyl group (-OH) is bound to a carbon atom, which in turn is bound to other hydrogen and/or carbon atoms. The general formula for a simple acyclic alcohol is $C_nH_{2n+1}OH$.
Carcinoma	Cancer that originates in the coverings of the body, such as the skin or the lining of the intestinal tract is a carcinoma.
Tumor	An abnormal mass of cells that forms within otherwise normal tissue is a tumor. This growth can be either malignant or benign
Lesion	A lesion is a non-specific term referring to abnormal tissue in the body. It can be caused by any disease process including trauma (physical, chemical, electrical), infection, neoplasm, metabolic and autoimmune.
Radiation	The emission of electromagnetic waves by all objects warmer than absolute zero is referred to as radiation.

Chapter 11. Diseases of the Digestive Tract

Chapter 11. Diseases of the Digestive Tract

Dysphagia	Dysphagia is the medical term for the symptom of difficulty in swallowing.
Varices	Varices in general refers to distended veins. It derives from the latin word for twisted, "varix".
Veins	Blood vessels that return blood toward the heart from the circulation are referred to as veins.
Vein	Vein in animals, is a vessel that returns blood to the heart. In plants, a vascular bundle in a leaf, composed of xylem and phloem.
Esophageal varices	In medicine (gastroenterology), esophageal varices are extreme dilations of sub-mucosal veins in the mucosa of the esophagus in diseases featuring portal hypertension, secondary to cirrhosis primarily.
Varicose veins	Varicose veins are veins on the leg which are large, twisted, and ropelike, and can cause pain, swelling, or itching. They are an extreme form of telangiectasia, or spider veins.
Cirrhosis	Cirrhosis is a chronic disease of the liver in which liver tissue is replaced by connective tissue, resulting in the loss of liver function. Cirrhosis is caused by damage from toxins (including alcohol), metabolic problems, chronic viral hepatitis or other causes
Portal vein	The portal vein is the largest vein in the human body draining blood from the digestive system and its associated glands. It is formed by the union of the splenic vein and superior mesenteric vein and divides into a right and a left branch, before entering the liver.
Tissue	A collection of interconnected cells that perform a similar function within an organism is called tissue.
Congestion	In medicine and pathology the term congestion is used to describe excessive accumulation of blood or other fluid in a particular part of the body.
Hemorrhage	Loss of blood from the circulatory system is referred to as a hemorrhage.
Inflammation	Inflammation is the first response of the immune system to infection or irritation and may be referred to as the innate cascade.
Inflammatory response	Inflammatory response refers to a complex sequence of events involving chemicals and immune cells that results in the isolation and destruction of antigens and tissues near the antigens.
Pain	Pain is an unpleasant sensation which may be associated with actual or potential tissue damage and which may have physical and emotional components.
Protrusion	Protrusion is the anterior movement of an object. This term is often applied to the jaw.
Hernia	Hernia refers to abnormal protrusion of an organ or a body part through the containing wall of its cavity. Commonly referred to as a rupture, a hernia often involves protrusion of the intestine through a break in the peritoneum.
Diaphragm	The diaphragm is a shelf of muscle extending across the bottom of the ribcage. It is critically important in respiration: in order to draw air into the lungs, the diaphragm contracts, thus enlarging the thoracic cavity and reducing intra-thoracic pressure.
Heartburn	A pain emanating from the esophagus, caused by stomach acid backing up into the esophagus and irritating the esophageal tissue is heartburn.
Gastritis	Gastritis is a medical term for inflammation of the lining of the stomach. It means that white blood cells move into the wall of the stomach as a response to some type of injury.
Blood vessel	A blood vessel is a part of the circulatory system and function to transport blood throughout the body. The most important types, arteries and veins, are so termed because they carry

Chapter 11. Diseases of the Digestive Tract

Chapter 11. Diseases of the Digestive Tract

	blood away from or towards the heart, respectively.
Acute	In medicine, an acute disease is a disease with either or both of: a rapid onset; and a short course (as opposed to a chronic course).
Mucosa	The mucosa is a lining of ectodermic origin, covered in epithelium, and involved in absorption and secretion. They line various body cavities that are exposed to the external environment and internal organs.
Intrinsic factor	A substance produced by the gastric glands that promotes absorption of vitamin is called an intrinsic factor.
Epidemiology	Epidemiology is the study of the distribution and determinants of disease and disorders in human populations, and the use of its knowledge to control health problems. Epidemiology is considered the cornerstone methodology in all of public health research, and is highly regarded in evidence-based clinical medicine for identifying risk factors for disease and determining optimal treatment approaches to clinical practice.
Helicobacter pylori	Helicobacter pylori is a bacterium that infects the mucus lining of the human stomach. This bacterium lives in the human stomach exclusively and is the only known organism that can thrive in that highly acidic environment..
Toxin	Toxin refers to a microbial product or component that can injure another cell or organism at low concentrations. Often the term refers to a poisonous protein, but toxins may be lipids and other substances.
Peptic ulcer	Peptic ulcer is an ulcer of one of those areas of the gastrointestinal tract that are usually acidic.
Gastric ulcer	An open sore in the lining of the stomach, resulting when pepsin and hydrochloric acid destroy the lining tissues faster than they can regenerate is a gastric ulcer.
Pepsin	Pepsin is a digestive protease released by the chief cells in the stomach that functions to degrade food proteins into peptides. It was the first animal enzyme to be discovered.
Infection	The invasion and multiplication of microorganisms in body tissues is called an infection.
Nerve	A nerve is an enclosed, cable-like bundle of nerve fibers or axons, which includes the glia that ensheath the axons in myelin.
Antibiotic	Antibiotic refers to substance such as penicillin or streptomycin that is toxic to microorganisms. Usually a product of a particular microorvanism or plant.
Shock	Circulatory shock, a state of cardiac output that is insufficient to meet the body's physiological needs, with consequences ranging from fainting to death is referred to as shock. Insulin shock, a state of severe hypoglycemia caused by administration of insulin.
Lead	Lead is a chemical element in the periodic table that has the symbol Pb and atomic number 82. A soft, heavy, toxic and malleable poor metal, lead is bluish white when freshly cut but tarnishes to dull gray when exposed to air. Lead is used in building construction, lead-acid batteries, bullets and shot, and is part of solder, pewter, and fusible alloys.
Artery	Vessel that takes blood away from the heart to the tissues and organs of the body is called an artery.
Base	The common definition of a base is a chemical compound that absorbs hydronium ions when dissolved in water (a proton acceptor). An alkali is a special example of a base, where in an aqueous environment, hydroxide ions are donated.
Stool	Stool is the waste matter discharged in a bowel movement.
Bacteria	The domain that contains procaryotic cells with primarily diacyl glycerol diesters in their

Chapter 11. Diseases of the Digestive Tract

Chapter 11. Diseases of the Digestive Tract

	membranes and with bacterial rRNA. Bacteria also is a general term for organisms that are composed of procaryotic cells and are not multicellular.
Scar	A scar results from the biologic process of wound repair in the skin and other tissues of the body. It is a connective tissue that fills the wound.
Gastrointestinal tract	The gastrointestinal tract is the system of organs within multicellular animals which takes in food, digests it to extract energy and nutrients, and expels the remaining waste.
Lifestyle	The culturally, socially, economically, and environmentally conditioned complex of actions characteristic of an individual, group, or community as a pattern of habituated behavior over time that is health related but not necessarily health directed is a lifestyle.
Stressor	A factor capable of stimulating a stress response is a stressor.
Gastroenteritis	Gastroenteritis is an illness of fever, diarrhea and vomiting caused by an infectious virus, bacterium or parasite. It usually is of acute onset, normally lasting less than 10 days and self-limiting.
Anorexia	Anorexia nervosa is an eating disorder characterized by voluntary starvation and exercise stress.
Diarrhea	Diarrhea or diarrhoea is a condition in which the sufferer has frequent and watery, chunky, or loose bowel movements.
Electrolyte	An electrolyte is a substance that dissociates into free ions when dissolved (or molten), to produce an electrically conductive medium. Because they generally consist of ions in solution, they are also known as ionic solutions.
Electrolytes	Electrolytes refers to compounds that separate into ions in water and, in turn, are able to conduct an electrical current. These include sodium, chloride, and potassium.
Salt	Salt is a term used for ionic compounds composed of positively charged cations and negatively charged anions, so that the product is neutral and without a net charge.
Intolerance	Intolerance refers to a type of interaction in which two or more drugs produce extremely uncomfortable symptoms.
Lactose	Lactose is a disaccharide that makes up around 2-8% of the solids in milk. Lactose is a disaccharide consisting of two subunits, a galactose and a glucose linked together.
Allergy	An allergy or Type I hypersensitivity is an immune malfunction whereby a person's body is hypersensitized to react immunologically to typically nonimmunogenic substances. When a person is hypersensitized, these substances are known as allergens.
Viral	Viral phenomena are objects or patterns able to replicate themselves or convert other objects into copies of themselves when these objects are exposed to them.
Lactose intolerance	Lactose intolerance is the condition in which lactase, an enzyme needed for proper metabolization of lactose (a constituent of milk and other dairy products), is not produced in adulthood.
Microorganism	A microorganism or microbe is an organism that is so small that it is microscopic (invisible to the naked eye).
Escherichia coli	Escherichia coli is one of the main species of bacteria that live in the lower intestines of warm-blooded animals, including birds and mammals. They are necessary for the proper digestion of food and are part of the intestinal flora. Its presence in groundwater is a common indicator of fecal contamination.
Syndrome	Syndrome is the association of several clinically recognizable features, signs, symptoms, phenomena or characteristics which often occur together, so that the presence of one feature

Chapter 11. Diseases of the Digestive Tract

Chapter 11. Diseases of the Digestive Tract

	alerts the physician to the presence of the others
Hemolytic uremic syndrome	Hemolytic uremic syndrome refers to a kidney disease characterized by blood in the urine and often by kidney failure.
Salmonella	Salmonella is a genus of rod-shaped Gram-negative enterobacteria that causes typhoid fever, paratyphoid and foodborne illness. It is motile in nature and produces hydrogen sulfide.
Egg	An egg is the zygote, resulting from fertilization of the ovum. It nourishes and protects the embryo.
Salmonellosis	Salmonellosis refers to an infection with certain species of the genus Salmonella, usually caused by ingestion of food containing salmonellae or their products.
Intervention	Intervention refers to a planned attempt to break through addicts' or abusers' denial and get them into treatment. Interventions most often occur when legal, workplace, health, relationship, or financial problems have become intolerable.
Elderly	Old age consists of ages nearing the average life span of human beings, and thus the end of the human life cycle. Euphemisms for older people include advanced adult, elderly, and senior or senior citizen.
Anemia	Anemia is a deficiency of red blood cells and/or hemoglobin. This results in a reduced ability of blood to transfer oxygen to the tissues, and this causes hypoxia; since all human cells depend on oxygen for survival, varying degrees of anemia can have a wide range of clinical consequences.
Biopsy	Removal of small tissue sample from the body for microscopic examination is called biopsy.
Etiology	The apparent causation and developmental history of an illness is an etiology.
Prognosis	Prognosis refers to the prospects for the future or outcome of a disease.
Constipation	Constipation is a condition of the digestive system where a person (or other animal) experiences hard feces that are difficult to eliminate; it may be extremely painful, and in severe cases (fecal impaction) lead to symptoms of bowel obstruction.
Abdomen	The abdomen is a part of the body. In humans, and in many other vertebrates, it is the region between the thorax and the pelvis. In fully developed insects, the abdomen is the third (or posterior) segment, after the head and thorax.
Fever	Fever (also known as pyrexia, or a febrile response, and archaically known as ague) is a medical symptom that describes an increase in internal body temperature to levels that are above normal (37°C, 98.6°F).
Pancreatitis	Pancreatitis is inflammation of the pancreas. The most common causes of pancreatitis are gallstones and frequent and excessive consumption of alcohol (80% of cases), and less common causes are drugs or medication.
Diagnosis	In medicine, diagnosis is the process of identifying a medical condition or disease by its signs, symptoms, and from the results of various diagnostic procedures.
Kidney	The kidney is a bean-shaped excretory organ in vertebrates. Part of the urinary system, the kidneys filter wastes (especially urea) from the blood and excrete them, along with water, as urine.
Gangrene	Gangrene is necrosis and subsequent decay of body tissues caused by infection or thrombosis or lack of blood flow. It is usually the result of critically insufficient blood supply sometimes caused by injury and subsequent contamination with bacteria.
Lipase	A lipase is a water-soluble enzyme that catalyzes the hydrolysis of ester bonds in water–insoluble, lipid substrates. Most lipases act at a specific position on the glycerol

Chapter 11. Diseases of the Digestive Tract

Chapter 11. Diseases of the Digestive Tract

	backbone of a lipid substrate (A1, A2 or A3).
Pancreatic duct	The pancreatic duct joins the pancreas to the bile duct to supply pancreatic juice which aid in digestion provided by the "exocrine pancreas".
Vitamin	An organic compound other than a carbohydrate, lipid, or protein that is needed for normal metabolism but that the body cannot synthesize in adequate amounts is called a vitamin.
Diverticulum	A diverticulum is an outpouching of a hollow (or a fluid filled) structure in the body. Its use implies that the structure is not normally present, although embryologically, some normal structures begin development as a diverticulum arising off of another structure.
Young adult	An young adult is someone between the ages of 20 and 40 years old.
Stress	Stress refers to a condition that is a response to factors that change the human systems normal state.
Exacerbation	Exacerbation is a period in an illness when the symptoms of the disease reappear.
Remission	Disappearance of the signs of a disease is called remission.
Corticosteroid	Any steroid hormone secreted by the adrenal cortex, such as aldosterone, cortisol, and sex steroids is called a corticosteroid.
Colon	The colon is the part of the intestine from the cecum to the rectum. Its primary purpose is to extract water from feces.
Ulcerative colitis	Ulcerative colitis (UC) is a form of inflammatory bowel disease (IBD) featuring systemic inflammation specifically causing episodic mucosal inflammation of the colon (large bowel).
Temperament	Temperament refers to a basic, innate disposition that emerges early in life.
Autoimmune	Autoimmune refers to immune reactions against normal body cells; self against self.
Antibody	An antibody is a protein used by the immune system to identify and neutralize foreign objects like bacteria and viruses. Each antibody recognizes a specific antigen unique to its target.
Autoimmune disease	Disease that results when the immune system mistakenly attacks the body's own tissues is referred to as autoimmune disease.
Rectum	The rectum is the final straight portion of the large intestine in some mammals, and the gut in others, terminating in the anus.
Fak	FAK is a protein tyrosine kinase recruited at focal adhesions, which are sites at cell membranes where cytoskeletal elements interact with extracellular matrix proteins. Cell migration and differentiation are initiated at these sites.
Freezing	Freezing is the process in which blood is frozen and all of the plasma and 99% of the WBCs are eliminated when thawing takes place and the nontransferable cryoprotectant is removed.
Chronic disease	Disease of long duration often not detected in its early stages and from which the patient will not recover is referred to as a chronic disease.
Autoimmunity	Autoimmunity is the failure of an organism to recognise its own constituent parts (down to the sub-molecular levels) as self, as a result of which it attempts to mount an immune response against its own cells and tissues.
Colostomy	A colostomy is a surgical procedure that involves connecting a part of the colon onto the anterior abdominal wall, leaving the patient with an opening on the abdomen called a stoma. This opening is formed from the end of the large intestine drawn out through the incision and sutured to the skin.
Colorectal	Colorectal cancer includes cancerous growths in the colon, rectum and appendix. It is the

Chapter 11. Diseases of the Digestive Tract

Chapter 11. Diseases of the Digestive Tract

cancer	third most common form of cancer and the second leading cause of death among cancers in the Western world.
Sigmoid colon	The sigmoid colon is the part of the large intestine after the descending colon and before the rectum. The walls of the sigmoid colon are muscular, and contract to increase the pressure inside the colon, causing the stool to move into the rectum.
Polyposis	Polyposis refers to condition of having many polyps in an organ or structure.
Fiber	Fibers used by man come from a wide variety of sources: Natural fiber include those made out of plants, animal and mineral sources. Natural fibers can be classified according to their origin.
Connective tissue	Connective tissue is any type of biological tissue with an extensive extracellular matrix and often serves to support, bind together, and protect organs.
Fibrous connective tissue	Any connective tissue with a preponderance of fiber, such as areolar, reticular, dense regular, and dense irregular connective tissues is referred to as the fibrous connective tissue.
Intussusception	An intussusception is a situation in which a part of the intestine has prolapsed into another section of intestine, similar to the way in which the parts of a collapsible telescope slide into one another. Also refers to the process whereby a new blood vessel is created by the splitting of an existing blood vessel in two.
Flatus	Gas or air in the gastrointestinal tract that may be expelled through the anus are referred to as flatus.
Irritable bowel syndrome	In gastroenterology, irritable bowel syndrome is a functional bowel disorder characterized by abdominal pain and changes in bowel habits which are not associated with any abnormalities seen on routine clinical testing.
Motility	Motility is the ability to move spontaneously and independently. The term can apply to single cells, or to multicellular organisms.
Laxatives	Medications used to soften stool and relieve constipation are referred to as laxatives.
Laxative	Laxative refers to a medication or other substance that stimulates evacuation of the intestinal tract.
Dysentery	Dysentery is an illness involving severe diarrhea that is often associated with blood in the feces. It is caused by ingestion of food containing bacteria, causing a disease in which inflammation of the intestines affect the body significantly.
Digestive system	The organ system that ingests food, breaks it down into smaller chemical units, and absorbs the nutrient molecules is referred to as the digestive system.
Medulla	Medulla in general means the inner part, and derives from the Latin word for 'marrow'. In medicine it is contrasted to the cortex.
Brain	The part of the central nervous system involved in regulating and controlling body activity and interpreting information from the senses transmitted through the nervous system is referred to as the brain.
Reabsorption	In physiology, reabsorption or tubular reabsorption is the flow of glomerular filtrate from the proximal tubule of the nephron into the peritubular capillaries. This happens as a result of sodium transport from the lumen into the blood by the Na+/K+ ATPase in the basolateral membrane of the epithelial cells.
Elimination	Elimination refers to the physiologic excretion of drugs and other substances from the body.
Defecation	Discharge of feces from the rectum through the anus is referred to as defecation.

Chapter 11. Diseases of the Digestive Tract

Chapter 11. Diseases of the Digestive Tract

Hemorrhoids	Hemorrhoids are varicosities or swelling and inflammation of veins in the rectum and anus.
Hemorrhoid	A pronounced swelling in a large vein, particularly veins found in the anal region is referred to as hemorrhoid.
Anus	In anatomy, the anus is the external opening of the rectum. Closure is controlled by sphincter muscles. Feces are expelled from the body through the anus during the act of defecation, which is the primary function of the anus.
External hemorrhoids	External hemorrhoids are hemorrhoids that occur outside of the anal verge (the distal end of the anal canal).
Heredity	Heredity refers to the transmission of genetic information from parent to offspring.
Uterus	The uterus is the major female reproductive organ of most mammals. One end, the cervix, opens into the vagina; the other is connected on both sides to the fallopian tubes. The main function is to accept a fertilized ovum which becomes implanted into the endometrium, and derives nourishment from blood vessels which develop exclusively for this purpose.
Suppository	A suppository is a medicine that is inserted either into the rectum (rectal suppository) or into the vagina (vaginal suppository) where it melts.
Inflammatory bowel disease	In medicine, inflammatory bowel disease is a group of inflammatory conditions of the large intestine and, in some cases, the small intestine. It should not be confused with IBS, irritable bowel syndrome, which is an inconvenient yet more innocent disease.
Fluoroscopy	Fluoroscopy is an imaging technique commonly used by physicians to obtain real-time images of the internal structures of a patient through the use of a fluoroscope.
Barium	Barium is a chemical element in the periodic table that has the symbol Ba and atomic number 56. A soft silvery metallic element, barium is an alkaline earth metal and melts at a very high temperature. Its oxide is historically known as baryta but is never found in nature in its pure form due to its reactivity with air.
Lens	The lens or crystalline lens is a transparent, biconvex structure in the eye that, along with the cornea, helps to refract light to focus on the retina. Its function is thus similar to a man-made optical lens.
Iron	Iron is essential to all organisms, except for a few bacteria. It is mostly stably incorporated in the inside of metalloproteins, because in exposed or in free form it causes production of free radicals that are generally toxic to cells.
Eye	An eye is an organ that detects light. Different kinds of light-sensitive organs are found in a variety of creatures. The simplest eyes do nothing but detect whether the surroundings are light or dark, while more complex eyes can distinguish shapes and colors.
Endoscopy	Endoscopy means looking inside and refers to looking inside the human body for medical reasons.
Chemotherapy	Chemotherapy is the use of chemical substances to treat disease. In its modern-day use, it refers almost exclusively to cytostatic drugs used to treat cancer. In its non-oncological use, the term may also refer to antibiotics.
Malnutrition	Malnutrition is a general term for the medical condition in a person or animal caused by an unbalanced diet—either too little or too much food, or a diet missing one or more important nutrients.
Floating	Floating is a technique used to advance the IV catheter into the vein, whereby the catheter is inserted halfway into the vein and the tourniquet and needle are removed. The cannula hub is then attached to the infusion tubing and the control clamp on the tubing is slowly opened, floating the catheter into the vein with the infusate.

Chapter 11. Diseases of the Digestive Tract

Chapter 11. Diseases of the Digestive Tract

Sedative	A sedative is a drug that depresses the central nervous system (CNS), which causes calmness, relaxation, reduction of anxiety, sleepiness, slowed breathing, slurred speech, staggering gait, poor judgment, and slow, uncertain reflexes.
Sternum	Sternum or breastbone is a long, flat bone located in the center of the thorax (chest). It connects to the rib bones via cartilage, forming the rib cage with them, and thus helps to protect the lungs and heart from physical trauma.
Esophageal cancer	Esophageal cancer is malignancy of the esophagus. There are various subtypes. Esophageal tumors usually lead to dysphagia (difficulty swallowing), pain and other symptoms, and is diagnosed with biopsy.

Go to **Cram101.com** for the Practice Tests for this Chapter.

Chapter 11. Diseases of the Digestive Tract

Chapter 12. Diseases of the Liver, Gallbladder, and Pancreas

Regeneration	Regeneration is the ability to restore lost or damaged tissues, organs or limbs. It is a common feature in invertebrates, but far more limited in most vertebrates.
Organ	Organ refers to a structure consisting of several tissues adapted as a group to perform specific functions.
Liver	The liver is an organ in vertebrates, including humans. It plays a major role in metabolism and has a number of functions in the body including drug detoxification, glycogen storage, and plasma protein synthesis. It also produces bile, which is important for digestion.
Portal vein	The portal vein is the largest vein in the human body draining blood from the digestive system and its associated glands. It is formed by the union of the splenic vein and superior mesenteric vein and divides into a right and a left branch, before entering the liver.
Blood	Blood is a circulating tissue composed of fluid plasma and cells. The main function of blood is to supply nutrients (oxygen, glucose) and constitutional elements to tissues and to remove waste products.
Vein	Vein in animals, is a vessel that returns blood to the heart. In plants, a vascular bundle in a leaf, composed of xylem and phloem.
Intestine	The intestine is the portion of the alimentary canal extending from the stomach to the anus and, in humans and mammals, consists of two segments, the small intestine and the large intestine. The intestine is the part of the body responsible for extracting nutrition from food.
Pancreas	The pancreas is a retroperitoneal organ that serves two functions: exocrine - it produces pancreatic juice containing digestive enzymes, and endocrine - it produces several important hormones, namely insulin.
Stomach	The stomach is an organ in the alimentary canal used to digest food. It's primary function is not the absorption of nutrients from digested food; rather, the main job of the stomach is to break down large food molecules into smaller ones, so that they can be absorbed into the blood more easily.
Spleen	The spleen is a ductless, vertebrate gland that is not necessary for life but is closely associated with the circulatory system, where it functions in the destruction of old red blood cells and removal of other debris from the bloodstream, and also in holding a reservoir of blood.
Glucose	Glucose, a simple monosaccharide sugar, is one of the most important carbohydrates and is used as a source of energy in animals and plants. Glucose is one of the main products of photosynthesis and starts respiration.
Glycogen	Glycogen refers to a complex, extensively branched polysaccharide of many glucose monomers; serves as an energy-storage molecule in liver and muscle cells.
Buffer	A chemical substance that resists changes in pH by accepting H^+ ions from or donating H^+ ions to solutions is called a buffer.
Protein	A protein is a complex, high-molecular-weight organic compound that consists of amino acids joined by peptide bonds. They are essential to the structure and function of all living cells and viruses. Many are enzymes or subunits of enzymes.
Enzyme	An enzyme is a protein that catalyzes, or speeds up, a chemical reaction. They are essential to sustain life because most chemical reactions in biological cells would occur too slowly, or would lead to different products, without them.
Albumin	Albumin refers generally to any protein with water solubility, which is moderately soluble in concentrated salt solutions, and experiences heat coagulation (protein denaturation).

Go to Cram101.com for the Practice Tests for this Chapter.

Chapter 12. Diseases of the Liver, Gallbladder, and Pancreas

Chapter 12. Diseases of the Liver, Gallbladder, and Pancreas

Plasma	Fluid portion of circulating blood is called plasma.
Blood vessel	A blood vessel is a part of the circulatory system and function to transport blood throughout the body. The most important types, arteries and veins, are so termed because they carry blood away from or towards the heart, respectively.
Tissue	A collection of interconnected cells that perform a similar function within an organism is called tissue.
Edema	Edema is swelling of any organ or tissue due to accumulation of excess fluid. Edema has many root causes, but its common mechanism is accumulation of fluid into the tissues.
Amino acid	An amino acid is any molecule that contains both amino and carboxylic acid functional groups. They are the basic structural building units of proteins. They form short polymer chains called peptides or polypeptides which in turn form structures called proteins.
Metabolism	Metabolism is the biochemical modification of chemical compounds in living organisms and cells. This includes the biosynthesis of complex organic molecules (anabolism) and their breakdown (catabolism).
Ammonia	Ammonia is a compound of nitrogen and hydrogen with the formula NH_3. At standard temperature and pressure ammonia is a gas. It is toxic and corrosive to some materials, and has a characteristic pungent odor.
Acid	An acid is a water-soluble, sour-tasting chemical compound that when dissolved in water, gives a solution with a pH of less than 7.
Urea	Urea is an organic compound of carbon, nitrogen, oxygen and hydrogen, CON_2H_4 or $(NH_2)_2CO$. Urea is essentially a waste product: it has no physiological function. It is dissolved in blood and excreted by the kidney.
Digestion	Digestion refers to the mechanical and chemical breakdown of food into molecules small enough for the body to absorb; the second main stage of food processing, following ingestion.
Lipid	Lipid is one class of aliphatic hydrocarbon-containing organic compounds essential for the structure and function of living cells. They are characterized by being water-insoluble but soluble in nonpolar organic solvents.
Small intestine	The small intestine is the part of the gastrointestinal tract between the stomach and the large intestine (colon). In humans over 5 years old it is about 7m long. It is divided into three structural parts: duodenum, jejunum and ileum.
Vitamin	An organic compound other than a carbohydrate, lipid, or protein that is needed for normal metabolism but that the body cannot synthesize in adequate amounts is called a vitamin.
Bile	Bile is a bitter, greenish-yellow alkaline fluid secreted by the liver of most vertebrates. In many species, it is stored in the gallbladder between meals and upon eating is discharged into the duodenum where it aids the process of digestion.
Bacteria	The domain that contains procaryotic cells with primarily diacyl glycerol diesters in their membranes and with bacterial rRNA. Bacteria also is a general term for organisms that are composed of procaryotic cells and are not multicellular.
Toxin	Toxin refers to a microbial product or component that can injure another cell or organism at low concentrations. Often the term refers to a poisonous protein, but toxins may be lipids and other substances.
Iron	Iron is essential to all organisms, except for a few bacteria. It is mostly stably incorporated in the inside of metalloproteins, because in exposed or in free form it causes production of free radicals that are generally toxic to cells.

Chapter 12. Diseases of the Liver, Gallbladder, and Pancreas

Chapter 12. Diseases of the Liver, Gallbladder, and Pancreas

Gallbladder	The gallbladder is a pear-shaped organ that stores bile until the body needs it for digestion. It is connected to the liver and the duodenum by the biliary tract.
Bile duct	A bile duct is any of a number of long tube-like structures that carry bile. The top half of the common bile duct is associated with the liver, while the bottom half of the common bile duct is associated with the pancreas, through which it passes on its way to the intestine. It opens in the part of the intestine called the duodenum into a structure called the ampulla of Vater.
Duodenum	The duodenum is a hollow jointed tube connecting the stomach to the jejunum. It is the first part of the small intestine. Two very important ducts open into the duodenum, namely the bile duct and the pancreatic duct. The duodenum is largely responsible for the breakdown of food in the small intestine.
Cholesterol	Cholesterol is a steroid, a lipid, and an alcohol, found in the cell membranes of all body tissues, and transported in the blood plasma of all animals. It is an important component of the membranes of cells, providing stability; it makes the membrane's fluidity stable over a bigger temperature interval.
Hemoglobin	Hemoglobin is the iron-containing oxygen-transport metalloprotein in the red cells of the blood in mammals and other animals. Hemoglobin transports oxygen from the lungs to the rest of the body, such as to the muscles, where it releases the oxygen load.
Bile salt	Bile salt is a steroid compound often conjugated with glycine and taurine, and act to some extent as a detergent, helping to emulsify fats, and thus aid in their absorption in the small intestine. The most important compounds are the salts of taurocholic acid and deoxycholic acid.
Bilirubin	A bile pigment produced from hemoglobin breakdown is bilirubin.
Salt	Salt is a term used for ionic compounds composed of positively charged cations and negatively charged anions, so that the product is neutral and without a net charge.
Hepatic duct	Hepatic duct refers to the duct that conveys bile from the liver to the gallbladder.
Cystic duct	The cystic duct is the short duct that joins the gall bladder to the common bile duct. It usually lies next to the cystic artery.
Common hepatic duct	The common hepatic duct is the duct formed by the junction of the right hepatic duct (which drains bile from the right functional lobe of the liver) and the left hepatic duct (which drains bile from the left functional lobe of the liver). The common hepatic duct then joins the cystic duct coming from the gallbladder to form the common bile duct.
Jaundice	Jaundice is yellowing of the skin, sclera (the white of the eyes) and mucous membranes caused by increased levels of bilirubin in the human body.
Skin	Skin is an organ of the integumentary system composed of a layer of tissues that protect underlying muscles and organs.
Eye	An eye is an organ that detects light. Different kinds of light-sensitive organs are found in a variety of creatures. The simplest eyes do nothing but detect whether the surroundings are light or dark, while more complex eyes can distinguish shapes and colors.
Gallstone	A gallstone is a crystalline body formed within the body by accretion or concretion of normal or abnormal bile components. They can occur anywhere within the biliary tree, including the gallbladder and the common bile duct.
Tumor	An abnormal mass of cells that forms within otherwise normal tissue is a tumor. This growth can be either malignant or benign
Urine	Concentrated filtrate produced by the kidneys and excreted via the bladder is called urine.

Go to **Cram101.com** for the Practice Tests for this Chapter.

Chapter 12. Diseases of the Liver, Gallbladder, and Pancreas

Chapter 12. Diseases of the Liver, Gallbladder, and Pancreas

Stool	Stool is the waste matter discharged in a bowel movement.
Inflammation	Inflammation is the first response of the immune system to infection or irritation and may be referred to as the innate cascade.
Infection	The invasion and multiplication of microorganisms in body tissues is called an infection.
Absorption	Absorption is a physical or chemical phenomenon or a process in which atoms, molecules, or ions enter some bulk phase - gas, liquid or solid material. In nutrition, amino acids are broken down through digestion, which begins in the stomach.
Hepatitis	Hepatitis is a gastroenterological disease, featuring inflammation of the liver. The clinical signs and prognosis, as well as the therapy, depend on the cause.
Cirrhosis	Cirrhosis is a chronic disease of the liver in which liver tissue is replaced by connective tissue, resulting in the loss of liver function. Cirrhosis is caused by damage from toxins (including alcohol), metabolic problems, chronic viral hepatitis or other causes
Etiology	The apparent causation and developmental history of an illness is an etiology.
Virus	Obligate intracellular parasite of living cells consisting of an outer capsid and an inner core of nucleic acid is referred to as virus. The term virus usually refers to those particles that infect eukaryotes whilst the term bacteriophage or phage is used to describe those infecting prokaryotes.
Hepatitis A	Hepatitis A is an enterovirus transmitted by the orofecal route, such as contaminated food. It causes an acute form of hepatitis and does not have a chronic stage.
Hepatitis B	Hepatitis B is caused by a doublestranded DNA virus formerly called the 'Dane particle.' The virus is transmitted by body fluids.
Viral	Viral phenomena are objects or patterns able to replicate themselves or convert other objects into copies of themselves when these objects are exposed to them.
Contamination	The introduction of microorganisms or particulate matter into a normally sterile environment is called contamination.
Epidemic	An epidemic is a disease that appears as new cases in a given human population, during a given period, at a rate that substantially exceeds what is "expected", based on recent experience.
Incubation	In problem solving, a hypothetical process that sometimes occurs when we stand back from a frustrating problem for a while and the solution 'suddenly' appears is an incubation.
Incubation period	The period after pathogen entry into a host and before signs and symptoms appear is called the incubation period.
Anorexia	Anorexia nervosa is an eating disorder characterized by voluntary starvation and exercise stress.
Fever	Fever (also known as pyrexia, or a febrile response, and archaically known as ague) is a medical symptom that describes an increase in internal body temperature to levels that are above normal (37°C, 98.6°F).
Prognosis	Prognosis refers to the prospects for the future or outcome of a disease.
Anemia	Anemia is a deficiency of red blood cells and/or hemoglobin. This results in a reduced ability of blood to transfer oxygen to the tissues, and this causes hypoxia; since all human cells depend on oxygen for survival, varying degrees of anemia can have a wide range of clinical consequences.
Serum	Serum is the same as blood plasma except that clotting factors (such as fibrin) have been

Chapter 12. Diseases of the Liver, Gallbladder, and Pancreas

Chapter 12. Diseases of the Liver, Gallbladder, and Pancreas

	removed. Blood plasma contains fibrinogen.
Lead	Lead is a chemical element in the periodic table that has the symbol Pb and atomic number 82. A soft, heavy, toxic and malleable poor metal, lead is bluish white when freshly cut but tarnishes to dull gray when exposed to air. Lead is used in building construction, lead-acid batteries, bullets and shot, and is part of solder, pewter, and fusible alloys.
Syringe	A device for injecting drugs directly into the body is a syringe.
Addict	A person with an overpowering physical or psychological need to continue taking a particular substance or drug is referred to as an addict.
Sexually transmitted disease	Infection transmitted from one individual to another by direct contact during sexual activity is referred to as a sexually transmitted disease.
Dialysis	Dialysis refers to separation and disposal of metabolic wastes from the blood by mechanical means; an artificial method of performing the functions of the kidneys.
Immunity	Resistance to the effects of specific disease-causing agents is called immunity.
Epidemiology	Epidemiology is the study of the distribution and determinants of disease and disorders in human populations, and the use of its knowledge to control health problems. Epidemiology is considered the cornerstone methodology in all of public health research, and is highly regarded in evidence-based clinical medicine for identifying risk factors for disease and determining optimal treatment approaches to clinical practice.
Hepatitis C	Hepatitis C is a blood-borne viral disease which can cause liver inflamation, fibrosis, cirrhosis and liver cancer.
Health	Health is a term that refers to a combination of the absence of illness, the ability to cope with everyday activities, physical fitness, and high quality of life.
Intravenous	Present or occurring within a vein, such as an intravenous blood clot is referred to as intravenous. Introduced directly into a vein, such as an intravenous injection or I.V. drip.
Interferon	Interferon is a natural protein produced by the cells of the immune systems of most animals in response to challenges by foreign agents such as viruses, bacteria, parasites and tumor cells. They belong to the large class of glycoproteins known as cytokines.
Injection	A method of rapid drug delivery that puts the substance directly in the bloodstream, in a muscle, or under the skin is called injection.
Alcoholism	A disorder that involves long-term, repeated, uncontrolled, compulsive, and excessive use of alcoholic beverages and that impairs the drinker's health and work and social relationships is called alcoholism.
Necrosis	Necrosis is the name given to unprogrammed death of cells/living tissue. There are many causes of necrosis including injury, infection, cancer, infarction, and inflammation. Necrosis is caused by special enzymes that are released by lysosomes.
Alcohol	Alcohol is a general term, applied to any organic compound in which a hydroxyl group (-OH) is bound to a carbon atom, which in turn is bound to other hydrogen and/or carbon atoms. The general formula for a simple acyclic alcohol is $C_nH_{2n+1}OH$.
Scar	A scar results from the biologic process of wound repair in the skin and other tissues of the body. It is a connective tissue that fills the wound.
Connective tissue	Connective tissue is any type of biological tissue with an extensive extracellular matrix and often serves to support, bind together, and protect organs.
Fibrous	Any connective tissue with a preponderance of fiber, such as areolar, reticular, dense

Go to Cram101.com for the Practice Tests for this Chapter.

Chapter 12. Diseases of the Liver, Gallbladder, and Pancreas

Chapter 12. Diseases of the Liver, Gallbladder, and Pancreas

connective tissue	regular, and dense irregular connective tissues is referred to as the fibrous connective tissue.
Malnutrition	Malnutrition is a general term for the medical condition in a person or animal caused by an unbalanced diet—either too little or too much food, or a diet missing one or more important nutrients.
Varices	Varices in general refers to distended veins. It derives from the latin word for twisted, "varix".
Veins	Blood vessels that return blood toward the heart from the circulation are referred to as veins.
Esophageal varices	In medicine (gastroenterology), esophageal varices are extreme dilations of sub-mucosal veins in the mucosa of the esophagus in diseases featuring portal hypertension, secondary to cirrhosis primarily.
Hemorrhage	Loss of blood from the circulatory system is referred to as a hemorrhage.
Abdomen	The abdomen is a part of the body. In humans, and in many other vertebrates, it is the region between the thorax and the pelvis. In fully developed insects, the abdomen is the third (or posterior) segment, after the head and thorax.
Adrenal	In mammals, the adrenal glands are the triangle-shaped endocrine glands that sit atop the kidneys. They are chiefly responsible for regulating the stress response through the synthesis of corticosteroids and catecholamines, including cortisol and adrenaline.
Gland	A gland is an organ in an animal's body that synthesizes a substance for release such as hormones, often into the bloodstream or into cavities inside the body or its outer surface.
Adrenal glands	The adrenal glands are the triangle-shaped endocrine glands that sit atop the kidneys; their name indicates that position. They are chiefly responsible for regulating the stress response through the synthesis of corticosteroids and catecholamines, including cortisol and adrenaline.
Adrenal gland	In mammals, the adrenal gland (also known as suprarenal glands or colloquially as kidney hats) are the triangle-shaped endocrine glands that sit atop the kidneys; their name indicates that position.
Estrogen	Estrogen is a steroid that functions as the primary female sex hormone. While present in both men and women, they are found in women in significantly higher quantities.
Gynecomastia	Gynecomastia is the development of abnormally large breasts on men. Gynecomastia is not simply a buildup of adipose tissue, but includes the development of glandular tissue as well.
Distribution	Distribution in pharmacology is a branch of pharmacokinetics describing reversible transfer of drug from one location to another within the body.
Atrophy	Atrophy is the partial or complete wasting away of a part of the body. Causes of atrophy include poor nourishment, poor circulation, loss of hormonal support, loss of nerve supply to the target organ, disuse or lack of exercise, or disease intrinsic to the tissue itself.
Cation	An ion with more protons than electrons and consequently a net positive charge is called a cation.
Affect	Affect is the scientific term used to describe a subject's externally displayed mood. This can be assesed by the nurse by observing facial expression, tone of voice, and body language.
Brain	The part of the central nervous system involved in regulating and controlling body activity and interpreting information from the senses transmitted through the nervous system is referred to as the brain.

Go to Cram101.com for the Practice Tests for this Chapter.

Chapter 12. Diseases of the Liver, Gallbladder, and Pancreas

Chapter 12. Diseases of the Liver, Gallbladder, and Pancreas

Tremor	Tremor is the rhythmic, oscillating shaking movement of the whole body or just a certain part of it, caused by problems of the neurons responsible from muscle action.
Cancer	Cancer is a class of diseases or disorders characterized by uncontrolled division of cells and the ability of these cells to invade other tissues, either by direct growth into adjacent tissue through invasion or by implantation into distant sites by metastasis.
Metastasis	The spread of cancer cells beyond their original site are called metastasis.
Colon	The colon is the part of the intestine from the cecum to the rectum. Its primary purpose is to extract water from feces.
Ascites	Serous fluid accumulation in the abdominal cavity is ascites.
Blocking	A sudden break or interuption in the flow of thinking or speech that is seen as an absence in thought is refered to as blocking.
Pain	Pain is an unpleasant sensation which may be associated with actual or potential tissue damage and which may have physical and emotional components.
Cholecystitis	Cholecystitis is inflammation of the gallbladder. It is commonly due to impaction (sticking) of a gallstone within the neck of the gall bladder, leading to inspiszation of bile, bile stasis, and infection by gut organisms.
Inflammatory response	Inflammatory response refers to a complex sequence of events involving chemicals and immune cells that results in the isolation and destruction of antigens and tissues near the antigens.
Infarction	The sudden death of tissue from a lack of blood perfusion is referred to as an infarction.
Gangrene	Gangrene is necrosis and subsequent decay of body tissues caused by infection or thrombosis or lack of blood flow. It is usually the result of critically insufficient blood supply sometimes caused by injury and subsequent contamination with bacteria.
Calcium	Calcium is the chemical element in the periodic table that has the symbol Ca and atomic number 20. Calcium is a soft grey alkaline earth metal that is used as a reducing agent in the extraction of thorium, zirconium and uranium. Calcium is also the fifth most abundant element in the Earth's crust.
Incidence	In epidemiological studies of a particular disorder, the rate at which new cases occur in a given place at a given time is called incidence.
Obesity	The state of being more than 20 percent above the average weight for a person of one's height is called obesity.
Extracorporeal	Extracorporeal refers to out of the body.
Sonography	Medical ultrasonography (sonography) is an ultrasound-based diagnostic imaging technique used to visualize muscles and internal organs, their size, structure and any pathological lesions, making them useful for scanning the organs. Obstetric sonography is commonly used during pregnancy.
Cholecystectomy	Cholecystectomy is the surgical removal of the gallbladder.
Common bile duct	The common bile duct begins at the junction of the common hepatic duct and the cystic duct and ends at the Ampulla of Vater which drains into the second part of the duodenum. It carries bile from the liver and gallbladder to the gastrointestinal tract.
Pancreatic duct	The pancreatic duct joins the pancreas to the bile duct to supply pancreatic juice which aid in digestion provided by the "exocrine pancreas".
Pancreatitis	Pancreatitis is inflammation of the pancreas. The most common causes of pancreatitis are

Chapter 12. Diseases of the Liver, Gallbladder, and Pancreas

Chapter 12. Diseases of the Liver, Gallbladder, and Pancreas

	gallstones and frequent and excessive consumption of alcohol (80% of cases), and less common causes are drugs or medication.
Insulin	Insulin is a polypeptide hormone that regulates carbohydrate metabolism. Apart from being the primary effector in carbohydrate homeostasis, it also has a substantial effect on small vessel muscle tone, controls storage and release of fat (triglycerides) and cellular uptake of both amino acids and some electrolytes.
Exocrine gland	Exocrine gland refers to glands that secrete their products via a duct. Typically, they include sweat glands, salivary glands, mammary glands and many glands of the digestive system.
Acute	In medicine, an acute disease is a disease with either or both of: a rapid onset; and a short course (as opposed to a chronic course).
Ulcer	An ulcer is an open sore of the skin, eyes or mucous membrane, often caused by an initial abrasion and generally maintained by an inflammation and/or an infection.
Ampulla	Base of a semicircular canal in the inner ear is called ampulla. The Ampulla also refers to a dilated segment in a tubular structure, and they are also the bulb-like structures above the tube feet in echinoderms.
Ampulla of Vater	The Ampulla of Vater, is an opening in the wall of the descending duodenum formed by the union of the pancreatic duct and the bile duct.
Idiopathic	Idiopathic is a medical adjective that indicates that a recognized cause has not yet been established.
Syndrome	Syndrome is the association of several clinically recognizable features, signs, symptoms, phenomena or characteristics which often occur together, so that the presence of one feature alerts the physician to the presence of the others
Diagnosis	In medicine, diagnosis is the process of identifying a medical condition or disease by its signs, symptoms, and from the results of various diagnostic procedures.
Amylase	Amylase is a digestive enzyme classified as a saccharidase. It is mainly a constituent of pancreatic juice and saliva, needed for the breakdown of long-chain carbohydrates (such as starch) into smaller units.
Mortality	The incidence of death in a population is mortality.
Mortality rate	Mortality rate is the number of deaths (from a disease or in general) per 1000 people and typically reported on an annual basis.
Calorie	Calorie refers to a unit used to measure heat energy and the energy contents of foods.
Oscilloscope	An oscilloscope is a piece of electronic test equipment that allows signal voltages to be viewed, usually as a two-dimensional graph of one or more electrical potential differences (vertical axis) plotted as a function of time or of some other voltage (horizontal axis).
Ultrasound	Ultrasound is sound with a frequency greater than the upper limit of human hearing, approximately 20 kilohertz. Medical use can visualise muscle and soft tissue, making them useful for scanning the organs, and obstetric ultrasonography is commonly used during pregnancy.
Pelvis	The pelvis is the bony structure located at the base of the spine (properly known as the caudal end). The pelvis incorporates the socket portion of the hip joint for each leg (in bipeds) or hind leg (in quadrupeds). It forms the lower limb (or hind-limb) girdle of the skeleton.
Computed	Computed tomography is an imaging method employing tomography where digital processing is

Chapter 12. Diseases of the Liver, Gallbladder, and Pancreas

Chapter 12. Diseases of the Liver, Gallbladder, and Pancreas

tomography	used to generate a three-dimensional image of the internals of an object from a large series of two-dimensional X-ray images taken around a single axis of rotation.
Digestive tract	The digestive tract is the system of organs within multicellular animals which takes in food, digests it to extract energy and nutrients, and expels the remaining waste.
Carcinoma	Cancer that originates in the coverings of the body, such as the skin or the lining of the intestinal tract is a carcinoma.
Critical thinking	Critical thinking consists of a mental process of analyzing or evaluating information, particularly statements or propositions that people have offered as true. It forms a process of reflecting upon the meaning of statements, examining the offered evidence and reasoning, and forming judgments about the facts.
Acute pancreatitis	Acute pancreatitis is a rapidly-onset inflammation of the pancreas. Depending on its severity, it can have severe complications and high mortality despite treatment.
Varicose veins	Varicose veins are veins on the leg which are large, twisted, and ropelike, and can cause pain, swelling, or itching. They are an extreme form of telangiectasia, or spider veins.
Chronic disease	Disease of long duration often not detected in its early stages and from which the patient will not recover is referred to as a chronic disease.
Liver failure	Liver failure is the final stage of liver disease. Liver failure is divided into types depending on the rapidity of onset.
Respiratory system	The respiratory system is the biological system of any organism that engages in gas exchange. In humans and other mammals, the respiratory system consists of the airways, the lungs, and the respiratory muscles that mediate the movement of air into and out of the body.

Chapter 12. Diseases of the Liver, Gallbladder, and Pancreas

Chapter 13. Diseases of the Respiratory System

Trachea	Trachea is an airway through which respiratory gas transport takes place in organisms. In terrestrial vertebrates, such as birds and humans, the trachea lets air move from the throat to the lungs. In terrestrial invertebrates, such as onychophorans and beetles, they conduct air from outside the organism directly to all of its internal tissues.
Larynx	The larynx is an organ in the neck of mammals involved in protection of the trachea and sound production. The larynx houses the vocal cords, and is situated at the point where the upper tract splits into the trachea and the esophagus.
Bronchioles	The bronchioles are the first airway branches that no longer contain cartilage. They are branches of the bronchi, and are smaller than one millimetre in diameter.
Bronchiole	The bronchiole is the first airway branch that no longer contains cartilage. They are branches of the bronchi, and are smaller than one millimetre in diameter.
Air sac	Air sac is an anatomical structure unique to the dinosaur and bird respiratory system that allows unidirectional flow of air into the lungs and through the body
Alveoli	Alveoli are anatomical structures that have the form of a hollow cavity. In the lung, the pulmonary alveoli are spherical outcroppings of the respiratory bronchioles and are the primary sites of gas exchange with the blood.
Lungs	Lungs are the essential organs of respiration in air-breathing vertebrates. Their principal function is to transport oxygen from the atmosphere into the bloodstream, and to excrete carbon dioxide from the bloodstream into the atmosphere.
Capillaries	Capillaries refer to the smallest of the blood vessels and the sites of exchange between the blood and tissue cells.
Capillary	A capillary is the smallest of a body's blood vessels, measuring 5-10 micro meters. They connect arteries and veins, and most closely interact with tissues. Their walls are composed of a single layer of cells, the endothelium. This layer is so thin that molecules such as oxygen, water and lipids can pass through them by diffusion and enter the tissues.
Blood	Blood is a circulating tissue composed of fluid plasma and cells. The main function of blood is to supply nutrients (oxygen, glucose) and constitutional elements to tissues and to remove waste products.
Oxygen	Oxygen is a chemical element in the periodic table. It has the symbol O and atomic number 8. Oxygen is the second most common element on Earth, composing around 46% of the mass of Earth's crust and 28% of the mass of Earth as a whole, and is the third most common element in the universe.
Hemoglobin	Hemoglobin is the iron-containing oxygen-transport metalloprotein in the red cells of the blood in mammals and other animals. Hemoglobin transports oxygen from the lungs to the rest of the body, such as to the muscles, where it releases the oxygen load.
Red blood cells	Red blood cells are the most common type of blood cell and are the vertebrate body's principal means of delivering oxygen from the lungs or gills to body tissues via the blood.
Red blood cell	The red blood cell is the most common type of blood cell and is the vertebrate body's principal means of delivering oxygen from the lungs or gills to body tissues via the blood.
Metabolism	Metabolism is the biochemical modification of chemical compounds in living organisms and cells. This includes the biosynthesis of complex organic molecules (anabolism) and their breakdown (catabolism).
Carbon	Carbon is a chemical element in the periodic table that has the symbol C and atomic number 6. An abundant nonmetallic, tetravalent element, carbon has several allotropic forms.
Carbon dioxide	Carbon dioxide is an atmospheric gas comprized of one carbon and two oxygen atoms. A very

Go to Cram101.com for the Practice Tests for this Chapter.

Chapter 13. Diseases of the Respiratory System

Chapter 13. Diseases of the Respiratory System

	widely known chemical compound, it is frequently called by its formula CO_2. In its solid state, it is commonly known as dry ice.
Respiratory system	The respiratory system is the biological system of any organism that engages in gas exchange. In humans and other mammals, the respiratory system consists of the airways, the lungs, and the respiratory muscles that mediate the movement of air into and out of the body.
Inspiration	Inspiration begins with the onset of contraction of the diaphragm, which results in expansion of the intrapleural space and an increase in negative pressure according to Boyle's Law.
Muscle	Muscle is a contractile form of tissue. It is one of the four major tissue types, the other three being epithelium, connective tissue and nervous tissue. Muscle contraction is used to move parts of the body, as well as to move substances within the body.
Expiration	In respiration, expiration is initiated by a decrease in volume and positive pressure exerted upon the intrapleural space upon diaphragm relaxation.
Intercostal muscles	Intercostal muscles are several groups of muscles that run between the ribs. They contract to pull the ribcage upwards and outwards, increasing the volume of the thorax and drawing in
Thoracic cavity	The thoracic cavity is the chamber of the human body (and other animal bodies) that is protected by the thoracic wall (thoracic cage and associated skin, muscle, and fascia).
Pleural cavity	The lungs are surrounded by two membranes, the pleura. The outer is attached to the chest wall and is known as the parietal pleura; the inner is attached to the lung and other visceral tissues and is known as the visceral pleura. In between the two is a thin space known as the pleural cavity or pleural space. It is filled with pleural fluid, a serous fluid produced by the pleura.
Hyperventilation	Hyperventilation is the state of breathing faster or deeper (hyper) than necessary, and thereby reducing the carbon dioxide concentration of the blood below normal. This causes various symptoms such as numbness or tingling in the hands, feet and lips, lightheadedness, dizziness, headache, chest pain and sometimes fainting.
Stimulus	Stimulus in a nervous system, a factor that triggers sensory transduction.
Brain	The part of the central nervous system involved in regulating and controlling body activity and interpreting information from the senses transmitted through the nervous system is referred to as the brain.
Respiratory center	The respiratory center regulates the rhythmic, alternating cycles of inspiration and expiration.
Blood vessel	A blood vessel is a part of the circulatory system and function to transport blood throughout the body. The most important types, arteries and veins, are so termed because they carry blood away from or towards the heart, respectively.
Epithelium	Epithelium is a tissue composed of a layer of cells. Epithelium can be found lining internal (e.g. endothelium, which lines the inside of blood vessels) or external (e.g. skin) free surfaces of the body. Functions include secretion, absorption and protection.
Respiratory tract	In humans the respiratory tract is the part of the anatomy that has to do with the process of respiration or breathing.
Projection	Attributing one's own undesirable thoughts, impulses, traits, or behaviors to others is referred to as projection.
Mucosa	The mucosa is a lining of ectodermic origin, covered in epithelium, and involved in absorption and secretion. They line various body cavities that are exposed to the external environment and internal organs.

Chapter 13. Diseases of the Respiratory System

Chapter 13. Diseases of the Respiratory System

Cilia	Microscopic, hairlike processes on the exposed surfaces of certain epithelial cells are cilia.
Infection	The invasion and multiplication of microorganisms in body tissues is called an infection.
Common cold	An acute, self-limiting, and highly contagious virus infection of the upper respiratory tract that produces inflammation, profuse discharge, and other symptoms is referred to as the common cold.
Immunity	Resistance to the effects of specific disease-causing agents is called immunity.
Virus	Obligate intracellular parasite of living cells consisting of an outer capsid and an inner core of nucleic acid is referred to as virus. The term virus usually refers to those particles that infect eukaryotes whilst the term bacteriophage or phage is used to describe those infecting prokaryotes.
Inflammation	Inflammation is the first response of the immune system to infection or irritation and may be referred to as the innate cascade.
Acute	In medicine, an acute disease is a disease with either or both of: a rapid onset; and a short course (as opposed to a chronic course).
Resistance	Resistance refers to a nonspecific ability to ward off infection or disease regardless of whether the body has been previously exposed to it. A force that opposes the flow of a fluid such as air or blood. Compare with immunity.
Viral	Viral phenomena are objects or patterns able to replicate themselves or convert other objects into copies of themselves when these objects are exposed to them.
Congestion	In medicine and pathology the term congestion is used to describe excessive accumulation of blood or other fluid in a particular part of the body.
Fever	Fever (also known as pyrexia, or a febrile response, and archaically known as ague) is a medical symptom that describes an increase in internal body temperature to levels that are above normal (37°C, 98.6°F).
Antihistamine	An antihistamine is a drug which serves to reduce or eliminate effects mediated by histamine, an endogenous chemical mediator released during allergic reactions, through action at the histamine receptor.
Sinusitis	Sinusitis is inflammation, either bacterial, fungal, viral, allergic or autoimmune, of the paranasal sinuses.
Blocking	A sudden break or interuption in the flow of thinking or speech that is seen as an absence in thought is refered to as blocking.
Sinus	A sinus is a pouch or cavity in any organ or tissue, or an abnormal cavity or passage caused by the destruction of tissue.
Hay fever	Hay fever is a collection of symptoms, predominantly in the nose and eyes, that occur after exposure to airborne particles of dust, dander, or the pollens of certain seasonal plants in people who are allergic to these substances.
Allergen	An allergen is any substance (antigen), most often eaten or inhaled, that is recognized by the immune system and causes an allergic reaction.
Allergic rhinitis	Allergic rhinitis is a collection of symptoms, predominantly in the nose and eyes, that occur after exposure to airborne particles of dust, dander, or the pollens of certain seasonal plants in people who are allergic to these substances
Mucus	Mucus is a slippery secretion of the lining of various membranes in the body (mucous membranes). Mucus aids in the protection of the lungs by trapping foreign particles that

Chapter 13. Diseases of the Respiratory System

Chapter 13. Diseases of the Respiratory System

	enter the nose during normal breathing. Additionally, it prevents tissues from drying out.
Eye	An eye is an organ that detects light. Different kinds of light-sensitive organs are found in a variety of creatures. The simplest eyes do nothing but detect whether the surroundings are light or dark, while more complex eyes can distinguish shapes and colors.
Injection	A method of rapid drug delivery that puts the substance directly in the bloodstream, in a muscle, or under the skin is called injection.
Allergy	An allergy or Type I hypersensitivity is an immune malfunction whereby a person's body is hypersensitized to react immunologically to typically nonimmunogenic substances. When a person is hypersensitized, these substances are known as allergens.
Antibody	An antibody is a protein used by the immune system to identify and neutralize foreign objects like bacteria and viruses. Each antibody recognizes a specific antigen unique to its target.
Antigen	An antigen is a substance that stimulates an immune response, especially the production of antibodies. They are usually proteins or polysaccharides, but can be any type of molecule, including small molecules (haptens) coupled to a protein (carrier).
Pharyngitis	Pharyngitis inflammation of the pharynx, often due to a S. pyogenes infection.
Tonsillitis	Tonsillitis is an inflammation of the tonsils, especially the palatine tonsils often due to S. pyogenes infection.
Bacteria	The domain that contains procaryotic cells with primarily diacyl glycerol diesters in their membranes and with bacterial rRNA. Bacteria also is a general term for organisms that are composed of procaryotic cells and are not multicellular.
Pathogen	A pathogen or infectious agent is a biological agent that causes disease or illness to its host. The term is most often used for agents that disrupt the normal physiology of a multicellular animal or plant.
Tissue	A collection of interconnected cells that perform a similar function within an organism is called tissue.
Lead	Lead is a chemical element in the periodic table that has the symbol Pb and atomic number 82. A soft, heavy, toxic and malleable poor metal, lead is bluish white when freshly cut but tarnishes to dull gray when exposed to air. Lead is used in building construction, lead-acid batteries, bullets and shot, and is part of solder, pewter, and fusible alloys.
Pain	Pain is an unpleasant sensation which may be associated with actual or potential tissue damage and which may have physical and emotional components.
Pharynx	The pharynx is the part of the digestive system and respiratory system of many animals immediately behind the mouth and in front of the esophagus.
Tonsils	The tonsils are areas of lymphoid tissue on either side of the throat. As with other organs of the lymphatic system, the tonsils act as part of the immune system to help protect against infection.
Tonsil	Tonsil refers to a patch of lymphatic tissue consisting of connective tissue that contains many lymphocytes; located in the pharynx and throat.
Purulent	Anything that creates or contains pus is purulent.
Culture	Culture, generally refers to patterns of human activity and the symbolic structures that give such activity significance.
Inhalation	Inhalation is the movement of air from the external environment, through the airways, into the alveoli during breathing.

Chapter 13. Diseases of the Respiratory System

Chapter 13. Diseases of the Respiratory System

Influenza	Influenza or flu refers to an acute viral infection of the respiratory tract, occurring in isolated cases, epidemics, and pandemics. Influenza is caused by three strains of influenza virus, labeled types A, B, and C, based on the antigens of their protein coats.
Pneumonia	Pneumonia is an illness of the lungs and respiratory system in which the microscopic, air-filled sacs (alveoli) responsible for absorbing oxygen from the atmosphere become inflamed and flooded with fluid.
Elderly	Old age consists of ages nearing the average life span of human beings, and thus the end of the human life cycle. Euphemisms for older people include advanced adult, elderly, and senior or senior citizen.
Vaccine	A harmless variant or derivative of a pathogen used to stimulate a host organism's immune system to mount a long-term defense against the pathogen is referred to as vaccine.
Antibiotic	Antibiotic refers to substance such as penicillin or streptomycin that is toxic to microorganisms. Usually a product of a particular microorvanism or plant.
Chronic obstructive pulmonary disease	Chronic obstructive pulmonary disease is an umbrella term for a group of respiratory tract diseases that are characterized by airflow obstruction or limitation. It is usually caused by tobacco smoking.
Bronchitis	Bronchitis is an obstructive pulmonary disease characterized by inflammation of the bronchi of the lungs.
Emphysema	Emphysema is a chronic lung disease. It is often caused by exposure to toxic chemicals or long-term exposure to tobacco smoke..
Asthma	Asthma is a complex disease characterized by bronchial hyperresponsiveness (BHR), inflammation, mucus production and intermittent airway obstruction.
Chronic bronchitis	A persistent lung infection characterized by coughing, swelling of the lining of the respiratory tract, an increase in mucus production, a decrease in the number and activity of cilia, and produces sputum for at least three months in two consecutive years is called chronic bronchitis.
Inflammatory response	Inflammatory response refers to a complex sequence of events involving chemicals and immune cells that results in the isolation and destruction of antigens and tissues near the antigens.
Dyspnea	Dyspnea or shortness of breath (SOB) is perceived difficulty breathing or pain on breathing. It is a common symptom of numerous medical disorders.
Medicine	Medicine is the branch of health science and the sector of public life concerned with maintaining or restoring human health through the study, diagnosis and treatment of disease and injury.
Sputum	The mucous secretion from the lungs, bronchi, and trachea that is ejected through the mouth is sputum.
Gland	A gland is an organ in an animal's body that synthesizes a substance for release such as hormones, often into the bloodstream or into cavities inside the body or its outer surface.
Hypertrophy	Hypertrophy is the increase of the size of an organ. It should be distinguished from hyperplasia which occurs due to cell division; hypertrophy occurs due to an increase in cell size rather than division. It is most commonly seen in muscle that has been actively stimulated, the most well-known method being exercise.
Hypoxia	Hypoxia is a pathological condition in which the body as a whole or region of the body is deprived of adequate oxygen supply.

Chapter 13. Diseases of the Respiratory System

Chapter 13. Diseases of the Respiratory System

Hypersensitivity	Hypersensitivity is an immune response that damages the body's own tissues. Four or five types of hypersensitivity are often described; immediate, antibody-dependent, immune complex, cell-mediated, and stimulatory.
Smooth muscle	Smooth muscle is a type of non-striated muscle, found within the "walls" of hollow organs; such as blood vessels, the bladder, the uterus, and the gastrointestinal tract. Smooth muscle is used to move matter within the body, via contraction; it generally operates "involuntarily", without nerve stimulation.
Wheezing	Wheezing is a continuous, coarse, whistling sound produced in the respiratory airways during breathing. For wheezing to occur, some part of the respiratory tree must be narrowed or obstructed, or airflow velocity within the respiratory tree must be heightened.
Aerosol	Liquid that is dispersed in the form of a fine mist is called aerosol.
Skin test	A skin test is a test to determine reactions to antigens or antibodies. Also used to determine sensitivity to allergens.
Skin	Skin is an organ of the integumentary system composed of a layer of tissues that protect underlying muscles and organs.
Lesion	A lesion is a non-specific term referring to abnormal tissue in the body. It can be caused by any disease process including trauma (physical, chemical, electrical), infection, neoplasm, metabolic and autoimmune.
Incidence	In epidemiological studies of a particular disorder, the rate at which new cases occur in a given place at a given time is called incidence.
Epinephrine	Epinephrine is a hormone and a neurotransmitter. Epinephrine plays a central role in the short-term stress reaction—the physiological response to threatening or exciting conditions (fight-or-flight response). It is secreted by the adrenal medulla.
Ephedrine	Ephedrine (EPH) is a sympathomimetic amine commonly used as a decongestant and to treat hypotension associated with regional anaesthesia. Chemically, it is an alkaloid derived from various plants in the genus Ephedra (family Ephedraceae).
Tracheotomy	A tracheotomy is a surgical procedure performed on the neck to open a direct airway through an incision in the trachea
Respiratory failure	Respiratory failure is a medical term for inadequate gas exchange by the respiratory system.
Infectious disease	In medicine, infectious disease or communicable disease is disease caused by a biological agent such as by a virus, bacterium or parasite. This is contrasted to physical causes, such as burns or chemical ones such as through intoxication.
Etiology	The apparent causation and developmental history of an illness is an etiology.
Fusion	Fusion refers to the combination of two atoms into a single atom as a result of a collision, usually accompanied by the release of energy.
Spirometer	A spirometer is an apparatus for measuring the volume of air inspired and expired by the lungs. It is a precision differential pressure transducer for the measurements of respiration flow rates.
Ozone	Ozone (O_3) is an allotrope of oxygen, the molecule consisting of three oxygen atoms, a triatomic molecule, instead of the more stable diatomic O_2. Ozone is a powerful oxidizing agent. It is also unstable, decaying to ordinary oxygen through the reaction: $2O_3 \rightarrow 3O_2$.
Abdomen	The abdomen is a part of the body. In humans, and in many other vertebrates, it is the region

Go to **Cram101.com** for the Practice Tests for this Chapter.

Chapter 13. Diseases of the Respiratory System

Chapter 13. Diseases of the Respiratory System

	between the thorax and the pelvis. In fully developed insects, the abdomen is the third (or posterior) segment, after the head and thorax.
Physical therapy	Physical therapy is a health profession concerned with the assessment, diagnosis, and treatment of disease and disability through physical means. It is based upon principles of medical science, and is generally held to be within the sphere of conventional medicine.
Exudate	An exudate is any fluid that filters from the circulatory system into leisions or areas of inflamation. Its composition varies but generally includes water and the disolved solutes of the blood, some or all plasma proteins, white blood cells, platelets and red blood cells.
Productive cough	A cough in which phlegm or mucus is dislodged, enabling a person to clear mucus from the lungs is a productive cough.
Affect	Affect is the scientific term used to describe a subject's externally displayed mood. This can be assesed by the nurse by observing facial expression, tone of voice, and body language.
Microorganism	A microorganism or microbe is an organism that is so small that it is microscopic (invisible to the naked eye).
Penicillin	Penicillin refers to a group of β-lactam antibiotics used in the treatment of bacterial infections caused by susceptible, usually Gram-positive, organisms.
Measles	Measles refers to a highly contagious skin disease that is endemic throughout the world. It is caused by a morbilli virus in the family Paramyxoviridae, which enters the body through the respiratory tract or through the conjunctiva.
Cancer	Cancer is a class of diseases or disorders characterized by uncontrolled division of cells and the ability of these cells to invade other tissues, either by direct growth into adjacent tissue through invasion or by implantation into distant sites by metastasis.
Young adult	An young adult is someone between the ages of 20 and 40 years old.
Conditioning	Processes by which behaviors can be learned or modified through interaction with the environment are conditioning.
Erythromycin	Erythromycin is a macrolide antibiotic which has an antimicrobial spectrum similar to or slightly wider than that of penicillin, and is often used for people who have an allergy to penicillins.
Immune system	The immune system is the system of specialized cells and organs that protect an organism from outside biological influences. When the immune system is functioning properly, it protects the body against bacteria and viral infections, destroying cancer cells and foreign substances.
Epidemic	An epidemic is a disease that appears as new cases in a given human population, during a given period, at a rate that substantially exceeds what is "expected", based on recent experience.
Tuberculosis	Tuberculosis is an infection caused by the bacterium Mycobacterium tuberculosis, which most commonly affects the lungs but can also affect the central nervous system, lymphatic system, circulatory system, genitourinary system, bones and joints.
Pleural membrane	The pleural membrane protects lungs and keeps moisture from escaping. They line the thoracic cavity and cover the external surface of the lungs.
Tumor	An abnormal mass of cells that forms within otherwise normal tissue is a tumor. This growth can be either malignant or benign
Necrosis	Necrosis is the name given to unprogrammed death of cells/living tissue. There are many causes of necrosis including injury, infection, cancer, infarction, and inflammation.

Go to **Cram101.com** for the Practice Tests for this Chapter.

Chapter 13. Diseases of the Respiratory System

Chapter 13. Diseases of the Respiratory System

	Necrosis is caused by special enzymes that are released by lysosomes.
Mycobacterium tuberculosis	Mycobacterium tuberculosis is the bacterium that causes most cases of tuberculosis. Its genome has been sequenced. It is an obligate aerobe mycobacterium (not gram positive/negative) that divides every 16 to 20 hours.
Mycobacterium	Mycobacterium is the a genus of actinobacteria, given its own family, the Mycobacteriaceae. It includes many pathogens known to cause serious diseases in mammals, including tuberculosis and leprosy.
Caseous lesion	Caseous lesion refers to a lesion resembling cheese or curd; cheesy. Most are caused by M. tuberculosis.
Fibrosis	Replacement of damaged tissue with fibrous scar tissue rather than by the original tissue type is called fibrosis.
Malnutrition	Malnutrition is a general term for the medical condition in a person or animal caused by an unbalanced diet—either too little or too much food, or a diet missing one or more important nutrients.
Stress	Stress refers to a condition that is a response to factors that change the human systems normal state.
Immunodeficiency	Immunodeficiency is a state in which the immune system's ability to fight infectious disease is compromised or entirely absent. Most cases of immunodeficiency are either congenital or acquired.
Leukocyte	A white blood cell is a leukocyte. They help to defend the body against infectious disease and foreign materials as part of the immune system.
Kidney	The kidney is a bean-shaped excretory organ in vertebrates. Part of the urinary system, the kidneys filter wastes (especially urea) from the blood and excrete them, along with water, as urine.
Organ	Organ refers to a structure consisting of several tissues adapted as a group to perform specific functions.
Lung cancer	Lung cancer is a malignant tumour of the lungs. Most commonly it is bronchogenic carcinoma (about 90%).
Carcinoma	Cancer that originates in the coverings of the body, such as the skin or the lining of the intestinal tract is a carcinoma.
Carcinogen	A carcinogen is any substance or agent that promotes cancer. A carcinogen is often, but not necessarily, a mutagen or teratogen.
Agent	Agent refers to an epidemiological term referring to the organism or object that transmits a disease from the environment to the host.
Bronchus	A bronchus is a caliber of airway in the respiratory tract that conducts air into the lungs. No gas exchange takes place in this part of the lungs.
Hemoptysis	Hemoptysis (or "coughing up blood") is the expectoration of blood or of blood-stained sputum from the bronchi, larynx, trachea, or lungs (e.g. in tuberculosis or other respiratory infections).
Anorexia	Anorexia nervosa is an eating disorder characterized by voluntary starvation and exercise stress.
Diagnosis	In medicine, diagnosis is the process of identifying a medical condition or disease by its signs, symptoms, and from the results of various diagnostic procedures.

Go to **Cram101.com** for the Practice Tests for this Chapter.

Chapter 13. Diseases of the Respiratory System

Chapter 13. Diseases of the Respiratory System

Biopsy	Removal of small tissue sample from the body for microscopic examination is called biopsy.
Bronchoscopy	Bronchoscopy is the visualization of the lower airways using a flexible or rigid endoscope.
Radiation	The emission of electromagnetic waves by all objects warmer than absolute zero is referred to as radiation.
Chemotherapy	Chemotherapy is the use of chemical substances to treat disease. In its modern-day use, it refers almost exclusively to cytostatic drugs used to treat cancer. In its non-oncological use, the term may also refer to antibiotics.
Reproductive system	A reproductive system is the ensembles and interactions of organs and or substances within an organism that stricly pertain to reproduction. As an example, this would include in the case of female mammals, the hormone estrogen, the womb and eggs but not the breast.
Cystic fibrosis	Cystic fibrosis is an autosomal recessive hereditary disease of the exocrine glands. It affects the lungs, sweat glands and the digestive system. It causes chronic respiratory and digestive problems.
Exocrine gland	Exocrine gland refers to glands that secrete their products via a duct. Typically, they include sweat glands, salivary glands, mammary glands and many glands of the digestive system.
Mortality	The incidence of death in a population is mortality.
Recessive gene	Recessive gene refers to a gene that will not be expressed if paired with a dominant gene but will be expressed if paired with another recessive gene.
Mortality rate	Mortality rate is the number of deaths (from a disease or in general) per 1000 people and typically reported on an annual basis.
Sweat gland	Gland responsible for the loss of a watery fluid, consisting mainly of sodium chloride (commonly known as salt) and urea in solution, that is secreted through the skin is a sweat gland.
Salt	Salt is a term used for ionic compounds composed of positively charged cations and negatively charged anions, so that the product is neutral and without a net charge.
Digestion	Digestion refers to the mechanical and chemical breakdown of food into molecules small enough for the body to absorb; the second main stage of food processing, following ingestion.
Stool	Stool is the waste matter discharged in a bowel movement.
Pancreas	The pancreas is a retroperitoneal organ that serves two functions: exocrine - it produces pancreatic juice containing digestive enzymes, and endocrine - it produces several important hormones, namely insulin.
Cyst	A cyst is a closed sac having a distinct membrane and developing abnormally in a cavity or structure of the body. They may occur as a result of a developmental error in the embryo during pregnancy or they may be caused by infections.
Enzyme	An enzyme is a protein that catalyzes, or speeds up, a chemical reaction. They are essential to sustain life because most chemical reactions in biological cells would occur too slowly, or would lead to different products, without them.
Electrolyte	An electrolyte is a substance that dissociates into free ions when dissolved (or molten), to produce an electrically conductive medium. Because they generally consist of ions in solution, they are also known as ionic solutions.
Diaphragm	The diaphragm is a shelf of muscle extending across the bottom of the ribcage. It is critically important in respiration: in order to draw air into the lungs, the diaphragm contracts, thus enlarging the thoracic cavity and reducing intra-thoracic pressure.

Go to Cram101.com for the Practice Tests for this Chapter.

Chapter 13. Diseases of the Respiratory System

Chapter 13. Diseases of the Respiratory System

Gas exchange	In humans and other mammals, respiratory gas exchange or ventilation is carried out by mechanisms of the lungs. The actual gas exchange occurs in the alveoli.
Arterial blood gas	Arterial blood gas measurement is a blood test that is performed to determine the concentration of oxygen, carbon dioxide and bicarbonate, as well as the pH, in the blood. Its main use is in pulmonology, as many lung diseases feature poor gas exchange, but it is also used in nephrology (kidney diseases) and electrolyte disturbances. As its name implies, the sample is taken from an artery, which is more uncomfortable and difficult than venipuncture.
Evaluation	The fifth step of the nursing process where nursing care and the patient's goal achievement are measured is the evaluation.
Ventilation	Ventilation refers to a mechanism that provides contact between an animal's respiratory surface and the air or water to which it is exposed. It is also called breathing.
Elimination	Elimination refers to the physiologic excretion of drugs and other substances from the body.
Absorption	Absorption is a physical or chemical phenomenon or a process in which atoms, molecules, or ions enter some bulk phase - gas, liquid or solid material. In nutrition, amino acids are broken down through digestion, which begins in the stomach.
Dysphagia	Dysphagia is the medical term for the symptom of difficulty in swallowing.
Cyanosis	Bluish skin coloration due to decreased blood oxygen concentration is called cyanosis.
Asymptomatic	A disease is asymptomatic when it is at a stage where the patient does not experience symptoms. By their nature, asymptomatic diseases are not usually discovered until the patient undergoes medical tests (X-rays or other investigations). Some diseases remain asymptomatic for a remarkably long time, including some forms of cancer.

Chapter 13. Diseases of the Respiratory System

Chapter 14. Diseases of the Endocrine System

Organ	Organ refers to a structure consisting of several tissues adapted as a group to perform specific functions.
Endocrine system	The endocrine system is a set of internal organs involved in the secretion of hormones into the blood. These glands are known as ductless, which means they do not have tubes inside them.
Hypothalamus	Located below the thalamus, the hypothalamus links the nervous system to the endocrine system by synthesizing and secreting neurohormones often called releasing hormones because they function by stimulating the secretion of hormones from the anterior pituitary gland.
Ovaries	Ovaries are egg-producing reproductive organs found in female organisms.
Thyroid	The thyroid is one of the larger endocrine glands in the body. It is located in the neck and produces hormones, principally thyroxine and triiodothyronine, that regulate the rate of metabolism and affect the growth and rate of function of many other systems in the body.
Adrenal	In mammals, the adrenal glands are the triangle-shaped endocrine glands that sit atop the kidneys. They are chiefly responsible for regulating the stress response through the synthesis of corticosteroids and catecholamines, including cortisol and adrenaline.
Testes	The testes are the male generative glands in animals. Male mammals have two testes, which are often contained within an extension of the abdomen called the scrotum.
Ovary	The primary reproductive organ of a female is called an ovary.
Gland	A gland is an organ in an animal's body that synthesizes a substance for release such as hormones, often into the bloodstream or into cavities inside the body or its outer surface.
Parathyroid gland	One of four endocrine glands embedded in the surface of the thyroid gland that secrete parathyroid hormone is called a parathyroid gland.
Pituitary gland	The pituitary gland or hypophysis is an endocrine gland about the size of a pea that sits in the small, bony cavity (sella turcica) at the base of the brain. Its posterior lobe is connected to a part of the brain called the hypothalamus via the infundibulum (or stalk), giving rise to the tuberoinfundibular pathway.
Adrenal glands	The adrenal glands are the triangle-shaped endocrine glands that sit atop the kidneys; their name indicates that position. They are chiefly responsible for regulating the stress response through the synthesis of corticosteroids and catecholamines, including cortisol and adrenaline.
Adrenal gland	In mammals, the adrenal gland (also known as suprarenal glands or colloquially as kidney hats) are the triangle-shaped endocrine glands that sit atop the kidneys; their name indicates that position.
Reproductive system	A reproductive system is the ensembles and interactions of organs and or substances within an organism that stricly pertain to reproduction. As an example, this would include in the case of female mammals, the hormone estrogen, the womb and eggs but not the breast.
Endocrine gland	An endocrine gland is one of a set of internal organs involved in the secretion of hormones into the blood. These glands are known as ductless, which means they do not have tubes inside them.
Affect	Affect is the scientific term used to describe a subject's externally displayed mood. This can be assesed by the nurse by observing facial expression, tone of voice, and body language.
Cholesterol	Cholesterol is a steroid, a lipid, and an alcohol, found in the cell membranes of all body tissues, and transported in the blood plasma of all animals. It is an important component of the membranes of cells, providing stability; it makes the membrane's fluidity stable over a bigger temperature interval.

Go to Cram101.com for the Practice Tests for this Chapter.

Chapter 14. Diseases of the Endocrine System

Chapter 14. Diseases of the Endocrine System

Amino acid	An amino acid is any molecule that contains both amino and carboxylic acid functional groups. They are the basic structural building units of proteins. They form short polymer chains called peptides or polypeptides which in turn form structures called proteins.
Protein	A protein is a complex, high-molecular-weight organic compound that consists of amino acids joined by peptide bonds. They are essential to the structure and function of all living cells and viruses. Many are enzymes or subunits of enzymes.
Steroid	A steroid is a lipid characterized by a carbon skeleton with four fused rings. Different steroids vary in the functional groups attached to these rings. Hundreds of distinct steroids have been identified in plants and animals. Their most important role in most living systems is as hormones.
Hormone	A hormone is a chemical messenger from one cell to another. All multicellular organisms produce hormones. The best known hormones are those produced by endocrine glands of vertebrate animals, but hormones are produced by nearly every organ system and tissue type in a human or animal body. Hormone molecules are secreted directly into the bloodstream, they move by circulation or diffusion to their target cells, which may be nearby cells in the same tissue or cells of a distant organ of the body.
Acid	An acid is a water-soluble, sour-tasting chemical compound that when dissolved in water, gives a solution with a pH of less than 7.
Glucagon	A peptide hormone secreted by islet cells in the pancreas that raises the level of glucose in the blood is referred to as glucagon. Glucagon is a 29 amino acid polypeptide acting as an important hormone in carbohydrate metabolism.
Insulin	Insulin is a polypeptide hormone that regulates carbohydrate metabolism. Apart from being the primary effector in carbohydrate homeostasis, it also has a substantial effect on small vessel muscle tone, controls storage and release of fat (triglycerides) and cellular uptake of both amino acids and some electrolytes.
Sugar	A sugar is the simplest molecule that can be identified as a carbohydrate. These include monosaccharides and disaccharides, trisaccharides and the oligosaccharides. The term "glyco-" indicates the presence of a sugar in an otherwise non-carbohydrate substance.
Blood	Blood is a circulating tissue composed of fluid plasma and cells. The main function of blood is to supply nutrients (oxygen, glucose) and constitutional elements to tissues and to remove waste products.
Negative feedback	Negative feedback refers to a control mechanism in which a chemical reaction, metabolic pathway, or hormonesecreting gland is inhibited by the products of the reaction, pathway, or gland.
Radiation	The emission of electromagnetic waves by all objects warmer than absolute zero is referred to as radiation.
Trauma	Trauma refers to a severe physical injury or wound to the body caused by an external force, or a psychological shock having a lasting effect on mental life.
Brain	The part of the central nervous system involved in regulating and controlling body activity and interpreting information from the senses transmitted through the nervous system is referred to as the brain.
Base	The common definition of a base is a chemical compound that absorbs hydronium ions when dissolved in water (a proton acceptor). An alkali is a special example of a base, where in an aqueous environment, hydroxide ions are donated.
Depression	In everyday language depression refers to any downturn in mood, which may be relatively transitory and perhaps due to something trivial. This is differentiated from Clinical

Chapter 14. Diseases of the Endocrine System

Chapter 14. Diseases of the Endocrine System

	depression which is marked by symptoms that last two weeks or more and are so severe that they interfere with daily living.
Skull	Skull refers to a bony protective encasement of the brain and the organs of hearing and equilibrium; includes the facial bones. Also called the cranium.
Hypophysis	The pituitary gland, or hypophysis, is an endocrine gland about the size of a pea that sits in the small, bony cavity (sella turcica) at the base of the brain.
Adenohypophysis	The adenohypophysis comprises the anterior lobe of the pituitary gland and is part of the endocrine system. Under the influence of the hypothalamus, the anterior pituitary produces and secretes several peptide hormones that regulate many physiological processes including stress, growth, and reproduction.
Blood vessel	A blood vessel is a part of the circulatory system and function to transport blood throughout the body. The most important types, arteries and veins, are so termed because they carry blood away from or towards the heart, respectively.
Anterior pituitary	The anterior pituitary comprises the anterior lobe of the pituitary gland and is part of the endocrine system. Under the influence of the hypothalamus, the anterior pituitary produces and secretes several peptide hormones that regulate many physiological processes including stress, growth, and reproduction.
Posterior pituitary	The posterior pituitary gland comprises the posterior lobe of the pituitary gland and is part of the endocrine system. Despite its name, the posterior pituitary gland is not a gland, rather, it is largely a collection of axonal projections from the hypothalamus that terminate behind the anterior pituitary gland.
Neurohypophysis	The neurohypophysis comprises the posterior lobe of the pituitary gland and is part of the endocrine system. Despite its name, the posterior pituitary gland is not a gland, rather, it is largely a collection of axonal projections from the hypothalamus that terminate behind the anterior pituitary gland.
Midbrain	Midbrain refers to one of three ancestral and embryonic regions of the vertebrate brain; develops into sensory integrating and relay centers that send sensory information to the cerebrum.
Nerve	A nerve is an enclosed, cable-like bundle of nerve fibers or axons, which includes the glia that ensheath the axons in myelin.
Fiber	Fibers used by man come from a wide variety of sources: Natural fiber include those made out of plants, animal and mineral sources. Natural fibers can be classified according to their origin.
Tropic hormone	A hormone that has another endocrine gland as a target for regulation is a tropic hormone.
Tissue	A collection of interconnected cells that perform a similar function within an organism is called tissue.
Growth hormone	Growth hormone is a polypeptide hormone synthesised and secreted by the anterior pituitary gland which stimulates growth and cell reproduction in humans and other vertebrate animals.
Puberty	A time in the life of a developing individual characterized by the increasing production of sex hormones, which cause it to reach sexual maturity is called puberty.
Liver	The liver is an organ in vertebrates, including humans. It plays a major role in metabolism and has a number of functions in the body including drug detoxification, glycogen storage, and plasma protein synthesis. It also produces bile, which is important for digestion.
Adolescence	Adolescence is the period of psychological and social transition between childhood and adulthood (gender-specific manhood, or womanhood). As a transitional stage of human

Go to **Cram101.com** for the Practice Tests for this Chapter.

Chapter 14. Diseases of the Endocrine System

Chapter 14. Diseases of the Endocrine System

	development it represents the period of time during which a juvenile matures into adulthood.
Thyroid stimulating hormone	Thyroid stimulating hormone is a hormone synthesized and secreted by thyrotrope cells in the anterior pituitary gland which regulates the endocrine function of the thyroid gland.
Medulla	Medulla in general means the inner part, and derives from the Latin word for 'marrow'. In medicine it is contrasted to the cortex.
Cortex	In anatomy and zoology the cortex is the outermost or superficial layer of an organ or the outer portion of the stem or root of a plant.
Gonadotropin	A hormone that stimulates the gonads is gonadotropin. They are protein hormones secreted by gonadotrope cells of the pituitary gland of vertebrates.
Adrenocortic-tropic hormone	Adrenocorticotropic hormone is a polypeptide hormone synthesised and secreted from corticotropes in the anterior lobe of the pituitary gland in response to the hormone corticotropin-releasing factor released by the hypothalamus. It stimulates the cortex of the adrenal gland and boosts the synthesis of corticosteroids, mainly glucocorticoids but also mineralcorticoids and sex steroids.
Adrenal cortex	Situated along the perimeter of the adrenal gland, the adrenal cortex mediates the stress response through the production of mineralocorticoids and glucocorticoids, including aldosterone and cortisol respectively. It is also a secondary site of androgen synthesis.
Gigantism	Gigantism is a condition characterized by excessive height growth. Gigantism is rarely used except to refer to the rare condition of pituitary gigantism due to prepubertal growth hormone excess.
Adenoma	Adenoma refers to a collection of growths of glandular origin. They can grow from many organs including the colon, adrenal, pituitary, thyroid, etc. These growths are benign, but some are known to have the potential, over time, to transform to malignancy
Tumor	An abnormal mass of cells that forms within otherwise normal tissue is a tumor. This growth can be either malignant or benign
Skin	Skin is an organ of the integumentary system composed of a layer of tissues that protect underlying muscles and organs.
Vertebrae	Vertebrae are the individual bones that make up the vertebral column (aka spine) - a flexuous and flexible column.
Acromegaly	Acromegaly is a hormonal disorder that results when the pituitary gland produces excess growth hormone (hGH). Most commonly it is a benign hGH producing tumor derived from a distinct type of cells (somatotrophs) and called pituitary adenoma.
Arthritis	Arthritis is a group of conditions that affect the health of the bone joints in the body. Arthritis can be caused from strains and injuries caused by repetitive motion, sports, overexertion, and falls. Unlike the autoimmune diseases, it largely affects older people and results from the degeneration of joint cartilage.
Cardiovascular disease	Cardiovascular disease refers to afflictions in the mechanisms, including the heart, blood vessels, and their controllers, that are responsible for transporting blood to the body's tissues and organs. Psychological factors may play important roles in such diseases and their treatments.
Population	Population refers to all members of a well-defined group of organisms, events, or things.
Mortality	The incidence of death in a population is mortality.
Mortality rate	Mortality rate is the number of deaths (from a disease or in general) per 1000 people and

Chapter 14. Diseases of the Endocrine System

Chapter 14. Diseases of the Endocrine System

	typically reported on an annual basis.
Hypopituitarism	Hypopituitarism is a medical term describing deficiency of one or more hormones of the pituitary gland.
Ischemia	Narrowing of arteries caused by plaque buildup within the arteries is called ischemia.
Infarction	The sudden death of tissue from a lack of blood perfusion is referred to as an infarction.
Atrophy	Atrophy is the partial or complete wasting away of a part of the body. Causes of atrophy include poor nourishment, poor circulation, loss of hormonal support, loss of nerve supply to the target organ, disuse or lack of exercise, or disease intrinsic to the tissue itself.
Metabolism	Metabolism is the biochemical modification of chemical compounds in living organisms and cells. This includes the biosynthesis of complex organic molecules (anabolism) and their breakdown (catabolism).
Salt	Salt is a term used for ionic compounds composed of positively charged cations and negatively charged anions, so that the product is neutral and without a net charge.
Gonadotropic hormone	Substance secreted by anterior pituitary that regulates the activity of the ovaries and testes is referred to as gonadotropic hormone.
Gonad	Gonad refers to a sex organ in an animal; an ovary or a testis. It is the organ that makes gametes.
Menstruation	Loss of blood and tissue from the uterine lining at the end of a female reproductive cycle are referred to as menstruation.
Sperm	Sperm refers to the male sex cell with three distinct parts at maturity: head, middle piece, and tail.
Pain	Pain is an unpleasant sensation which may be associated with actual or potential tissue damage and which may have physical and emotional components.
Thyroxine	The thyroid hormone thyroxine is a tyrosine-based hormone produced by the thyroid gland. An important component in the synthesis is iodine. It acts on the body to increase the basal metabolic rate, affect protein synthesis and increase the body's sensitivity to catecholamines.
Injection	A method of rapid drug delivery that puts the substance directly in the bloodstream, in a muscle, or under the skin is called injection.
Optic nerve	The optic nerve is the nerve that transmits visual information from the retina to the brain. The blind spot of the eye is produced by the absence of retina where the optic nerve leaves the eye. This is because there are no photoreceptors in this area.
Abdomen	The abdomen is a part of the body. In humans, and in many other vertebrates, it is the region between the thorax and the pelvis. In fully developed insects, the abdomen is the third (or posterior) segment, after the head and thorax.
Vasopressin	Vasopressin is a human hormone that is mainly released when the body is low on water; it causes the kidneys to conserve water by concentrating the urine. It has also various functions in the brain.
Oxytocin	Oxytocin is a hormone, found in humans and other mammals, which is involved in the facilitation of birth and breastfeeding as well as in bonding and the formation of trust between people.
Uterus	The uterus is the major female reproductive organ of most mammals. One end, the cervix, opens into the vagina; the other is connected on both sides to the fallopian tubes. The main function is to accept a fertilized ovum which becomes implanted into the endometrium, and

Go to Cram101.com for the Practice Tests for this Chapter.

Chapter 14. Diseases of the Endocrine System

Chapter 14. Diseases of the Endocrine System

	derives nourishment from blood vessels which develop exclusively for this purpose.
Muscle	Muscle is a contractile form of tissue. It is one of the four major tissue types, the other three being epithelium, connective tissue and nervous tissue. Muscle contraction is used to move parts of the body, as well as to move substances within the body.
Antidiuretic hormone	Antidiuretic hormone is a hormone that is mainly released when the body is low on water; it causes the kidneys to save water by concentrating the urine and is also involved in the creation of thirst. It is a peptide hormone produced by the hypothalamus, and stored in the posterior part of the pituitary gland.
Smooth muscle	Smooth muscle is a type of non-striated muscle, found within the "walls" of hollow organs; such as blood vessels, the bladder, the uterus, and the gastrointestinal tract. Smooth muscle is used to move matter within the body, via contraction; it generally operates "involuntarily", without nerve stimulation.
Hemorrhage	Loss of blood from the circulatory system is referred to as a hemorrhage.
Kidney	The kidney is a bean-shaped excretory organ in vertebrates. Part of the urinary system, the kidneys filter wastes (especially urea) from the blood and excrete them, along with water, as urine.
Diabetes	Diabetes is a medical disorder characterized by varying or persistent elevated blood sugar levels, especially after eating. All types of diabetes share similar symptoms and complications at advanced stages: dehydration and ketoacidosis, cardiovascular disease, chronic renal failure, retinal damage which can lead to blindness, nerve damage which can lead to erectile dysfunction, gangrene with risk of amputation of toes, feet, and even legs.
Urine	Concentrated filtrate produced by the kidneys and excreted via the bladder is called urine.
Polydipsia	Polydipsia is a medical term meaning abnormally large intake of fluids through the mouth.
Polyuria	Excessive output of urine is called polyuria.
Dehydration	Dehydration is the removal of water from an object. Medically, dehydration is a serious and potentially life-threatening condition in which the body contains an insufficient volume of water for normal functioning.
Lead	Lead is a chemical element in the periodic table that has the symbol Pb and atomic number 82. A soft, heavy, toxic and malleable poor metal, lead is bluish white when freshly cut but tarnishes to dull gray when exposed to air. Lead is used in building construction, lead-acid batteries, bullets and shot, and is part of solder, pewter, and fusible alloys.
Calorie	Calorie refers to a unit used to measure heat energy and the energy contents of foods.
Metabolic rate	Energy expended by the body per unit time is called metabolic rate.
Oxygen	Oxygen is a chemical element in the periodic table. It has the symbol O and atomic number 8. Oxygen is the second most common element on Earth, composing around 46% of the mass of Earth's crust and 28% of the mass of Earth as a whole, and is the third most common element in the universe.
Obesity	The state of being more than 20 percent above the average weight for a person of one's height is called obesity.
Trachea	Trachea is an airway through which respiratory gas transport takes place in organisms. In terrestrial vertebrates, such as birds and humans, the trachea lets air move from the throat to the lungs. In terrestrial invertebrates, such as onychophorans and beetles, they conduct air from outside the organism directly to all of its internal tissues.
Isthmus	An isthmus is a narrow strip of land that is bordered on two sides by water and connects two

Go to **Cram101.com** for the Practice Tests for this Chapter.

Chapter 14. Diseases of the Endocrine System

Chapter 14. Diseases of the Endocrine System

	larger land masses. It is the inverse of a strait (which lies between two land masses and connects two larger bodies of water).
Protrusion	Protrusion is the anterior movement of an object. This term is often applied to the jaw.
Larynx	The larynx is an organ in the neck of mammals involved in protection of the trachea and sound production. The larynx houses the vocal cords, and is situated at the point where the upper tract splits into the trachea and the esophagus.
Follicle	Follicle refers to a cluster of cells surrounding, protecting, and nourishing a developing egg cell in the ovary; also secretes estrogen. In botany, a follicle is a type of simple dry fruit produced by certain flowering plants. It is regarded as one the most primitive types of fruits, and derives from a simple pistil or carpel.
Thyroid hormones	The thyroid hormones, thyroxine (T4) and triiodothyronine (T3), are tyrosine-based hormones produced by the thyroid gland. An important component in the synthesis is iodine. They act on the body to increase the basal metabolic rate, affect protein synthesis and increase the body's sensitivity to catecholamines.
Triiodothyronine	A hormone produced by the thyroid gland that speeds up the metabolic rate is called triiodothyronine.
Capillaries	Capillaries refer to the smallest of the blood vessels and the sites of exchange between the blood and tissue cells.
Capillary	A capillary is the smallest of a body's blood vessels, measuring 5-10 micro meters. They connect arteries and veins, and most closely interact with tissues. Their walls are composed of a single layer of cells, the endothelium. This layer is so thin that molecules such as oxygen, water and lipids can pass through them by diffusion and enter the tissues.
Iodine	Iodine is a chemical element in the periodic table that has the symbol I and atomic number 53. It is required as a trace element for most living organisms. Chemically, iodine is the least reactive of the halogens, and the most electropositive halogen. Iodine is primarily used in medicine, photography and in dyes.
Plasma	Fluid portion of circulating blood is called plasma.
Serum	Serum is the same as blood plasma except that clotting factors (such as fibrin) have been removed. Blood plasma contains fibrinogen.
Absorption	Absorption is a physical or chemical phenomenon or a process in which atoms, molecules, or ions enter some bulk phase - gas, liquid or solid material. In nutrition, amino acids are broken down through digestion, which begins in the stomach.
Hyperactivity	Hyperactivity can be described as a state in which a individual is abnormally easily excitable and exuberant. Strong emotional reactions and a very short span of attention is also typical for the individual.
Cartilage	Cartilage is a type of dense connective tissue. Cartilage is composed of cells called chondrocytes which are dispersed in a firm gel-like ground substance, called the matrix. Cartilage is avascular (contains no blood vessels) and nutrients are diffused through the matrix.
Thyroid cartilage	Thyroid cartilage refers to largest laryngeal cartilage. It forms the laryngeal prominence, or Adam's apple.
Basal metabolic rate	Basal metabolic rate, is the rate of metabolism that occurs when an individual is at rest in a warm environment and is in the post absorptive state, and has not eaten for at least 12 hours.
Carbon	Carbon is a chemical element in the periodic table that has the symbol C and atomic number 6.

Chapter 14. Diseases of the Endocrine System

Chapter 14. Diseases of the Endocrine System

	An abundant nonmetallic, tetravalent element, carbon has several allotropic forms.
Carbon dioxide	Carbon dioxide is an atmospheric gas comprized of one carbon and two oxygen atoms. A very widely known chemical compound, it is frequently called by its formula CO_2. In its solid state, it is commonly known as dry ice.
Circulatory system	The circulatory system or cardiovascular system is the organ system which circulates blood around the body of most animals.
Cardiac output	Cardiac output is the volume of blood being pumped by the heart in a minute. It is equal to the heart rate multiplied by the stroke volume.
Respiratory center	The respiratory center regulates the rhythmic, alternating cycles of inspiration and expiration.
Digestive tract	The digestive tract is the system of organs within multicellular animals which takes in food, digests it to extract energy and nutrients, and expels the remaining waste.
Intestine	The intestine is the portion of the alimentary canal extending from the stomach to the anus and, in humans and mammals, consists of two segments, the small intestine and the large intestine. The intestine is the part of the body responsible for extracting nutrition from food.
Carbohydrate	Carbohydrate is a chemical compound that contains oxygen, hydrogen, and carbon atoms. They consist of monosaccharide sugars of varying chain lengths and that have the general chemical formula $C_n(H_2O)_n$ or are derivatives of such.
Inhibition	The ability to prevent from making some cognitive or behavioral response is called inhibition.
Goiter	Goiter refers to an enlargement of the thyroid gland resulting from a dietary iodine deficiency.
Colloid	Colloid refers to a mixture that contains dispersed particles larger than molecules but small enough so that they do not settle out.
Hypothyroidism	Hypothyroidism refers to slower metabolism and sluggishness caused by an underactive thyroid gland.
Esophagus	The esophagus, or gullet is the muscular tube in vertebrates through which ingested food passes from the mouth area to the stomach. Food is passed through the esophagus by using the process of peristalsis.
Hyperthyroidism	Hyperthyroidism is the clinical syndrome caused by an excess of circulating free thyroxine (T4) or free triiodothyronine (T3), or both.
Elderly	Old age consists of ages nearing the average life span of human beings, and thus the end of the human life cycle. Euphemisms for older people include advanced adult, elderly, and senior or senior citizen.
Pulse	The rhythmic stretching of the arteries caused by the pressure of blood forced through the arteries by contractions of the ventricles during systole is a pulse.
Eye	An eye is an organ that detects light. Different kinds of light-sensitive organs are found in a variety of creatures. The simplest eyes do nothing but detect whether the surroundings are light or dark, while more complex eyes can distinguish shapes and colors.
Edema	Edema is swelling of any organ or tissue due to accumulation of excess fluid. Edema has many root causes, but its common mechanism is accumulation of fluid into the tissues.
Reabsorption	In physiology, reabsorption or tubular reabsorption is the flow of glomerular filtrate from the proximal tubule of the nephron into the peritubular capillaries. This happens as a result

Go to **Cram101.com** for the Practice Tests for this Chapter.

Chapter 14. Diseases of the Endocrine System

Chapter 14. Diseases of the Endocrine System

	of sodium transport from the lumen into the blood by the Na+/K+ ATPase in the basolateral membrane of the epithelial cells.
Diarrhea	Diarrhea or diarrhoea is a condition in which the sufferer has frequent and watery, chunky, or loose bowel movements.
Large intestine	In anatomy of the digestive system, the colon, also called the large intestine or large bowel, is the part of the intestine from the cecum ('caecum' in British English) to the rectum. Its primary purpose is to extract water from feces.
Palpitation	A palpitation is an awareness of the beating of the heart, whether it is too slow, too fast, irregular, or at its normal frequency; brought on by overexertion, adrenaline, alcohol, disease or drugs, or as a symptom of panic disorder.
Tachycardia	Tachycardia is an abnormally rapid beating of the heart, defined as a resting heart rate of over 100 beats per minute. Common causes are autonomic nervous system or endocrine system activity, hemodynamic responses, and various forms of cardiac arrhythmia.
Autoimmune	Autoimmune refers to immune reactions against normal body cells; self against self.
Antibody	An antibody is a protein used by the immune system to identify and neutralize foreign objects like bacteria and viruses. Each antibody recognizes a specific antigen unique to its target.
Antigen	An antigen is a substance that stimulates an immune response, especially the production of antibodies. They are usually proteins or polysaccharides, but can be any type of molecule, including small molecules (haptens) coupled to a protein (carrier).
Tolerance	Drug tolerance occurs when a subject's reaction to a drug decreases so that larger doses are required to achieve the same effect.
Heart rate	Heart rate is a term used to describe the frequency of the cardiac cycle. It is considered one of the four vital signs. Usually it is calculated as the number of contractions of the heart in one minute and expressed as "beats per minute".
Lipid	Lipid is one class of aliphatic hydrocarbon-containing organic compounds essential for the structure and function of living cells. They are characterized by being water-insoluble but soluble in nonpolar organic solvents.
Digestive system	The organ system that ingests food, breaks it down into smaller chemical units, and absorbs the nutrient molecules is referred to as the digestive system.
Atherosclerosis	Process by which a fatty substance or plaque builds up inside arteries to form obstructions is called atherosclerosis.
Constipation	Constipation is a condition of the digestive system where a person (or other animal) experiences hard feces that are difficult to eliminate; it may be extremely painful, and in severe cases (fecal impaction) lead to symptoms of bowel obstruction.
Excitability	The ability of a cell to respond to a stimulus, especially the ability of nerve and muscle cells to produce membrane voltage changes in response to stimuli is excitability.
Insomnia	Insomnia is a sleep disorder characterized by an inability to sleep and/or to remain asleep for a reasonable period during the night.
Tremor	Tremor is the rhythmic, oscillating shaking movement of the whole body or just a certain part of it, caused by problems of the neurons responsible from muscle action.
Mental retardation	Mental retardation refers to having significantly below-average intellectual functioning and limitations in at least two areas of adaptive functioning. Many categorize retardation as mild, moderate, severe, or profound.
Cretinism	Cretinism is a condition of severely stunted physical and mental growth due to untreated

Chapter 14. Diseases of the Endocrine System

Chapter 14. Diseases of the Endocrine System

	congenital deficiency of thyroid hormones (hypothyroidism).
Prognosis	Prognosis refers to the prospects for the future or outcome of a disease.
Steroid hormones	Steroid hormones are steroids which act as hormones. They can be grouped into five groups by the receptors to which they bind: glucocorticoids, mineralocorticoids, androgens, estrogens, and progestagens.
Mineralocort-coids	Hormones the adrenal cortex secretes that influence the concentrations of electrolytes in body fluids are called mineralocorticoids.
Mineralocort-coid	Mineralocorticoid is a class of steroids characterized by their similarity to aldosterone and their influence on salt and water metabolism.
Aldosterone	Aldosterone is a steroid hormone synthesized from cholesterol by the enzyme aldosterone synthase. It helps regulate the body's electrolyte balance by acting on the mineralocorticoid receptor. It diminishes the secretion of sodium ions and therefore, water and stimulates the secretion of potassium ions through the kidneys.
Potassium	Potassium is a chemical element in the periodic table. It has the symbol K (L. kalium) and atomic number 19. Potassium is a soft silvery-white metallic alkali metal that occurs naturally bound to other elements in seawater and many minerals.
Sodium	Sodium is the chemical element in the periodic table that has the symbol Na (Natrium in Latin) and atomic number 11. Sodium is a soft, waxy, silvery reactive metal belonging to the alkali metals that is abundant in natural compounds (especially halite). It is highly reactive.
Glucocorticoid	Glucocorticoid is a class of steroid hormones characterized by the ability to bind with the cortisol receptor and trigger similar effects. They are distinguished from mineralocorticoids and sex steroids by the specific receptors, target cells, and effects.
Cortisol	Cortisol is a corticosteroid hormone that is involved in the response to stress; it increases blood pressure and blood sugar levels and suppresses the immune system.
Anabolic steroid	An anabolic steroid is a class of natural and synthetic steroid hormones that promote cell growth and division, resulting in growth of muscle tissue and sometimes bone size and strength. They act in different ways on the body to promote muscle growth, and each has androgenic and anabolic properties.
Testosterone	Testosterone is a steroid hormone from the androgen group. Testosterone is secreted in the testes of men and the ovaries of women. It is the principal male sex hormone and the "original" anabolic steroid. In both males and females, it plays key roles in health and well-being.
Irritability	Irritability is an excessive response to stimuli. Irritability takes many forms, from the contraction of a unicellular organism when touched to complex reactions involving all the senses of higher animals.
Androgen	Androgen is the generic term for any natural or synthetic compound, usually a steroid hormone, that stimulates or controls the development and maintenance of masculine characteristics in vertebrates by binding to androgen receptors.
Epinephrine	Epinephrine is a hormone and a neurotransmitter. Epinephrine plays a central role in the short-term stress reaction—the physiological response to threatening or exciting conditions (fight-or-flight response). It is secreted by the adrenal medulla.
Adrenal medulla	Composed mainly of hormone-producing chromaffin cells, the adrenal medulla is the principal site of the conversion of the amino acid tyrosine into the catecholamines epinephrine and norepinephrine.

Chapter 14. Diseases of the Endocrine System

Chapter 14. Diseases of the Endocrine System

Norepinephrine	Norepinephrine is a catecholamine and a phenethylamine with chemical formula $C_8H_{11}NO_3$. It is released from the adrenal glands as a hormone into the blood, but it is also a neurotransmitter in the nervous system where it is released from noradrenergic neurons during synaptic transmission.
Regression	Return to a form of behavior characteristic of an earlier stage of development is a regression.
Vasoconstriction	Vasoconstriction refers to a decrease in the diameter of a blood vessel.
Shunt	In medicine, a shunt is a hole or passage which moves, or allows movement of, fluid from one part of the body to another. The term may describe either congenital or acquired shunts; and acquired shunts may be either biological or mechanical.
Hyperplasia	Hyperplasia is a general term for an increase in the number of the cells of an organ or tissue causing it to increase in size.
Tuberculosis	Tuberculosis is an infection caused by the bacterium Mycobacterium tuberculosis, which most commonly affects the lungs but can also affect the central nervous system, lymphatic system, circulatory system, genitourinary system, bones and joints.
Corticosteroid	Any steroid hormone secreted by the adrenal cortex, such as aldosterone, cortisol, and sex steroids is called a corticosteroid.
Syndrome	Syndrome is the association of several clinically recognizable features, signs, symptoms, phenomena or characteristics which often occur together, so that the presence of one feature alerts the physician to the presence of the others
Elevation	Elevation refers to upward movement of a part of the body.
Glucose	Glucose, a simple monosaccharide sugar, is one of the most important carbohydrates and is used as a source of energy in animals and plants. Glucose is one of the main products of photosynthesis and starts respiration.
Hyperglycemia	Hyperglycemia is a condition in which an excessive amount of glucose circulates in the blood plasma.
Striae	In medicine, striae are most commonly seen as stretch marks on the skin with a silvery white
Infection	The invasion and multiplication of microorganisms in body tissues is called an infection.
Wound	A wound is type of physical trauma wherein the skin is torn, cut or punctured, or where blunt force trauma causes a contusion.
Hypertension	Hypertension is a medical condition where the blood pressure in the arteries is chronically elevated. Persistent hypertension is one of the risk factors for strokes, heart attacks, heart failure and arterial aneurysm, and is a leading cause of chronic renal failure.
Clitoris	The clitoris is a sexual organ in the body of female mammals. The visible knob-like portion is located near the anterior junction of the labia minora, above the opening of the vagina. Unlike its male counterpart, the penis, the clitoris has no urethra, is not involved in urination, and its sole function is to induce sexual pleasure.
Distribution	Distribution in pharmacology is a branch of pharmacokinetics describing reversible transfer of drug from one location to another within the body.
Hirsutism	Hirsutism is the excessive growth of hair, particularly on a woman's face, torso and limbs, and is generally caused by increased androgens.
Masculinization	Prenatal virilization, or masculinization, of a genetically female fetus can occur when an excessive amount of androgen is produced by the fetal adrenal glands or is present in maternal blood.

Chapter 14. Diseases of the Endocrine System

Chapter 14. Diseases of the Endocrine System

Genitalia	The Latin term genitalia is used to describe the sex organs, and in the English language this term and genital area are most often used to describe the externally visible sex organs or external genitalia: in males the penis and scrotum, in females the vulva.
Androgenital syndrome	A disorder in which genetic females become masculinized as a result of prenatal exposure to male hormones is androgenital syndrome.
Penis	The penis is the male reproductive organ and for mammals additionally serves as the external male organ of urination.
Genitals	Genitals refers to the internal and external reproductive organs.
Ovulation	Ovulation is the process in the menstrual cycle by which a mature ovarian follicle ruptures and discharges an ovum (also known as an oocyte, female gamete, or casually, an egg) that participates in reproduction.
Cancer	Cancer is a class of diseases or disorders characterized by uncontrolled division of cells and the ability of these cells to invade other tissues, either by direct growth into adjacent tissue through invasion or by implantation into distant sites by metastasis.
Idiopathic	Idiopathic is a medical adjective that indicates that a recognized cause has not yet been established.
Shock	Circulatory shock, a state of cardiac output that is insufficient to meet the body's physiological needs, with consequences ranging from fainting to death is referred to as shock. Insulin shock, a state of severe hypoglycemia caused by administration of insulin.
Melanin	Broadly, melanin is any of the polyacetylene, polyaniline, and polypyrrole "blacks" or their mixed copolymers. The most common form of biological melanin is a polymer of either or both of two monomer molecules: indolequinone, and dihydroxyindole carboxylic acid.
Areola	In anatomy, the term areola is used to describe any small circular area such as the colored skin surrounding the nipple.
Scar	A scar results from the biologic process of wound repair in the skin and other tissues of the body. It is a connective tissue that fills the wound.
Excretion	Excretion is the biological process by which an organism chemically separates waste products from its body. The waste products are then usually expelled from the body by elimination.
Parathyroid hormone	Parathyroid hormone is secreted by the parathyroid glands as a polypeptide containing 84 amino acids. It acts to increase the concentration of calcium in the blood, whereas calcitonin (a hormone produced by the thyroid gland) acts to decrease calcium concentration.
Phosphate	A phosphate is a polyatomic ion or radical consisting of one phosphorus atom and four oxygen. In the ionic form, it carries a -3 formal charge, and is denoted PO_4^{3-}.
Calcium	Calcium is the chemical element in the periodic table that has the symbol Ca and atomic number 20. Calcium is a soft grey alkaline earth metal that is used as a reducing agent in the extraction of thorium, zirconium and uranium. Calcium is also the fifth most abundant element in the Earth's crust.
Muscle contraction	A muscle contraction occurs when a muscle cell (called a muscle fiber) shortens. There are three general types: skeletal, heart, and smooth.
Constant	A behavior or characteristic that does not vary from one observation to another is referred to as a constant.
Osteoblast	An osteoblast is a mononucleate cell that produces a protein that produces osteoid.
Vitamin	An organic compound other than a carbohydrate, lipid, or protein that is needed for normal metabolism but that the body cannot synthesize in adequate amounts is called a vitamin.

Go to Cram101.com for the Practice Tests for this Chapter.

Chapter 14. Diseases of the Endocrine System

Chapter 14. Diseases of the Endocrine System

Hypercalcemia	Hypercalcemia refers to an excess of calcium ions in the blood.
Cyst	A cyst is a closed sac having a distinct membrane and developing abnormally in a cavity or structure of the body. They may occur as a result of a developmental error in the embryo during pregnancy or they may be caused by infections.
Nervous system	The nervous system of an animal coordinates the activity of the muscles, monitors the organs, constructs and processes input from the senses, and initiates actions.
Lactation	Lactation describes the secretion of milk from the mammary glands, the process of providing that milk to the young, and the period of time that a mother lactates to feed her young. The process occurs in all female mammals, and in humans it is called breastfeeding.
Traction	Traction refers to the set of mechanisms for straightening broken bones or relieving pressure on the skeletal system. It is largely replaced now by more modern techniques, but certain approaches are still used today for hip fractures.
Tetany	Tetany is the point at which signals from nerves are arriving to a single skeletal muscle rapidly enough in succession to cause a steady contraction, and not just a series of individual twitches. In multiple mussels, it is diseases and other conditions that increase action potential frequency cause unwanted contraction of muscles.
Respiratory tract	In humans the respiratory tract is the part of the anatomy that has to do with the process of respiration or breathing.
Hypocalcemia	In medicine, hypocalcaemia is the presence of low serum calcium levels in the blood, usually taken as less than 2.2 mmol/L or 9mg/dl or an ionized calcium level of less than 1.1 mmol/L (4.5 mg/dL).
Skeletal muscle	Skeletal muscle is a type of striated muscle, attached to the skeleton. They are used to facilitate movement, by applying force to bones and joints; via contraction. They generally contract voluntarily (via nerve stimulation), although they can contract involuntarily.
Gastrointestinal tract	The gastrointestinal tract is the system of organs within multicellular animals which takes in food, digests it to extract energy and nutrients, and expels the remaining waste.
Pancreas	The pancreas is a retroperitoneal organ that serves two functions: exocrine - it produces pancreatic juice containing digestive enzymes, and endocrine - it produces several important hormones, namely insulin.
Glycogen	Glycogen refers to a complex, extensively branched polysaccharide of many glucose monomers; serves as an energy-storage molecule in liver and muscle cells.
Target cell	Specific cell on which a hormone exerts its effect is a target cell.
Diabetes mellitus	Diabetes mellitus is a medical disorder characterized by varying or persistent hyperglycemia (elevated blood sugar levels), especially after eating. All types of diabetes mellitus share similar symptoms and complications at advanced stages.
Glycosuria	The presence of glucose in the urine, typically indicative of a kidney disease, diabetes mellitus, or other endocrine disorder is called glycosuria.
Fatty acid	A fatty acid is a carboxylic acid (or organic acid), often with a long aliphatic tail (long chains), either saturated or unsaturated.
Ketone bodies	Ketone bodies are three chemicals that are produced as by-products when fatty acids are broken down for energy. Any production of ketone bodies is called ketogenesis, and this is necessary in small amounts. But when excess ketone bodies accumulate, this abnormal state is called ketosis.
Bladder	A hollow muscular storage organ for storing urine is a bladder.

Chapter 14. Diseases of the Endocrine System

Chapter 14. Diseases of the Endocrine System

Susceptibility	The degree of resistance of a host to a pathogen is susceptibility.
Occlusion	The term occlusion is often used to refer to blood vessels, arteries or veins which have become totally blocked to any blood flow.
Gangrene	Gangrene is necrosis and subsequent decay of body tissues caused by infection or thrombosis or lack of blood flow. It is usually the result of critically insufficient blood supply sometimes caused by injury and subsequent contamination with bacteria.
Artery	Vessel that takes blood away from the heart to the tissues and organs of the body is called an artery.
Retina	The retina is a thin layer of cells at the back of the eyeball of vertebrates and some cephalopods; it is the part of the eye which converts light into nervous signals.
Diabetic retinopathy	Diabetic retinopathy is retinopathy (damage to the retina) caused by complications of diabetes mellitus, which could eventually lead to blindness. It is an ocular manifestation of systemic disease which affects up to 80% of all diabetics who have had diabetes for 15 years or more.
Retinal	Retinal is fundamental in the transduction of light into visual signals in the photoreceptor level of the retina.
Paralysis	Paralysis is the complete loss of muscle function for one or more muscle groups. Paralysis may be localized, or generalized, or it may follow a certain pattern.
Stress	Stress refers to a condition that is a response to factors that change the human systems normal state.
Diuretic	A diuretic is any drug that elevates the rate of bodily urine excretion.
Acidosis	Acidosis is an increased acidity (i.e. hydrogen ion concentration) of blood plasma. Generally acidosis is said to occur when arterial pH falls below 7.35, while its counterpart (alkalosis) occurs at a pH over 7.45.
Ketoacidosis	Ketoacidosis is a type of metabolic acidosis which is caused by high concentrations of keto acids, formed by the deamination of amino acids. This is most common in untreated type 1 diabetes mellitus, when the liver breaks down fat and proteins in response to a perceived need for respiratory substrate.
Diabetic ketoacidosis	Diabetic ketoacidosis (DKA) is one consequence of severe, out-of-control diabetes mellitus (chronic high blood sugar, or hyperglycemia). In a diabetes sufferer, DKA begins with relative deficiency in insulin.
Electrolyte	An electrolyte is a substance that dissociates into free ions when dissolved (or molten), to produce an electrically conductive medium. Because they generally consist of ions in solution, they are also known as ionic solutions.
Electrolytes	Electrolytes refers to compounds that separate into ions in water and, in turn, are able to conduct an electrical current. These include sodium, chloride, and potassium.
Double vision	Diplopia, colloquially known as double vision, is the perception of two images from a single object. The images may be horizontal, vertical, or diagonal.
Consciousness	Consciousness refers to the ability to perceive, communicate, remember, understand, appreciate, and initiate voluntary movements; a functioning sensorium.
Intravenous	Present or occurring within a vein, such as an intravenous blood clot is referred to as intravenous. Introduced directly into a vein, such as an intravenous injection or I.V. drip.
Intravenous injection	The introduction of drugs directly into a vein is an intravenous injection.

Chapter 14. Diseases of the Endocrine System

Chapter 14. Diseases of the Endocrine System

Hemoglobin	Hemoglobin is the iron-containing oxygen-transport metalloprotein in the red cells of the blood in mammals and other animals. Hemoglobin transports oxygen from the lungs to the rest of the body, such as to the muscles, where it releases the oxygen load.
Solution	Solution refers to homogenous mixture formed when a solute is dissolved in a solvent.
Value	Value is worth in general, and it is thought to be connected to reasons for certain practices, policies, actions, beliefs or emotions. Value is "that which one acts to gain and/or keep."
Agent	Agent refers to an epidemiological term referring to the organism or object that transmits a disease from the environment to the host.
Insulin reaction	Insulin reaction is an excessively low blood sugar caused by insulin overload. It results in too-rapid metabolism of the body's glucose; insulin shock:; hypoglycemia.
Estrogen	Estrogen is a steroid that functions as the primary female sex hormone. While present in both men and women, they are found in women in significantly higher quantities.
Hypogonadism	Hypogonadism is a medical term for a defect of the reproductive system which results in lack of function of the gonads (ovaries or testes).
Masculinity	A culture value reflecting an emphasis on achievement as opposed to on the well-being of others is a masculinity.
Epiphyses	Epiphyses refers to ends of long bones. The epiphyseal plate-sometimes referred to as the growth plate-is made of cartilage and allows growth of the bone to occur. During childhood, the cartilage cells multiply and absorb calcium, to develop into bone.
Osmotic pressure	Osmotic pressure is the pressure produced by a solution in a space that is enclosed by a differentially permeable membrane.
Carcinoma	Cancer that originates in the coverings of the body, such as the skin or the lining of the intestinal tract is a carcinoma.
Precocious puberty	Precocious puberty means early puberty.
Hypoglycemia	An abnormally low level of glucose in the blood that results when the pancreas secretes too much insulin into the blood is called hypoglycemia.
Urinalysis	A urinalysis (or "UA") is an array of tests performed on urine and one of the most common methods of medical diagnosis. A part of a urinalysis can be performed by using urine dipsticks, in which the test results can be read as color changes.
Connective tissue	Connective tissue is any type of biological tissue with an extensive extracellular matrix and often serves to support, bind together, and protect organs.
Polyphagia	Polyphagia is a medical term meaning excessive hunger and abnormally large intake of solids through the mouth.
Nerve cell	A cell specialized to originate or transmit nerve impulses is referred to as nerve cell.
Complaint	Complaint refers to report made by the police or some other agency to the court that initiates the intake process.
Critical thinking	Critical thinking consists of a mental process of analyzing or evaluating information, particularly statements or propositions that people have offered as true. It forms a process of reflecting upon the meaning of statements, examining the offered evidence and reasoning, and forming judgments about the facts.
Secondary sex	Secondary sex characteristics are traits that distinguish the two sexes of a species, but

Chapter 14. Diseases of the Endocrine System

Chapter 14. Diseases of the Endocrine System

characteristics	that are not directly part of the reproductive system.
Blood pressure	Blood pressure is the pressure exerted by the blood on the walls of the blood vessels.
Inflammatory response	Inflammatory response refers to a complex sequence of events involving chemicals and immune cells that results in the isolation and destruction of antigens and tissues near the antigens.
Fetus	Fetus refers to a developing human from the ninth week of gestation until birth; has all the major structures of an adult.
Embryo	A prenatal stage of development after germ layers form but before the rudiments of all organs are present is referred to as an embryo.
Fertilization	Fertilization is fusion of gametes to form a new organism. In animals, the process involves a sperm fusing with an ovum, which eventually leads to the development of an embryo.

Chapter 14. Diseases of the Endocrine System

Chapter 15. Diseases of the Reproductive Systems and Sexually Transmitted Infections

Mons pubis	In human anatomy or in mammals in general, the mons pubis is the soft mound of flesh present in both genders just above the genitals, raised above the surrounding area due to a pad of fat lying just beneath it which protects the pubic bone.
Clitoris	The clitoris is a sexual organ in the body of female mammals. The visible knob-like portion is located near the anterior junction of the labia minora, above the opening of the vagina. Unlike its male counterpart, the penis, the clitoris has no urethra, is not involved in urination, and its sole function is to induce sexual pleasure.
Follicle	Follicle refers to a cluster of cells surrounding, protecting, and nourishing a developing egg cell in the ovary; also secretes estrogen. In botany, a follicle is a type of simple dry fruit produced by certain flowering plants. It is regarded as one the most primitive types of fruits, and derives from a simple pistil or carpel.
Sagittal	A sagittal plane is an X-Z plane, perpendicular to the ground and to the coronal plane, which separates left from right. The midsagittal plane is the specific sagittal plane that is exactly in the middle of the body.
Ovaries	Ovaries are egg-producing reproductive organs found in female organisms.
Vagina	The vagina is the tubular tract leading from the uterus to the exterior of the body in female placental mammals and marsupials, or to the cloaca in female birds, monotremes, and some reptiles. Female insects and other invertebrates also have a vagina, which is the terminal part of the oviduct.
Uterus	The uterus is the major female reproductive organ of most mammals. One end, the cervix, opens into the vagina; the other is connected on both sides to the fallopian tubes. The main function is to accept a fertilized ovum which becomes implanted into the endometrium, and derives nourishment from blood vessels which develop exclusively for this purpose.
Pelvis	The pelvis is the bony structure located at the base of the spine (properly known as the caudal end). The pelvis incorporates the socket portion of the hip joint for each leg (in bipeds) or hind leg (in quadrupeds). It forms the lower limb (or hind-limb) girdle of the skeleton.
Pubis	The pubis, the anterior part of the hip bone, is divisible into a body, a superior and an inferior ramus.
Ovary	The primary reproductive organ of a female is called an ovary.
Organ	Organ refers to a structure consisting of several tissues adapted as a group to perform specific functions.
Vulva	The outer features of the female reproductive anatomy is referred to as vulva.
Reproductive system	A reproductive system is the ensembles and interactions of organs and or substances within an organism that stricly pertain to reproduction. As an example, this would include in the case of female mammals, the hormone estrogen, the womb and eggs but not the breast.
Fallopian tube	The Fallopian tube is one of two very fine tubes leading from the ovaries of female mammals into the uterus. They deliver the ovum to the uterus.
Anatomy	Anatomy is the branch of biology that deals with the structure and organization of living things. It can be divided into animal anatomy (zootomy) and plant anatomy (phytonomy).
Cervix	The cervix is actually the lower, narrow portion of the uterus where it joins with the top end of the vagina. It is cylindrical or conical in shape and protrudes through the upper anterior vaginal wall.
Endometrium	The endometrium is the inner uterine membrane in mammals which is developed in preparation for the implantation of a fertilized egg upon its arrival into the uterus.

Chapter 15. Diseases of the Reproductive Systems and Sexually Transmitted Infections

Chapter 15. Diseases of the Reproductive Systems and Sexually Transmitted Infections

Muscle	Muscle is a contractile form of tissue. It is one of the four major tissue types, the other three being epithelium, connective tissue and nervous tissue. Muscle contraction is used to move parts of the body, as well as to move substances within the body.
Smooth muscle	Smooth muscle is a type of non-striated muscle, found within the "walls" of hollow organs; such as blood vessels, the bladder, the uterus, and the gastrointestinal tract. Smooth muscle is used to move matter within the body, via contraction; it generally operates "involuntarily", without nerve stimulation.
Ovum	An ovum is a female sex cell or gamete. It is a mature egg cell released during ovulation from an ovary.
Projection	Attributing one's own undesirable thoughts, impulses, traits, or behaviors to others is referred to as projection.
Ligament	A ligament is a short band of tough fibrous connective tissue composed mainly of long, stringy collagen fibres. They connect bones to other bones to form a joint. (They do not connect muscles to bones.)
Gland	A gland is an organ in an animal's body that synthesizes a substance for release such as hormones, often into the bloodstream or into cavities inside the body or its outer surface.
Labia majora	A pair of outer thickened folds of skin that protect the female genital region is the labia majora.
Labia minora	The labia minora are two soft folds of skin within the labia majora and to either side of the opening of the vagina.
Genitalia	The Latin term genitalia is used to describe the sex organs, and in the English language this term and genital area are most often used to describe the externally visible sex organs or external genitalia: in males the penis and scrotum, in females the vulva.
Puberty	A time in the life of a developing individual characterized by the increasing production of sex hormones, which cause it to reach sexual maturity is called puberty.
Tissue	A collection of interconnected cells that perform a similar function within an organism is called tissue.
Anus	In anatomy, the anus is the external opening of the rectum. Closure is controlled by sphincter muscles. Feces are expelled from the body through the anus during the act of defecation, which is the primary function of the anus.
Hymen	The hymen is a ring of tissue around the vaginal opening. Although many people believe that the hymen completely occludes the vaginal opening in human females, this is quite rare. The hymen has great symbolic significance as an indicator of a woman's virginity.
Mucus	Mucus is a slippery secretion of the lining of various membranes in the body (mucous membranes). Mucus aids in the protection of the lungs by trapping foreign particles that enter the nose during normal breathing. Additionally, it prevents tissues from drying out.
Reproduction	Biological reproduction is the biological process by which new individual organisms are produced. Reproduction is a fundamental feature of all known life; each individual organism exists as the result of reproduction by an antecedent.
Skin	Skin is an organ of the integumentary system composed of a layer of tissues that protect underlying muscles and organs.
Connective tissue	Connective tissue is any type of biological tissue with an extensive extracellular matrix and often serves to support, bind together, and protect organs.
Areola	In anatomy, the term areola is used to describe any small circular area such as the colored

Chapter 15. Diseases of the Reproductive Systems and Sexually Transmitted Infections

Chapter 15. Diseases of the Reproductive Systems and Sexually Transmitted Infections

	skin surrounding the nipple.
Physiology	The study of the function of cells, tissues, and organs is referred to as physiology.
Hypothalamus	Located below the thalamus, the hypothalamus links the nervous system to the endocrine system by synthesizing and secreting neurohormones often called releasing hormones because they function by stimulating the secretion of hormones from the anterior pituitary gland.
Progesterone	Progesterone is a C-21 steroid hormone involved in the female menstrual cycle, pregnancy (supports gestation) and embryogenesis of humans and other species.
Estrogen	Estrogen is a steroid that functions as the primary female sex hormone. While present in both men and women, they are found in women in significantly higher quantities.
Hormone	A hormone is a chemical messenger from one cell to another. All multicellular organisms produce hormones. The best known hormones are those produced by endocrine glands of vertebrate animals, but hormones are produced by nearly every organ system and tissue type in a human or animal body. Hormone molecules are secreted directly into the bloodstream, they move by circulation or diffusion to their target cells, which may be nearby cells in the same tissue or cells of a distant organ of the body.
Brain	The part of the central nervous system involved in regulating and controlling body activity and interpreting information from the senses transmitted through the nervous system is referred to as the brain.
Gonadotropic hormone	Substance secreted by anterior pituitary that regulates the activity of the ovaries and testes is referred to as gonadotropic hormone.
Anterior pituitary	The anterior pituitary comprises the anterior lobe of the pituitary gland and is part of the endocrine system. Under the influence of the hypothalamus, the anterior pituitary produces and secretes several peptide hormones that regulate many physiological processes including stress, growth, and reproduction.
Pituitary gland	The pituitary gland or hypophysis is an endocrine gland about the size of a pea that sits in the small, bony cavity (sella turcica) at the base of the brain. Its posterior lobe is connected to a part of the brain called the hypothalamus via the infundibulum (or stalk), giving rise to the tuberoinfundibular pathway.
Central nervous system	The central nervous system comprized of the brain and spinal cord, represents the largest part of the nervous system. Together with the peripheral nervous system, it has a fundamental role in the control of behavior.
Nervous system	The nervous system of an animal coordinates the activity of the muscles, monitors the organs, constructs and processes input from the senses, and initiates actions.
Menstruation	Loss of blood and tissue from the uterine lining at the end of a female reproductive cycle are referred to as menstruation.
Menopause	Menopause is the physiological cessation of menstrual cycles associated with advancing age in species that experience such cycles. Menopause is sometimes referred to as change of life or climacteric.
Menarche	Menarche is the first menstrual period as a girl's body progresses through the changes of puberty. Menarche usually occurs about two years after the first changes of breast development.
Ovarian follicle	Ovarian follicle is the roughly spherical cell aggregation in the ovary containing an ovum and from which the egg is released during ovulation.
Ovulation	Ovulation is the process in the menstrual cycle by which a mature ovarian follicle ruptures and discharges an ovum (also known as an oocyte, female gamete, or casually, an egg) that

Chapter 15. Diseases of the Reproductive Systems and Sexually Transmitted Infections

Chapter 15. Diseases of the Reproductive Systems and Sexually Transmitted Infections

	participates in reproduction.
Blood	Blood is a circulating tissue composed of fluid plasma and cells. The main function of blood is to supply nutrients (oxygen, glucose) and constitutional elements to tissues and to remove waste products.
Corpus luteum	The corpus luteum is a small, temporary endocrine structure in animals. It develops from an ovarian follicle during the luteal phase of the estrous cycle, following the release of a mature egg from the follicle during ovulation. While the egg traverses the Fallopian tube into the uterus, the corpus luteum remains in the ovary.
Fertilization	Fertilization is fusion of gametes to form a new organism. In animals, the process involves a sperm fusing with an ovum, which eventually leads to the development of an embryo.
Placenta	The placenta is an organ present only in female placental mammals during gestation. It is composed of two parts, one genetically and biologically part of the fetus, the other part of the mother. It is implanted in the wall of the uterus, where it receives nutrients and oxygen from the mother's blood and passes out waste.
Implantation	Implantation refers to attachment and penetration of the embryo into the lining of the uterus.
Chorion	In animals, the outermost extraembryonic membrane, which becomes the mammalian embryo's part of the placenta is referred to as the chorion.
Artery	Vessel that takes blood away from the heart to the tissues and organs of the body is called an artery.
Oxygen	Oxygen is a chemical element in the periodic table. It has the symbol O and atomic number 8. Oxygen is the second most common element on Earth, composing around 46% of the mass of Earth's crust and 28% of the mass of Earth as a whole, and is the third most common element in the universe.
Umbilical artery	An umbilical artery carries deoxygenated blood from the fetus to the placenta in the umbilical cord. There are usually two, but occasionally there is only one umbilical artery present together with one umbilical vein in the cord.
Chorionic villi	The chorion develops chorionic villi, which are finger-like projections on its surface. The chorionic villi extend downward through the uterine lining into the maternal blood supply to help supply the developing embryo with oxygen and nutrients.
Diffusion	Random movement of molecules from a region of higher concentration toward one of lower concentration is referred to as diffusion.
Blood vessel	A blood vessel is a part of the circulatory system and function to transport blood throughout the body. The most important types, arteries and veins, are so termed because they carry blood away from or towards the heart, respectively.
Fetus	Fetus refers to a developing human from the ninth week of gestation until birth; has all the major structures of an adult.
Vein	Vein in animals, is a vessel that returns blood to the heart. In plants, a vascular bundle in a leaf, composed of xylem and phloem.
Umbilical vein	The umbilical vein is a blood vessel present during fetal development that carries oxygenated blood from the placenta to the growing fetus. Within a week of birth, the infant's umbilical vein is completely obliterated and is replaced by a fibrous cord called the round ligament.
Infection	The invasion and multiplication of microorganisms in body tissues is called an infection.
Tumor	An abnormal mass of cells that forms within otherwise normal tissue is a tumor. This growth

Chapter 15. Diseases of the Reproductive Systems and Sexually Transmitted Infections

Chapter 15. Diseases of the Reproductive Systems and Sexually Transmitted Infections

	can be either malignant or benign
Cyst	A cyst is a closed sac having a distinct membrane and developing abnormally in a cavity or structure of the body. They may occur as a result of a developmental error in the embryo during pregnancy or they may be caused by infections.
Menstrual cycle	The menstrual cycle is the set of recurring physiological changes in a female's body that are under the control of the reproductive hormone system and necessary for reproduction. Besides humans, only other great apes exhibit menstrual cycles, in contrast to the estrus cycle of most mammalian species.
Gonorrhea	Gonorrhea refers to an acute infectious sexually transmitted disease of the mucous membranes of the genitourinary tract, eye, rectum, and throat. It is caused by Neisseria gonorrhoeae.
Pelvic inflammatory disease	Pelvic inflammatory disease is a generic term for infection of the female uterus, fallopian tubes, and/or ovaries as it progresses to scar formation with adhesions to nearby tissues and organs.
Chlamydia	A sexually transmitted disease, caused by a bacterium, that causes inflammation of the urethra in males and of the urethra and cervix in females is referred to as chlamydia.
Abortion	An abortion is the termination of a pregnancy associated with the death of an embryo or a fetus.
Fever	Fever (also known as pyrexia, or a febrile response, and archaically known as ague) is a medical symptom that describes an increase in internal body temperature to levels that are above normal (37°C, 98.6°F).
Pain	Pain is an unpleasant sensation which may be associated with actual or potential tissue damage and which may have physical and emotional components.
Infertility	The inability to conceive after one year of regular, unprotected intercourse is infertility.
Antibiotic	Antibiotic refers to substance such as penicillin or streptomycin that is toxic to microorganisms. Usually a product of a particular microorvanism or plant.
Inflammation	Inflammation is the first response of the immune system to infection or irritation and may be referred to as the innate cascade.
Salpingitis	Salpingitis is inflammation of the fallopian tubes due to infection.
Sexually transmitted disease	Infection transmitted from one individual to another by direct contact during sexual activity is referred to as a sexually transmitted disease.
Affect	Affect is the scientific term used to describe a subject's externally displayed mood. This can be assesed by the nurse by observing facial expression, tone of voice, and body language.
Ectopic pregnancy	An ectopic pregnancy is one in which the fertilized ovum is implanted in any tissue other than the uterine wall.
Vaginitis	Vaginitis is an inflammation of the vaginal mucosa usually caused by a Candida albicans (a yeast), Trichomonas vaginalis (a protozoan) or Gardnerella (a bacterium), and rarely by other pathogens.
Agent	Agent refers to an epidemiological term referring to the organism or object that transmits a disease from the environment to the host.
Causative agent	In the chain of infection, the organism capable of producing an infection is called a causative agent.
Normal flora	The bacteria and fungi that live on animal body surfaces without causing disease is normal

Go to Cram101.com for the Practice Tests for this Chapter.

Chapter 15. Diseases of the Reproductive Systems and Sexually Transmitted Infections

Chapter 15. Diseases of the Reproductive Systems and Sexually Transmitted Infections

	flora.
Microorganism	A microorganism or microbe is an organism that is so small that it is microscopic (invisible to the naked eye).
Fungi	Fungi refers to simple parasitic life forms, including molds, mildews, yeasts, and mushrooms. They live on dead or decaying organic matter. Fungi can grow as single cells, like yeast, or as multicellular colonies, as seen with molds.
Atrophy	Atrophy is the partial or complete wasting away of a part of the body. Causes of atrophy include poor nourishment, poor circulation, loss of hormonal support, loss of nerve supply to the target organ, disuse or lack of exercise, or disease intrinsic to the tissue itself.
Mucosa	The mucosa is a lining of ectodermic origin, covered in epithelium, and involved in absorption and secretion. They line various body cavities that are exposed to the external environment and internal organs.
Steroid	A steroid is a lipid characterized by a carbon skeleton with four fused rings. Different steroids vary in the functional groups attached to these rings. Hundreds of distinct steroids have been identified in plants and animals. Their most important role in most living systems is as hormones.
Childbirth	Childbirth (also called labour, birth, partus or parturition) is the culmination of a human pregnancy with the emergence of a newborn infant from its mother's uterus.
Sepsis	Sepsis is a serious medical condition caused by a severe infection. The more critical subsets of sepsis include severe sepsis and septic shock. If a proven source of infection is lacking but the other criteria of sepsis are met the condition is known as systemic inflammatory response syndrome.
Puerperium	Puerperium is the period beginning immediately after the birth of a child and extending for about six weeks.
Trauma	Trauma refers to a severe physical injury or wound to the body caused by an external force, or a psychological shock having a lasting effect on mental life.
Necrosis	Necrosis is the name given to unprogrammed death of cells/living tissue. There are many causes of necrosis including injury, infection, cancer, infarction, and inflammation. Necrosis is caused by special enzymes that are released by lysosomes.
Blood clot	A blood clot is the final product of the blood coagulation step in hemostasis. It is achieved via the aggregation of platelets that form a platelet plug, and the activation of the humoral coagulation system
Septicemia	Septicemia is sepsis of the bloodstream caused by bacteremia, which is the presence of bacteria in the bloodstream. It is also called blood poisoning.
Abdomen	The abdomen is a part of the body. In humans, and in many other vertebrates, it is the region between the thorax and the pelvis. In fully developed insects, the abdomen is the third (or posterior) segment, after the head and thorax.
Diagnosis	In medicine, diagnosis is the process of identifying a medical condition or disease by its signs, symptoms, and from the results of various diagnostic procedures.
Neoplasm	Neoplasm refers to abnormal growth of cells; often used to mean a tumor.
Cancer	Cancer is a class of diseases or disorders characterized by uncontrolled division of cells and the ability of these cells to invade other tissues, either by direct growth into adjacent tissue through invasion or by implantation into distant sites by metastasis.
Carcinoma	Cancer that originates in the coverings of the body, such as the skin or the lining of the

Chapter 15. Diseases of the Reproductive Systems and Sexually Transmitted Infections

Chapter 15. Diseases of the Reproductive Systems and Sexually Transmitted Infections

	intestinal tract is a carcinoma.
Incidence	In epidemiological studies of a particular disorder, the rate at which new cases occur in a given place at a given time is called incidence.
Biopsy	Removal of small tissue sample from the body for microscopic examination is called biopsy.
Lesion	A lesion is a non-specific term referring to abnormal tissue in the body. It can be caused by any disease process including trauma (physical, chemical, electrical), infection, neoplasm, metabolic and autoimmune.
Bladder	A hollow muscular storage organ for storing urine is a bladder.
Rectum	The rectum is the final straight portion of the large intestine in some mammals, and the gut in others, terminating in the anus.
Radiation	The emission of electromagnetic waves by all objects warmer than absolute zero is referred to as radiation.
Radiation therapy	Treatment for cancer in which parts of the body that have cancerous tumors are exposed to high-energy radiation to disrupt cell division of the cancer cells is called radiation therapy.
Human papillomavirus	Human papillomavirus is a member of a group of viruses in the genus Papillomavirus that can infect humans and cause changes in cells leading to abnormal tissue growth.
Benign tumor	A benign tumor does not invade neighboring tissues and do not seed metastases, but may locally grow to great size. They usually do not return after surgical removal.
Fibroids	Uterine fibroids are the most common neoplasm in females, and may affect about of 25 % of white and 50% of black women during the reproductive years. Fibroids may be removed simply by means of a hysterectomy, but much more favourably by a myomectomy or by uterine artery embolization, which preserve the uterus.
Nerve	A nerve is an enclosed, cable-like bundle of nerve fibers or axons, which includes the glia that ensheath the axons in myelin.
Hysterectomy	A hysterectomy is the surgical removal of the uterus, usually done by a gynecologist. Hysterectomy may be total (removing the body and cervix of the uterus) or partial. In many cases, surgical removal of the ovaries (oophorectomy) is performed concurrent with a hysterectomy.
Primary tumor	Primary tumor is the nomenclature used when the tumor has originated in the same organ, and has not metastasized to it.
Chemotherapy	Chemotherapy is the use of chemical substances to treat disease. In its modern-day use, it refers almost exclusively to cytostatic drugs used to treat cancer. In its non-oncological use, the term may also refer to antibiotics.
Hair follicle	A hair follicle is part of the skin that grows hair by packing old cells together. Attached to the follicle is a sebaceous gland, a tiny sebum-producing gland found everywhere except on the palms and soles of the feet.
Hydatidiform mole	A hydatidiform mole (or mola hydatidiforma) is a disease of trophoblastic proliferation. It can mimic pregnancy, causes high human chorionic gonadotropin (HCG) levels and therefore gives false positive readings of pregnancy tests.
Choriocarcinoma	Choriocarcinoma is a malignant and aggressive cancer of the placenta. It is characterized by early hematogenous spread to the lungs.
Urine	Concentrated filtrate produced by the kidneys and excreted via the bladder is called urine.

Chapter 15. Diseases of the Reproductive Systems and Sexually Transmitted Infections

Chapter 15. Diseases of the Reproductive Systems and Sexually Transmitted Infections

Gonadotropin	A hormone that stimulates the gonads is gonadotropin. They are protein hormones secreted by gonadotrope cells of the pituitary gland of vertebrates.
Chorionic gonadotropin	A hormone, secreted by the chorion, that maintains the integrity of the corpus luteum during early pregnancy is called chorionic gonadotropin.
Diethylstilbstrol	Diethylstilbestrol is a drug, a synthetic estrogen that was developed to supplement a woman's natural estrogen production. First prescribed by physicians in 1938 for women who experienced miscarriages or premature deliveries, it was originally considered effective and safe for both the pregnant woman and the developing baby.
Epididymis	The epididymis is part of the human male reproductive system and is present in all male mammals. It is a narrow, tightly-coiled tube connecting the efferent ducts from the rear of each testicle to its vas deferens.
Testes	The testes are the male generative glands in animals. Male mammals have two testes, which are often contained within an extension of the abdomen called the scrotum.
National Cancer Institute	The National Cancer Institute (NCI) is the United States federal government's principal agency for cancer research and training, and the first institute of the present-day National Institutes of Health. The NCI is a federally funded research and development center, one of eight agencies that compose the Public Health Service in the United States Department of Health and Human Services. The Institute coordinates the National Cancer Program.
Dense fibrous connective tissue	Dense fibrous connective tissue has collagen fibers as its main matrix element. Crowded between the collagen fibers are rows of fibroblasts, fiber-forming cells, that manufacture the fibers. Dense fibrous connective tissue forms strong, rope-like structures such as tendons and ligaments.
Fibrous connective tissue	Any connective tissue with a preponderance of fiber, such as areolar, reticular, dense regular, and dense irregular connective tissues is referred to as the fibrous connective tissue.
Lymph node	A lymph node acts as a filter, with an internal honeycomb of connective tissue filled with lymphocytes that collect and destroy bacteria and viruses. When the body is fighting an infection, these lymphocytes multiply rapidly and produce a characteristic swelling of the lymph node.
Lymph	Lymph originates as blood plasma lost from the circulatory system, which leaks out into the surrounding tissues. The lymphatic system collects this fluid by diffusion into lymph capillaries, and returns it to the circulatory system.
Lungs	Lungs are the essential organs of respiration in air-breathing vertebrates. Their principal function is to transport oxygen from the atmosphere into the bloodstream, and to excrete carbon dioxide from the bloodstream into the atmosphere.
Liver	The liver is an organ in vertebrates, including humans. It plays a major role in metabolism and has a number of functions in the body including drug detoxification, glycogen storage, and plasma protein synthesis. It also produces bile, which is important for digestion.
Mammography	Mammography is the process of using low-dose X-rays (usually around 0.7 mSv) to examine the human breast. It is used to look for different types of tumors and cysts.
Mastectomy	Surgical removal of a breast. Radical mastectomy involves removal of the breast, muscle tissue, and lymph nodes in the armpit. Simple mastectomy involves removal of the breast only.
Axillary lymph node	A lymph node in the armpit region that drains lymph channels from the breast is the axillary lymph node.
Prognosis	Prognosis refers to the prospects for the future or outcome of a disease.

Chapter 15. Diseases of the Reproductive Systems and Sexually Transmitted Infections

Chapter 15. Diseases of the Reproductive Systems and Sexually Transmitted Infections

Lumpectomy	Lumpectomy is a common surgical procedure designed to remove a discrete lump (usually a tumour, benign or otherwise) from an affected woman's breast.
Hyperplasia	Hyperplasia is a general term for an increase in the number of the cells of an organ or tissue causing it to increase in size.
Amenorrhea	Amenorrhea is the absence of a menstrual period in a woman of reproductive age. Physiologic states of amenorrhea are seen during pregnancy and lactation (breastfeeding).
Depression	In everyday language depression refers to any downturn in mood, which may be relatively transitory and perhaps due to something trivial. This is differentiated from Clinical depression which is marked by symptoms that last two weeks or more and are so severe that they interfere with daily living.
Stress	Stress refers to a condition that is a response to factors that change the human systems normal state.
Eating disorders	Psychological disorders characterized by distortion of the body image and gross disturbances in eating patterns are called eating disorders.
Metrorrhagia	Metrorrhagia refers to vaginal bleeding that among premenopausal women that is not synchronized with their menstrual period.
Syndrome	Syndrome is the association of several clinically recognizable features, signs, symptoms, phenomena or characteristics which often occur together, so that the presence of one feature alerts the physician to the presence of the others
Shock	Circulatory shock, a state of cardiac output that is insufficient to meet the body's physiological needs, with consequences ranging from fainting to death is referred to as shock. Insulin shock, a state of severe hypoglycemia caused by administration of insulin.
Staphylococcus aureus	Staphylococcus aureus (which is occasionally given the nickname golden staph) is a bacterium, frequently living on the skin or in the nose of a healthy person, that can cause illnesses ranging from minor skin infections (such as pimples, boils, and cellulitis) and abscesses, to life-threatening diseases such as pneumonia, meningitis, endocarditis and septicemia.
Toxic shock syndrome	Toxic shock syndrome (TSS) is a rare but potentially fatal disease caused by a bacterial toxin. Different bacterial toxins may cause toxic shock syndrome, depending on the situation. The causative agent is Staphylococcus aureus.
Staphylococcus	Staphylococcus is a genus of gram-positive bacteria. Under the microscope they appear round (cocci), and form in grape-like clusters.
Blood pressure	Blood pressure is the pressure exerted by the blood on the walls of the blood vessels.
Toxin	Toxin refers to a microbial product or component that can injure another cell or organism at low concentrations. Often the term refers to a poisonous protein, but toxins may be lipids and other substances.
Fiber	Fibers used by man come from a wide variety of sources: Natural fiber include those made out of plants, animal and mineral sources. Natural fibers can be classified according to their origin.
Magnesium	Magnesium is the chemical element in the periodic table that has the symbol Mg and atomic number 12 and an atomic mass of 24.31.
Bacteria	The domain that contains procaryotic cells with primarily diacyl glycerol diesters in their membranes and with bacterial rRNA. Bacteria also is a general term for organisms that are composed of procaryotic cells and are not multicellular.
Premenstrual	Premenstrual Syndrome is stress which is a physical symptom prior to the onset of

Chapter 15. Diseases of the Reproductive Systems and Sexually Transmitted Infections

Chapter 15. Diseases of the Reproductive Systems and Sexually Transmitted Infections

syndrome	menstruation. It is not dysmenorrhea (increasingly painful periods), in spite of the two conditions being commonly confused in usage. It occurs prior to the onset of menstrual bleeding, while dysmenorrha occurs during the period of bleeding.
Constipation	Constipation is a condition of the digestive system where a person (or other animal) experiences hard feces that are difficult to eliminate; it may be extremely painful, and in severe cases (fecal impaction) lead to symptoms of bowel obstruction.
Irritability	Irritability is an excessive response to stimuli. Irritability takes many forms, from the contraction of a unicellular organism when touched to complex reactions involving all the senses of higher animals.
Anxiety	Anxiety is a complex combination of the feeling of fear, apprehension and worry often accompanied by physical sensations such as palpitations, chest pain and/or shortness of breath.
Binge	Binge refers to relatively brief episode of uncontrolled, excessive consumption.
Neurotransmitter	A neurotransmitter is a chemical that is used to relay, amplify and modulate electrical signals between a neuron and another cell.
Aerobic	An aerobic organism is an organism that has an oxygen based metabolism. Aerobes, in a process known as cellular respiration, use oxygen to oxidize substrates (for example sugars and fats) in order to obtain energy.
Aerobic exercise	Exercise in which oxygen is used to produce ATP is aerobic exercise.
Management techniques	Combining praise, recognition, approval, rules, and reasoning to enforce child discipline are referred to as management techniques.
Stress management	Stress management encompasses techniques intended to equip a person with effective coping mechanisms for dealing with psychological stress.
Endometriosis	Endometriosis is a common medical condition where the tissue lining the uterus is found outside of the uterus, typically affecting other organs in the pelvis.
Dyspareunia	Dyspareunia is painful sexual intercourse, due to medical or psychological causes. The term is used almost exclusively in women, although the problem may occur in men.
Dysmenorrhea	Dysmenorrhea, cramps or painful menstruation, involves menstrual periods that are accompanied by either sharp, intermittent pain or dull, aching pain, usually in the pelvis or lower abdomen.
Hot flash	A hot flash is a symptom of menopause and changing hormone levels which typically expresses itself at night as periods of intense heat with sweating and rapid heartbeat and may typically last from two to thirty minutes on each occasion.
Complaint	Complaint refers to report made by the police or some other agency to the court that initiates the intake process.
Vasodilation	An increase in the diameter of superficial blood vessels triggered by nerve signals that relax the smooth muscles of the vessel walls is referred to as vasodilation.
Hemorrhage	Loss of blood from the circulatory system is referred to as a hemorrhage.
Embryo	A prenatal stage of development after germ layers form but before the rudiments of all organs are present is referred to as an embryo.
Miscarriage	Miscarriage or spontaneous abortion is the natural or accidental termination of a pregnancy at a stage where the embryo or the fetus is incapable of surviving, generally defined at a gestation of prior to 20 weeks.

Chapter 15. Diseases of the Reproductive Systems and Sexually Transmitted Infections

Chapter 15. Diseases of the Reproductive Systems and Sexually Transmitted Infections

Spontaneous abortion	Spontaneous abortion is the natural or accidental termination of a pregnancy at a stage where the embryo or the fetus is incapable of surviving, generally defined at a gestation less than 20 weeks.
Genetic abnormality	Any abnormality in the genes, including missing genes, extra genes, or defective genes is called genetic abnormality.
Trimester	In human development, one of three 3-mnonth-long periods of pregnancy is called trimester.
Toxemia	Toxemia is another term for blood poisoning, or the presence in the bloodstream of quantities of bacteria or bacterial toxins sufficient to cause serious illness.
Hypertension	Hypertension is a medical condition where the blood pressure in the arteries is chronically elevated. Persistent hypertension is one of the risk factors for strokes, heart attacks, heart failure and arterial aneurysm, and is a leading cause of chronic renal failure.
Albuminuria	Albuminuria is a pathological condition where albumin is present in the urine. The kidneys normally filter out large molecules from the urine, so albuminuria can be an indicator of damage to the kidneys.
Edema	Edema is swelling of any organ or tissue due to accumulation of excess fluid. Edema has many root causes, but its common mechanism is accumulation of fluid into the tissues.
Convulsions	Involuntary muscle spasms, often severe, that can be caused by stimulant overdose or by depressant withdrawal are called convulsions.
Eclampsia	Eclampsia is a serious complication of pregnancy and is characterised by convulsions.
Albumin	Albumin refers generally to any protein with water solubility, which is moderately soluble in concentrated salt solutions, and experiences heat coagulation (protein denaturation).
Preeclampsia	A complication in pregnancy characterized by high blood pressure, protein in the urine, and edema is referred to as preeclampsia.
Diuretic	A diuretic is any drug that elevates the rate of bodily urine excretion.
Salt	Salt is a term used for ionic compounds composed of positively charged cations and negatively charged anions, so that the product is neutral and without a net charge.
Anticonvulsant	The anticonvulsant belong to a diverse group of pharmaceuticals used in prevention of the occurrence of epileptic seizures. The goal of an anticonvulsant is to suppress the rapid and excessive firing of neurons that start a seizure.
Penis	The penis is the male reproductive organ and for mammals additionally serves as the external male organ of urination.
Sperm	Sperm refers to the male sex cell with three distinct parts at maturity: head, middle piece, and tail.
Scrotum	In some male mammals the scrotum is an external bag of skin and muscle containing the testicles. It is an extension of the abdomen, and is located between the penis and anus.
Seminiferous tubule	Highly coiled duct within the male testes that produces and transports sperm is the seminiferous tubule.
Vas deferens	Sperm are transferred from the vas deferens, muscular tubes, into the urethra, collecting fluids from the male accessory sex glands en route.
Base	The common definition of a base is a chemical compound that absorbs hydronium ions when dissolved in water (a proton acceptor). An alkali is a special example of a base, where in an aqueous environment, hydroxide ions are donated.
Ejaculatory duct	The Ejaculatory duct is a part of the human male anatomy, which causes the reflex action of

Chapter 15. Diseases of the Reproductive Systems and Sexually Transmitted Infections

Chapter 15. Diseases of the Reproductive Systems and Sexually Transmitted Infections

	ejaculation. Each male has two of them. They begin at the vas deferens, pass through the prostate, and empty into the urethra at the Colliculus seminalis.
Urinary bladder	In the anatomy of mammals, the urinary bladder is the organ that collects urine excreted by the kidneys prior to disposal by urination. Urine enters the bladder via the ureters and exits via the urethra.
Prostate	The prostate is a gland that is part of male mammalian sex organs. Its main function is to secrete and store a clear, slightly basic fluid that is part of semen. The prostate differs considerably between species anatomically, chemically and physiologically.
Urethra	In anatomy, the urethra is a tube which connects the urinary bladder to the outside of the body. The urethra has an excretory function in both sexes, to pass urine to the outside, and also a reproductive function in the male, as a passage for sperm.
Bulbourethral gland	The bulbourethral gland is a small, rounded, and somewhat lobulated body, of a yellow color, about the size of a pea, placed behind and lateral to the membranous portion of the urethra, between the two layers of the fascia of the urogenital diaphragm. They secrete a clear fluid known as pre-ejaculate.
Glans penis	The glans penis is the sensitive erectile tip of the penis. It is wholly or partially covered by the foreskin, except when the foreskin is retracted, such as during sexual intercourse while the penis is erect, or when the foreskin has been removed by circumcision.
Glan	A glan is a structure internally composed of corpus spongiosum in males or of corpus cavernosa and vestibular tissue in females that is located at the tip of homologous genital structures involved in sexual arousal.
Prepuce	The prepuce is a retractable piece of skin which covers part of the genitals of primates and other mammals. On a male, this covers the head of the penis (the glans penis). On a female, it surrounds and protects the clitoris.
Circumcision	Circumcision is the removal of some or all of the foreskin (prepuce) from the penis.
Spermatogenesis	Spermatogenesis refers to the creation, or genesis, of spermatozoa, which occurs in the male gonads.
Motility	Motility is the ability to move spontaneously and independently. The term can apply to single cells, or to multicellular organisms.
Semen	Semen is a fluid that contains spermatozoa. It is secreted by the gonads (sexual glands) of male or hermaphroditic animals including humans for fertilization of female ova. Semen discharged by an animal or human is known as ejaculate, and the process of discharge is called ejaculation.
Fructose	Fructose is a simple sugar (monosaccharide) found in many foods and one of the three most important blood sugars along with glucose and galactose.
Vesicle	Membranous, cytoplasmic sac formed by an infolding of the cell membrane is called a vesicle.
Seminal vesicles	The seminal vesicles are a pair of glands on the posterior surface of the urinary bladder of males. They secrete a significant proportion of the fluid that ultimately becomes semen.
Prostaglandin	A prostaglandin is any member of a group of lipid compounds that are derived from fatty acids and have important functions in the animal body.
Buffer	A chemical substance that resists changes in pH by accepting H^+ ions from or donating H^+ ions to solutions is called a buffer.
Veins	Blood vessels that return blood toward the heart from the circulation are referred to as veins.

Chapter 15. Diseases of the Reproductive Systems and Sexually Transmitted Infections

Chapter 15. Diseases of the Reproductive Systems and Sexually Transmitted Infections

Sugar	A sugar is the simplest molecule that can be identified as a carbohydrate. These include monosaccharides and disaccharides, trisaccharides and the oligosaccharides. The term "glyco-" indicates the presence of a sugar in an otherwise non-carbohydrate substance.
Urinary tract infection	A urinary tract infection is an infection anywhere from the kidneys to the ureters to the bladder to the urethra.
Urination	Urination is the process of disposing urine from the urinary bladder through the urethra to the outside of the body. The process of urination is usually under voluntary control.
Penicillin	Penicillin refers to a group of β-lactam antibiotics used in the treatment of bacterial infections caused by susceptible, usually Gram-positive, organisms.
Hypersensitivity	Hypersensitivity is an immune response that damages the body's own tissues. Four or five types of hypersensitivity are often described; immediate, antibody-dependent, immune complex, cell-mediated, and stimulatory.
Cystitis	Cystitis is the inflammation of the bladder. The condition primarily affects women, but can affect all age groups from either sex.
Residual urine	Any urine left in the bladder following urination is residual urine.
Hydroureter	An enlargement of the ureter caused by any obstruction that prevent urine from entering the bladder is hydroureter.
Ureter	A ureter is a duct that carries urine from the kidneys to the urinary bladder. They are muscular tubes that can propel urine along by the motions of peristalsis.
Testosterone	Testosterone is a steroid hormone from the androgen group. Testosterone is secreted in the testes of men and the ovaries of women. It is the principal male sex hormone and the "original" anabolic steroid. In both males and females, it plays key roles in health and well-being.
Adrenal	In mammals, the adrenal glands are the triangle-shaped endocrine glands that sit atop the kidneys. They are chiefly responsible for regulating the stress response through the synthesis of corticosteroids and catecholamines, including cortisol and adrenaline.
Cortex	In anatomy and zoology the cortex is the outermost or superficial layer of an organ or the outer portion of the stem or root of a plant.
Ratio	In number and more generally in algebra, a ratio is the linear relationship between two quantities.
Adrenal cortex	Situated along the perimeter of the adrenal gland, the adrenal cortex mediates the stress response through the production of mineralocorticoids and glucocorticoids, including aldosterone and cortisol respectively. It is also a secondary site of androgen synthesis.
Asymptomatic	A disease is asymptomatic when it is at a stage where the patient does not experience symptoms. By their nature, asymptomatic diseases are not usually discovered until the patient undergoes medical tests (X-rays or other investigations). Some diseases remain asymptomatic for a remarkably long time, including some forms of cancer.
Antigen	An antigen is a substance that stimulates an immune response, especially the production of antibodies. They are usually proteins or polysaccharides, but can be any type of molecule, including small molecules (haptens) coupled to a protein (carrier).
Urinary incontinence	Urinary incontinence is the involuntary excretion of urine from one's body. It is often temporary, and it almost always results from an underlying medical condition.
Bilateral	In medicine, the term "bilateral" indicates a condition or disease that affects both sides of the body.

Chapter 15. Diseases of the Reproductive Systems and Sexually Transmitted Infections

Chapter 15. Diseases of the Reproductive Systems and Sexually Transmitted Infections

Outcome	Outcome is the impact of care provided to a patient. They can be positive, such as the ability to walk freely as a result of rehabilitation, or negative, such as the occurrence of bedsores as a result of lack of mobility of a patient.
Joint	A joint (articulation) is the location at which two bones make contact (articulate). They are constructed to both allow movement and provide mechanical support.
Scar	A scar results from the biologic process of wound repair in the skin and other tissues of the body. It is a connective tissue that fills the wound.
Alcohol	Alcohol is a general term, applied to any organic compound in which a hydroxyl group (-OH) is bound to a carbon atom, which in turn is bound to other hydrogen and/or carbon atoms. The general formula for a simple acyclic alcohol is $C_nH_{2n+1}OH$.
Viral	Viral phenomena are objects or patterns able to replicate themselves or convert other objects into copies of themselves when these objects are exposed to them.
Mumps	Mumps is a viral disease of humans. Prior to the development of vaccination, it was a common childhood disease worldwide, and is still a significant threat to health in the third world.
Parotid	The parotid gland is the largest of the salivary glands. It is found in the subcutaneous tissue of the face, overlying the mandibular ramus and anterior and inferior to the external
Salivary gland	The salivary gland produces saliva, which keeps the mouth and other parts of the digestive system moist. It also helps break down carbohydrates and lubricates the passage of food down from the oro-pharynx to the esophagus to the stomach.
Irradiation	A process in which radiation energy is applied to foods, creating compounds within the food that destroy cell membranes, break down DNA, link proteins together, limit enzyme activity, and alter a variety of other proteins and cell functions is referred to as irradiation.
Radiotherapy	Radiotherapy is the medical use of ionising radiation as part of cancer treatment to control malignant cells (not to be confused with radiology, the use of radiation in medical imaging and diagnosis).
Impotence	Erectile dysfunction, also known as impotence, is a sexual dysfunction characterized by the inability to develop or maintain an erection of the penis for satisfactory sexual intercourse regardless of the capability of ejaculation.
Engorgement	Breast engorgement occurs in the mammary glands when too much breast milk is contained within them. It is caused by insufficient breastfeeding and/or blocked milk ducts.
Lead	Lead is a chemical element in the periodic table that has the symbol Pb and atomic number 82. A soft, heavy, toxic and malleable poor metal, lead is bluish white when freshly cut but tarnishes to dull gray when exposed to air. Lead is used in building construction, lead-acid batteries, bullets and shot, and is part of solder, pewter, and fusible alloys.
Autonomic nervous system	The autonomic nervous system is the part of the nervous system that is not consciously controlled. It is commonly divided into two usually antagonistic subsystems: the sympathetic and parasympathetic nervous system.
Diabetes	Diabetes is a medical disorder characterized by varying or persistent elevated blood sugar levels, especially after eating. All types of diabetes share similar symptoms and complications at advanced stages: dehydration and ketoacidosis, cardiovascular disease, chronic renal failure, retinal damage which can lead to blindness, nerve damage which can lead to erectile dysfunction, gangrene with risk of amputation of toes, feet, and even legs.
Premature ejaculation	Premature ejaculation is the most common sexual problem in men, characterized by a lack of voluntary control over ejaculation
Diabetes	Diabetes mellitus is a medical disorder characterized by varying or persistent hyperglycemia

Chapter 15. Diseases of the Reproductive Systems and Sexually Transmitted Infections

Chapter 15. Diseases of the Reproductive Systems and Sexually Transmitted Infections

mellitus	(elevated blood sugar levels), especially after eating. All types of diabetes mellitus share similar symptoms and complications at advanced stages.
Alcoholism	A disorder that involves long-term, repeated, uncontrolled, compulsive, and excessive use of alcoholic beverages and that impairs the drinker's health and work and social relationships is called alcoholism.
Drug abuse	Drug abuse has a wide range of definitions, all of them relating either to the misuse or overuse of a psychoactive drug or performance enhancing drug for a non-therapeutic or non-medical effect, or referring to any use of illegal drug in the absence of a required, yet practically impossible to get, license from a government authority.
Adolescence	Adolescence is the period of psychological and social transition between childhood and adulthood (gender-specific manhood, or womanhood). As a transitional stage of human development it represents the period of time during which a juvenile matures into adulthood.
Cardiovascular disease	Cardiovascular disease refers to afflictions in the mechanisms, including the heart, blood vessels, and their controllers, that are responsible for transporting blood to the body's tissues and organs. Psychological factors may play important roles in such diseases and their treatments.
HIV	The virus that causes AIDS is HIV (human immunodeficiency virus).
Genitals	Genitals refers to the internal and external reproductive organs.
Reservoir	Reservoir is the source of infection. It is the environment in which microorganisms are able to live and grow.
Acute	In medicine, an acute disease is a disease with either or both of: a rapid onset; and a short course (as opposed to a chronic course).
Abscess	An abscess is a collection of pus collected in a cavity formed by the tissue on the basis of an infectious process (usually caused by bacteria or parasites) or other foreign materials (e.g. splinters or bullet wounds). It is a defensive reaction of the tissue to prevent the spread of infectious materials to other parts of the body.
Fibrosis	Replacement of damaged tissue with fibrous scar tissue rather than by the original tissue type is called fibrosis.
Conjunctiva	Conjunctiva refers to a mucous membrane that helps keep the eye moist; lines the inner surface of the eyelids and covers the front of the eyeball, except the cornea.
Purulent	Anything that creates or contains pus is purulent.
Conjunctivitis	Conjunctivitis refers to serious inflammation of the eye caused by any number of pathogens or irritants; can be caused by stds such as chlamydia.
Cornea	The cornea is the transparent front part of the eye that covers the iris, pupil, and anterior chamber and provides most of an eye's optical power.
Eye	An eye is an organ that detects light. Different kinds of light-sensitive organs are found in a variety of creatures. The simplest eyes do nothing but detect whether the surroundings are light or dark, while more complex eyes can distinguish shapes and colors.
Erythromycin	Erythromycin is a macrolide antibiotic which has an antimicrobial spectrum similar to or slightly wider than that of penicillin, and is often used for people who have an allergy to penicillins.
Abstinence	Abstinence has diverse forms. In its oldest sense it is sexual, as in the practice of continence, chastity, and celibacy.
Condom	Sheath used to cover the penis during sexual intercourse is referred to as condom.

Chapter 15. Diseases of the Reproductive Systems and Sexually Transmitted Infections

Chapter 15. Diseases of the Reproductive Systems and Sexually Transmitted Infections

Syphilis	Syphilis is a sexually transmitted disease that is caused by a spirochaete bacterium, Treponema pallidum. If not treated, syphilis can cause serious effects such as damage to the nervous system, heart, or brain. Untreated syphilis can be ultimately fatal.
Treponema pallidum	Treponema pallidum is a spirochaete bacterium. It is a motile spirochaete that is generally acquired by close sexual contact, entering the host via breaches in squamous or columnar epithelium.
Chancre	The primary lesion of syphilis, occurring at the site of initial exposure to the bacterium, often on the penis, vagina or rectum is referred to as the chancre.
Systemic infection	Systemic infection is a generic term for infection caused by microorganisms in animals or plants, where the causal agent (the microbe) has spread actively or passively in the host's anatomy and is disseminated throughout several organs in different systems of the host.
Cardiovascular system	The circulatory system or cardiovascular system is the organ system which circulates blood around the body of most animals.
Aorta	The largest artery in the human body, the aorta originates from the left ventricle of the heart and brings oxygenated blood to all parts of the body in the systemic circulation.
Inflammatory response	Inflammatory response refers to a complex sequence of events involving chemicals and immune cells that results in the isolation and destruction of antigens and tissues near the antigens.
Mental disorder	Mental disorder refers to a disturbance in a person's emotions, drives, thought processes, or behavior that involves serious and relatively prolonged distress and/or impairment in ability to function, is not simply a normal response to some event or set of events in the person's environment.
Cerebral cortex	The cerebral cortex is a brain structure in vertebrates. It is the outermost layer of the cerebrum and has a grey color. In the "higher" animals, the surface becomes folded. The cerebral cortex, made up of four lobes, is involved in many complex brain functions including memory, attention, perceptual awareness, "thinking", language and consciousness.
Spinal cord	The spinal cord is a part of the vertebrate nervous system that is enclosed in and protected by the vertebral column (it passes through the spinal canal). It consists of nerve cells. The spinal cord carries sensory signals and motor innervation to most of the skeletal muscles in the body.
Paralysis	Paralysis is the complete loss of muscle function for one or more muscle groups. Paralysis may be localized, or generalized, or it may follow a certain pattern.
Mental retardation	Mental retardation refers to having significantly below-average intellectual functioning and limitations in at least two areas of adaptive functioning. Many categorize retardation as mild, moderate, severe, or profound.
Health	Health is a term that refers to a combination of the absence of illness, the ability to cope with everyday activities, physical fitness, and high quality of life.
Reagin	Antibody that mediates immediate hypersensitivity reactions. IgE is the major reagin in humans.
Plasma	Fluid portion of circulating blood is called plasma.
Public health	Public health is concerned with threats to the overall health of a community based on population health analysis.
Antibody	An antibody is a protein used by the immune system to identify and neutralize foreign objects like bacteria and viruses. Each antibody recognizes a specific antigen unique to its target.

Chapter 15. Diseases of the Reproductive Systems and Sexually Transmitted Infections

Chapter 15. Diseases of the Reproductive Systems and Sexually Transmitted Infections

Immobilization	A mechanical action of preventing movement of a joint to allow for healing to occur is immobilization.
Genital herpes	Genital herpes refers to a sexually transmitted disease, caused by a virus, that can cause painful blisters on the genitals and surrounding skin.
Affinity	Chemical affinity results from electronic properties by which dissimilar substances are capable of forming chemical compounds. Specifically, the term refers to the tendency of an atom or compound to combine by chemical reaction with atoms or compounds of unlike composition.
Virus	Obligate intracellular parasite of living cells consisting of an outer capsid and an inner core of nucleic acid is referred to as virus. The term virus usually refers to those particles that infect eukaryotes whilst the term bacteriophage or phage is used to describe those infecting prokaryotes.
Cold sore	Cold sore refers to a lesion caused by the herpes simplex virus; usually occurs on the border of the lips or nares. Also known as a fever blister or herpes labialis.
Herpes simplex virus	The herpes simplex virus is a virus that manifests itself in two common viral infections, each marked by painful, watery blisters in the skin or mucous membranes (such as the mouth or lips) or on the genitals. The disease is contagious, particularly during an outbreak, and is incurable.
Herpes simplex	Herpes simplex refers to two common types of viruses, herpes simplex virus 1 and herpes simplex virus 2. Herpes simplex virus 2 is responsible for the STD known as genital herpes.
Resistance	Resistance refers to a nonspecific ability to ward off infection or disease regardless of whether the body has been previously exposed to it. A force that opposes the flow of a fluid such as air or blood. Compare with immunity.
Culture	Culture, generally refers to patterns of human activity and the symbolic structures that give such activity significance.
Activation	As reflected by facial expressions, the degree of arousal a person is experiencing is referred to as activation.
Wart	A wart is a generally small, rough, cauliflower-like growth, of viral origin, typically on hands and feet.
Human papilloma virus	Human papilloma virus is a member of a group of viruses in the genus Papillomavirus that can infect humans and cause changes in cells leading to abnormal tissue growth.
Genital warts	A sexually transmitted disease, caused by a virus, that forms growths or bumps on the external genitalia, in or around the vagina or anus, or on the cervix in females or penis, scrotum, groin, or thigh in males are called genital warts.
Peritoneum	In higher vertebrates, the peritoneum is the serous membrane that forms the lining of the abdominal cavity - it covers most of the intra-abdominal organs. The peritoneum both supports the abdominal organs and serves as a conduit for their blood and lymph vessels and nerves.
Risk factor	A risk factor is a variable associated with an increased risk of disease or infection but risk factors are not necessarily causal.
Cervical cancer	Cervical cancer is a malignancy of the cervix. Worldwide, it is the second most common cancer of women.
Freezing	Freezing is the process in which blood is frozen and all of the plasma and 99% of the WBCs are eliminated when thawing takes place and the nontransferable cryoprotectant is removed.

Go to **Cram101.com** for the Practice Tests for this Chapter.

Chapter 15. Diseases of the Reproductive Systems and Sexually Transmitted Infections

Chapter 15. Diseases of the Reproductive Systems and Sexually Transmitted Infections

Chlamydia trachomatis	Chlamydia trachomatis is a species of the chlamydiae, a group of obligately intracellular bacteria. It causes chlamydia, a sexually transmitted disease, and trachoma, an eye infection that is a frequent cause of blindness.
Carrier	Person in apparent health whose chromosomes contain a pathologic mutant gene that may be transmitted to his or her children is a carrier.
Asymptomatic carrier	An asymptomatic carrier, is a person who is infected with an infectious disease or carries the abnormal gene of a recessive genetic disorder, but displays no symptoms.
Infectious disease	In medicine, infectious disease or communicable disease is disease caused by a biological agent such as by a virus, bacterium or parasite. This is contrasted to physical causes, such as burns or chemical ones such as through intoxication.
Centers for Disease Control and Prevention	The Centers for Disease Control and Prevention in Atlanta, Georgia, is recognized as the lead United States agency for protecting the public health and safety of people by providing credible information to enhance health decisions, and promoting health through strong partnerships with state health departments and other organizations.
Superinfection	Superinfection describes the process by which a cell that has previously been infected by one virus gets coinfected with another virus at a later point in time. In medicine, superinfection is an infection following a previous infection, especially when caused by microorganisms that are resistant or have become resistant to the antibiotics used earlier.
Ultrasound	Ultrasound is sound with a frequency greater than the upper limit of human hearing, approximately 20 kilohertz. Medical use can visualise muscle and soft tissue, making them useful for scanning the organs, and obstetric ultrasonography is commonly used during pregnancy.
Intervention	Intervention refers to a planned attempt to break through addicts' or abusers' denial and get them into treatment. Interventions most often occur when legal, workplace, health, relationship, or financial problems have become intolerable.
Aspiration	In medicine, aspiration is the entry of secretions or foreign material into the trachea and lungs.
Palpation	Palpation is a method of examination in which the examiner feels the size or shape or firmness or location of something.
Acyclovir	Acyclovir is one of the main antiviral drugs: a synthetic purine nucleoside derivative with antiviral activity against herpes simplex virus.
Perineum	The perineum is the region between the genital area and the anus in both sexes.
Crisis	A crisis is a temporary state of high anxiety where the persons usual coping mechanisims cease to work. This may have a result of disorganization or possibly personality growth.
Gumma	A soft, gummy tumor occurring in tertiary syphilis is called gumma. Though they don't always develop, they occur singly, in groups, or exhibit a diffuse distribution. They have a firm center that may become partly hyalinized.
Critical thinking	Critical thinking consists of a mental process of analyzing or evaluating information, particularly statements or propositions that people have offered as true. It forms a process of reflecting upon the meaning of statements, examining the offered evidence and reasoning, and forming judgments about the facts.

Go to **Cram101.com** for the Practice Tests for this Chapter.

Chapter 15. Diseases of the Reproductive Systems and Sexually Transmitted Infections

Chapter 16. Diseases of the Nervous System

Spinal nerve	The spinal nerve is usually a mized nerve, formed from the dorsal and ventral roots that come out of the spinal cord.
Spinal cord	The spinal cord is a part of the vertebrate nervous system that is enclosed in and protected by the vertebral column (it passes through the spinal canal). It consists of nerve cells. The spinal cord carries sensory signals and motor innervation to most of the skeletal muscles in the body.
Cranial	In the limbs of most animals, the terms cranial and caudal are used in the regions proximal to the carpus (the wrist, in the forelimb) and the tarsus (the ankle in the hindlimb). Objects and surfaces closer to or facing towards the head are cranial; those facing away or further from the head are caudal.
Nerve	A nerve is an enclosed, cable-like bundle of nerve fibers or axons, which includes the glia that ensheath the axons in myelin.
Cranial nerves	Cranial nerves are nerves that emerge from the brainstem instead of the spinal cord. In human anatomy, there are exactly 12 pairs of them, traditionally abbreviated by the corresponding Roman numerals.
Cranial nerve	A cranial nerve is a nerve that emerges from the brainstem instead of the spinal cord. Nerves I and II are named as such, but are technically not nerves, as they are continuations of the central nervous system.
Nerve cell	A cell specialized to originate or transmit nerve impulses is referred to as nerve cell.
Neuron	The neuron is a major class of cells in the nervous system. In vertebrates, they are found in the brain, the spinal cord and in the nerves and ganglia of the peripheral nervous system, and their primary role is to process and transmit neural information.
Nervous system	The nervous system of an animal coordinates the activity of the muscles, monitors the organs, constructs and processes input from the senses, and initiates actions.
Extension	Movement increasing the angle between parts at a joint is referred to as extension.
Fiber	Fibers used by man come from a wide variety of sources: Natural fiber include those made out of plants, animal and mineral sources. Natural fibers can be classified according to their origin.
Axon	An axon is a long slender projection of a nerve cell, or neuron, which conducts electrical impulses away from the neuron's cell body or soma. They are in effect the primary transmission lines of the nervous system, and as bundles they help make up nerves.
Brain	The part of the central nervous system involved in regulating and controlling body activity and interpreting information from the senses transmitted through the nervous system is referred to as the brain.
Myelin	Myelin is an electrically insulating fatty layer that surrounds the axons of many neurons, especially those in the peripheral nervous system. It is an outgrowth of glial cells: Schwann cells supply the myelin for peripheral neurons while oligodendrocytes supply it to those of the central nervous system.
Lipid	Lipid is one class of aliphatic hydrocarbon-containing organic compounds essential for the structure and function of living cells. They are characterized by being water-insoluble but soluble in nonpolar organic solvents.
Multiple sclerosis	Multiple sclerosis affects neurons, the cells of the brain and spinal cord that carry information, create thought and perception, and allow the brain to control the body. Surrounding and protecting these neurons is a layer of fat, called myelin, which helps neurons carry electrical signals. MS causes gradual destruction of myelin (demyelination) in

Go to Cram101.com for the Practice Tests for this Chapter.

Chapter 16. Diseases of the Nervous System

Chapter 16. Diseases of the Nervous System

	patches throughout the brain and/or spinal cord, causing various symptoms depending upon which signals are interrupted.
Brain tumor	A brain tumor is any intracranial mass created by an abnormal and uncontrolled growth of cells either normally found in the brain itself: neurons, glial cells (astrocytes, oligodendrocytes, ependymal cells), lymphatic tissue, blood vessels), in the cranial nerves, in the brain envelopes (meninges), skull, pituitary and pineal gland, or spread from cancers primarily located in other organs.
Tumor	An abnormal mass of cells that forms within otherwise normal tissue is a tumor. This growth can be either malignant or benign
Depression	In everyday language depression refers to any downturn in mood, which may be relatively transitory and perhaps due to something trivial. This is differentiated from Clinical depression which is marked by symptoms that last two weeks or more and are so severe that they interfere with daily living.
Elevation	Elevation refers to upward movement of a part of the body.
Cortex	In anatomy and zoology the cortex is the outermost or superficial layer of an organ or the outer portion of the stem or root of a plant.
White matter	White matter is composed of nerve cell processes, or axons, which connect various grey matter areas of the brain to each other and carry nerve impulses between neurons.
Basal ganglia	The basal ganglia are a group of nuclei in the brain associated with motor and learning functions.
Ventricle	In the heart, a ventricle is a heart chamber which collects blood from an atrium (another heart chamber) and pumps it out of the heart.
Cerebrospinal fluid	Cerebrospinal fluid is a clear bodily fluid that occupies the subarachnoid space in the brain (the space between the skull and the cerebral cortex). It is basically a saline solution and acts as a "cushion" or buffer for the cortex.
Central canal	The central canal is the cerebrospinal fluid-filled space that runs longitudinally through the length of the entire spinal cord. The central canal is contiguous with the ventricular system of the brain.
Dura mater	The dura mater is the tough and inflexible outermost of the three layers of the meninges surrounding the brain. The other two meninges are the pia mater and the arachnoid mater. The dura mater envelops and protects the brain and spinal cord.
Hydrocephalus	Hydrocephalus is an abnormal accumulation of cerebrospinal fluid in the ventricles of the brain. This increase in intracranial volume results in elevated intracranial pressure and compression of the brain.
Brain stem	The brain stem refers to a composite substructure of the brain. It includes the midbrain, the pons and the medulla oblongata. It is the major route for communication between the forebrain, the spinal cord, and peripheral nerves. It also controls various functions including respiration, regulation of heart rhythms, and primary aspects of sound localization.
Muscle	Muscle is a contractile form of tissue. It is one of the four major tissue types, the other three being epithelium, connective tissue and nervous tissue. Muscle contraction is used to move parts of the body, as well as to move substances within the body.
Gland	A gland is an organ in an animal's body that synthesizes a substance for release such as hormones, often into the bloodstream or into cavities inside the body or its outer surface.
Vertebral column	In human anatomy, the vertebral column is a column of vertebrae situated in the dorsal aspect

Chapter 16. Diseases of the Nervous System

Chapter 16. Diseases of the Nervous System

	of the abdomen. It houses the spinal cord in its spinal canal.
Nerve tissue	Nerve tissue refers the specialized tissue making up the central and peripheral nervous systems; consists of neurons and glial cells.
Meninges	The meninges are the system of membranes that envelop the central nervous system. The meninges consist of three layers, the dura mater, the arachnoid mater, and the pia mater.
Tissue	A collection of interconnected cells that perform a similar function within an organism is called tissue.
Pia mater	The pia mater is the delicate innermost layer of the meninges - the membranes surrounding the brain and spinal cord.
Inflammation	Inflammation is the first response of the immune system to infection or irritation and may be referred to as the innate cascade.
Meningitis	Meningitis is inflammation of the membranes covering the brain and the spinal cord. Although the most common causes are infection (bacterial, viral, fungal or parasitic), chemical agents and even tumor cells may cause meningitis.
Autonomic nervous system	The autonomic nervous system is the part of the nervous system that is not consciously controlled. It is commonly divided into two usually antagonistic subsystems: the sympathetic and parasympathetic nervous system.
Sympathetic	The sympathetic nervous system activates what is often termed the "fight or flight response". It is an automatic regulation system, that is, one that operates without the intervention of conscious thought.
Parasympathetic nervous system	The parasympathetic nervous system is one of two divisions of the autonomic nervous system. It conserves energy as it slows the heart rate, increases intestinal and gland activity, and relaxes sphincter muscles in the gastro-intestinal tract. In other words, it acts to reverse the effects of the sympathetic nervous system.
Hypothalamus	Located below the thalamus, the hypothalamus links the nervous system to the endocrine system by synthesizing and secreting neurohormones often called releasing hormones because they function by stimulating the secretion of hormones from the anterior pituitary gland.
Central nervous system	The central nervous system comprized of the brain and spinal cord, represents the largest part of the nervous system. Together with the peripheral nervous system, it has a fundamental role in the control of behavior.
Heart rate	Heart rate is a term used to describe the frequency of the cardiac cycle. It is considered one of the four vital signs. Usually it is calculated as the number of contractions of the heart in one minute and expressed as "beats per minute".
Blood	Blood is a circulating tissue composed of fluid plasma and cells. The main function of blood is to supply nutrients (oxygen, glucose) and constitutional elements to tissues and to remove waste products.
Blood pressure	Blood pressure is the pressure exerted by the blood on the walls of the blood vessels.
Stress	Stress refers to a condition that is a response to factors that change the human systems normal state.
Ulcer	An ulcer is an open sore of the skin, eyes or mucous membrane, often caused by an initial abrasion and generally maintained by an inflammation and/or an infection.
Ulcerative colitis	Ulcerative colitis (UC) is a form of inflammatory bowel disease (IBD) featuring systemic inflammation specifically causing episodic mucosal inflammation of the colon (large bowel).
Digestive system	The organ system that ingests food, breaks it down into smaller chemical units, and absorbs

Go to Cram101.com for the Practice Tests for this Chapter.

Chapter 16. Diseases of the Nervous System

Chapter 16. Diseases of the Nervous System

	the nutrient molecules is referred to as the digestive system.
Tendon	A tendon or sinew is a tough band of fibrous connective tissue that connects muscle to bone. They are similar to ligaments except that ligaments join one bone to another.
Organ	Organ refers to a structure consisting of several tissues adapted as a group to perform specific functions.
Skin	Skin is an organ of the integumentary system composed of a layer of tissues that protect underlying muscles and organs.
Sensory neuron	Sensory neuron refers to nerve cell that transmits nerve impulses to the central nervous system after a sensory receptor has been stimulated.
Simple reflex	Simple reflex is a reflex involving a single muscle.
Synapse	A junction, or relay point, between two neurons, or between a neuron and an effector cell. Electrical and chemical signals are relayed from one cell to another at a synapse.
Cerebellum	The cerebellum is a region of the brain that plays an important role in the integration of sensory perception and motor output. The cerebellum integrates these two functions, using the constant feedback on body position to fine-tune motor movements.
Cerebral cortex	The cerebral cortex is a brain structure in vertebrates. It is the outermost layer of the cerebrum and has a grey color. In the "higher" animals, the surface becomes folded. The cerebral cortex, made up of four lobes, is involved in many complex brain functions including memory, attention, perceptual awareness, "thinking", language and consciousness.
Abdomen	The abdomen is a part of the body. In humans, and in many other vertebrates, it is the region between the thorax and the pelvis. In fully developed insects, the abdomen is the third (or posterior) segment, after the head and thorax.
Olfactory	Pertaining to the sense of smell is referred to as olfactory.
Auditory	Pertaining to the ear or to the sense of hearing is called auditory.
Sensory input	The conduction of signals from sensory receptors to processing centers in the central nervous system is sensory input.
Motor cortex	Motor cortex refers to the section of cortex that lies in the frontal lobe, just across the central fissure from the sensory cortex. Neural impulses in the motor cortex are linked to muscular responses throughout the body.
Sulcus	A sulcus is a depression or fissure in the surface of an organ, most especially the brain. In the brain it surrounds the gyri, creating the characteristic appearance of the brain.
Primary motor cortex	The primary motor cortex is a group of networked cells in mammalian brains that controls movements of specific body parts associated with cell groups in that area of the brain. The area is closely linked by neural networks to corresponding areas in the primary somatosensory cortex.
Skeletal muscle	Skeletal muscle is a type of striated muscle, attached to the skeleton. They are used to facilitate movement, by applying force to bones and joints; via contraction. They generally contract voluntarily (via nerve stimulation), although they can contract involuntarily.
Central sulcus	The central sulcus is a prominent landmark of the brain, separating the parietal lobe from the frontal lobe. The central sulcus is the site of the primary motor cortex in mammals, a group of cells that controls voluntary movements of the body.
Medulla	Medulla in general means the inner part, and derives from the Latin word for 'marrow'. In medicine it is contrasted to the cortex.

Chapter 16. Diseases of the Nervous System

Chapter 16. Diseases of the Nervous System

Affect	Affect is the scientific term used to describe a subject's externally displayed mood. This can be assesed by the nurse by observing facial expression, tone of voice, and body language.
Premotor cortex	Mirror neurons are cells located in the premotor cortex, the part of the brain relevant to the planning, selection and execution of actions. It is a part of the Cerebral cortex.
Blood clot	A blood clot is the final product of the blood coagulation step in hemostasis. It is achieved via the aggregation of platelets that form a platelet plug, and the activation of the humoral coagulation system
Hemorrhage	Loss of blood from the circulatory system is referred to as a hemorrhage.
Infection	The invasion and multiplication of microorganisms in body tissues is called an infection.
Ischemia	Narrowing of arteries caused by plaque buildup within the arteries is called ischemia.
Trauma	Trauma refers to a severe physical injury or wound to the body caused by an external force, or a psychological shock having a lasting effect on mental life.
Lesion	A lesion is a non-specific term referring to abnormal tissue in the body. It can be caused by any disease process including trauma (physical, chemical, electrical), infection, neoplasm, metabolic and autoimmune.
Lead	Lead is a chemical element in the periodic table that has the symbol Pb and atomic number 82. A soft, heavy, toxic and malleable poor metal, lead is bluish white when freshly cut but tarnishes to dull gray when exposed to air. Lead is used in building construction, lead-acid batteries, bullets and shot, and is part of solder, pewter, and fusible alloys.
Seizure	A seizure is a temporary alteration in brain function expressed as a changed mental state, tonic or clonic movements and various other symptoms. They are due to temporary abnormal electrical activity of a group of brain cells.
Cerebral hemorrhage	Cerebral hemorrhage is a form of stroke that occurs when a blood vessel in the brain ruptures or bleeds. Hemorrhagic strokes are deadlier than their more common counterpart, ischemic strokes.
Amphetamine	Amphetamine is a synthetic stimulant used to suppress the appetite, control weight, and treat disorders including narcolepsy and ADHD. It is also used recreationally and for performance enhancement.
Stimulant	A stimulant is a drug which increases the activity of the sympathetic nervous system and produces a sense of euphoria or awakeness.
Paranoia	In popular culture, the term paranoia is usually used to describe excessive concern about one's own well-being, sometimes suggesting a person holds persecutory beliefs concerning a threat to themselves or their property and is often linked to a belief in conspiracy theories.
Hallucination	Hallucination refers to a perception in the absence of sensory stimulation that is confused with reality.
Barbiturate	A barbiturate is a drug that acts as a central nervous system (CNS) depressant, and by virtue of this produces a wide spectrum of effects, from mild sedation to anesthesia.
Hypnotic	Hypnotic drugs are a class of drugs that induce sleep, used in the treatment of severe insomnia.
Sedative	A sedative is a drug that depresses the central nervous system (CNS), which causes calmness, relaxation, reduction of anxiety, sleepiness, slowed breathing, slurred speech, staggering gait, poor judgment, and slow, uncertain reflexes.
Affinity	Chemical affinity results from electronic properties by which dissimilar substances are

Chapter 16. Diseases of the Nervous System

Chapter 16. Diseases of the Nervous System

	capable of forming chemical compounds. Specifically, the term refers to the tendency of an atom or compound to combine by chemical reaction with atoms or compounds of unlike composition.
Virus	Obligate intracellular parasite of living cells consisting of an outer capsid and an inner core of nucleic acid is referred to as virus. The term virus usually refers to those particles that infect eukaryotes whilst the term bacteriophage or phage is used to describe those infecting prokaryotes.
Agent	Agent refers to an epidemiological term referring to the organism or object that transmits a disease from the environment to the host.
Infectious disease	In medicine, infectious disease or communicable disease is disease caused by a biological agent such as by a virus, bacterium or parasite. This is contrasted to physical causes, such as burns or chemical ones such as through intoxication.
Causative agent	In the chain of infection, the organism capable of producing an infection is called a causative agent.
Bacteria	The domain that contains procaryotic cells with primarily diacyl glycerol diesters in their membranes and with bacterial rRNA. Bacteria also is a general term for organisms that are composed of procaryotic cells and are not multicellular.
Toxin	Toxin refers to a microbial product or component that can injure another cell or organism at low concentrations. Often the term refers to a poisonous protein, but toxins may be lipids and other substances.
Wound	A wound is type of physical trauma wherein the skin is torn, cut or punctured, or where blunt force trauma causes a contusion.
Systemic infection	Systemic infection is a generic term for infection caused by microorganisms in animals or plants, where the causal agent (the microbe) has spread actively or passively in the host's anatomy and is disseminated throughout several organs in different systems of the host.
Acute	In medicine, an acute disease is a disease with either or both of: a rapid onset; and a short course (as opposed to a chronic course).
Young adult	An young adult is someone between the ages of 20 and 40 years old.
Middle ear	Middle ear refers to one of three main regions of the vertebrate ear; a chamber containing three small bones that convey vibrations from the eardrum to the inner ear.
Lungs	Lungs are the essential organs of respiration in air-breathing vertebrates. Their principal function is to transport oxygen from the atmosphere into the bloodstream, and to excrete carbon dioxide from the bloodstream into the atmosphere.
Carrier	Person in apparent health whose chromosomes contain a pathologic mutant gene that may be transmitted to his or her children is a carrier.
Mumps	Mumps is a viral disease of humans. Prior to the development of vaccination, it was a common childhood disease worldwide, and is still a significant threat to health in the third world.
Viral	Viral phenomena are objects or patterns able to replicate themselves or convert other objects into copies of themselves when these objects are exposed to them.
Herpes simplex	Herpes simplex refers to two common types of viruses, herpes simplex virus 1 and herpes simplex virus 2. Herpes simplex virus 2 is responsible for the STD known as genital herpes.
Fever	Fever (also known as pyrexia, or a febrile response, and archaically known as ague) is a medical symptom that describes an increase in internal body temperature to levels that are above normal (37°C, 98.6°F).

Chapter 16. Diseases of the Nervous System

Chapter 16. Diseases of the Nervous System

Intracranial pressure	Intracranial pressure is the pressure of the brain, Cerebrospinal fluid (CSF), and the brain's blood supply within the intracranial space.
Pain	Pain is an unpleasant sensation which may be associated with actual or potential tissue damage and which may have physical and emotional components.
Convulsions	Involuntary muscle spasms, often severe, that can be caused by stimulant overdose or by depressant withdrawal are called convulsions.
Lumbar	In anatomy, lumbar is an adjective that means of or pertaining to the abdominal segment of the torso, between the diaphragm and the sacrum (pelvis). The five vertebra in the lumbar region are the largest and strongest in the spinal column.
Sacrum	The sacrum is a large, triangular bone at the base of the vertebral column and at the upper and back part of the pelvic cavity, where it is inserted like a wedge between the two hip bones. Its upper part or base articulates with the last lumbar vertebra, its apex with the coccyx.
Lumbar puncture	In medicine, a lumbar puncture (colloquially known as a spinal tap) is a diagnostic procedure that is done to collect a sample of cerebrospinal fluid (CSF) for biochemical, microbiological and cytological analysis, or rarely to relieve increased CSF pressure.
Diagnosis	In medicine, diagnosis is the process of identifying a medical condition or disease by its signs, symptoms, and from the results of various diagnostic procedures.
Protein	A protein is a complex, high-molecular-weight organic compound that consists of amino acids joined by peptide bonds. They are essential to the structure and function of all living cells and viruses. Many are enzymes or subunits of enzymes.
Glucose	Glucose, a simple monosaccharide sugar, is one of the most important carbohydrates and is used as a source of energy in animals and plants. Glucose is one of the main products of photosynthesis and starts respiration.
Sugar	A sugar is the simplest molecule that can be identified as a carbohydrate. These include monosaccharides and disaccharides, trisaccharides and the oligosaccharides. The term "glyco-" indicates the presence of a sugar in an otherwise non-carbohydrate substance.
Prognosis	Prognosis refers to the prospects for the future or outcome of a disease.
Antibiotic	Antibiotic refers to substance such as penicillin or streptomycin that is toxic to microorganisms. Usually a product of a particular microorvanism or plant.
Paralysis	Paralysis is the complete loss of muscle function for one or more muscle groups. Paralysis may be localized, or generalized, or it may follow a certain pattern.
Mental retardation	Mental retardation refers to having significantly below-average intellectual functioning and limitations in at least two areas of adaptive functioning. Many categorize retardation as mild, moderate, severe, or profound.
Epidemic	An epidemic is a disease that appears as new cases in a given human population, during a given period, at a rate that substantially exceeds what is "expected", based on recent experience.
Encephalitis	Encephalitis is an acute inflammation of the brain, commonly caused by a viral infection.
Sleeping sickness	Sleeping sickness or African trypanosomiasis is a parasitic disease in people and in animals. Caused by protozoa of genus Trypanosoma and transmitted by the tsetse fly, the disease is endemic in certain regions of Sub-Saharan Africa, covering about 36 countries and 60 million people.
Delirium	Delirium is a medical term used to describe an acute decline in attention and cognition.

Go to Cram101.com for the Practice Tests for this Chapter.

Chapter 16. Diseases of the Nervous System

	Delirium is probably the single most common acute disorder affecting adults in general hospitals. It affects 10-20% of all adults in hospital, and 30-40% of older patients.
Measles	Measles refers to a highly contagious skin disease that is endemic throughout the world. It is caused by a morbilli virus in the family Paramyxoviridae, which enters the body through the respiratory tract or through the conjunctiva.
Electrolyte	An electrolyte is a substance that dissociates into free ions when dissolved (or molten), to produce an electrically conductive medium. Because they generally consist of ions in solution, they are also known as ionic solutions.
Kidney	The kidney is a bean-shaped excretory organ in vertebrates. Part of the urinary system, the kidneys filter wastes (especially urea) from the blood and excrete them, along with water, as urine.
Rehabilitation	Rehabilitation is the restoration of lost capabilities, or the treatment aimed at producing it. Also refers to treatment for dependency on psychoactive substances such as alcohol, prescription drugs, and illicit drugs such as cocaine, heroin or amphetamines.
Vaccine	A harmless variant or derivative of a pathogen used to stimulate a host organism's immune system to mount a long-term defense against the pathogen is referred to as vaccine.
Poliomyelitis	Poliomyelitis refers to an acute, contagious viral disease that attacks the central nervous system, injuring or destroying the nerve cells that control the muscles and sometimes causing paralysis; also called polio or infantile paralysis.
Immunization	Use of a vaccine to protect the body against specific disease-causing agents is called immunization.
Motor nerve	A motor nerve enables the brain to stimulate muscle contraction. A motor nerve is an efferent nerve that exclusively contains the axons of motorneurons, which innervate skeletal muscle.
Medulla oblongata	Medulla oblongata refers to part of the vertebrate hindbrain continuous with the spinal cord; passes data between the spinal cord and forebrain and controls autonomic, homeostatic functions, including breathing, heart rate, swallowing, and digestion.
Value	Value is worth in general, and it is thought to be connected to reasons for certain practices, policies, actions, beliefs or emotions. Value is "that which one acts to gain and/or keep."
Antibody	An antibody is a protein used by the immune system to identify and neutralize foreign objects like bacteria and viruses. Each antibody recognizes a specific antigen unique to its target.
Centers for Disease Control and Prevention	The Centers for Disease Control and Prevention in Atlanta, Georgia, is recognized as the lead United States agency for protecting the public health and safety of people by providing credible information to enhance health decisions, and promoting health through strong partnerships with state health departments and other organizations.
Rabies	Rabies refers to an acute infectious disease of the central nervous system, which affects all warmblooded animals, It is caused by an ssRNA virus belonging to the genus Lv.ssaviru.s in the family Rhahdoviridae.
Saliva	Saliva is the moist, clear, and usually somewhat frothy substance produced in the mouths of some animals, including humans.
Incubation	In problem solving, a hypothetical process that sometimes occurs when we stand back from a frustrating problem for a while and the solution 'suddenly' appears is an incubation.
Incubation period	The period after pathogen entry into a host and before signs and symptoms appear is called the incubation period.

Chapter 16. Diseases of the Nervous System

Chapter 16. Diseases of the Nervous System

Tetanus	Tetanus is a serious and often fatal disease caused by the neurotoxin tetanospasmin which is produced by the Gram-positive, obligate anaerobic bacterium Clostridium tetani. Tetanus also refers to a state of muscle tension.
Injection	A method of rapid drug delivery that puts the substance directly in the bloodstream, in a muscle, or under the skin is called injection.
Immunity	Resistance to the effects of specific disease-causing agents is called immunity.
Serum	Serum is the same as blood plasma except that clotting factors (such as fibrin) have been removed. Blood plasma contains fibrinogen.
Passive immunity	Passive immunity refers to temporary immunity obtained by acquiring ready-made antibodies or immune cells; lasts only a few weeks or months because the immune system has not been stimulated by antigens.
Temperament	Temperament refers to a basic, innate disposition that emerges early in life.
Anxiety	Anxiety is a complex combination of the feeling of fear, apprehension and worry often accompanied by physical sensations such as palpitations, chest pain and/or shortness of breath.
Shingles	A reactivated form of chickenpox caused by the varicella-zoster virus is shingles. It leads to a crop of painful blisters over the area of a dermatome.
Optic nerve	The optic nerve is the nerve that transmits visual information from the retina to the brain. The blind spot of the eye is produced by the absence of retina where the optic nerve leaves the eye. This is because there are no photoreceptors in this area.
Conjunctivitis	Conjunctivitis refers to serious inflammation of the eye caused by any number of pathogens or irritants; can be caused by stds such as chlamydia.
Cornea	The cornea is the transparent front part of the eye that covers the iris, pupil, and anterior chamber and provides most of an eye's optical power.
Tuberculosis	Tuberculosis is an infection caused by the bacterium Mycobacterium tuberculosis, which most commonly affects the lungs but can also affect the central nervous system, lymphatic system, circulatory system, genitourinary system, bones and joints.
Pneumonia	Pneumonia is an illness of the lungs and respiratory system in which the microscopic, air-filled sacs (alveoli) responsible for absorbing oxygen from the atmosphere become inflamed and flooded with fluid.
Syndrome	Syndrome is the association of several clinically recognizable features, signs, symptoms, phenomena or characteristics which often occur together, so that the presence of one feature alerts the physician to the presence of the others
Influenza	Influenza or flu refers to an acute viral infection of the respiratory tract, occurring in isolated cases, epidemics, and pandemics. Influenza is caused by three strains of influenza virus, labeled types A, B, and C, based on the antigens of their protein coats.
Encephalopathy	Encephalopathy is a nonspecific term describing a syndrome affecting the brain. Generally, it refers to involvement of large parts of the brain (or the whole organ), instead of identifiable changes confined to parts of the brain.
Intestine	The intestine is the portion of the alimentary canal extending from the stomach to the anus and, in humans and mammals, consists of two segments, the small intestine and the large intestine. The intestine is the part of the body responsible for extracting nutrition from food.
Bacillus	Bacillus is a genus of rod-shaped bacteria.

Chapter 16. Diseases of the Nervous System

Chapter 16. Diseases of the Nervous System

Asphyxiation	Asphyxia or asphyxiation is a condition of severely deficient supply of oxygen to the body. In the absence of remedial action it will very rapidly lead to unconsciousness and death.
Toxoid	A bacterial exotoxmn that has been modified so that it is no longer toxic but will still stimulate antitoxin formation when injected into a person or animal is a toxoid.
Oxygen	Oxygen is a chemical element in the periodic table. It has the symbol O and atomic number 8. Oxygen is the second most common element on Earth, composing around 46% of the mass of Earth's crust and 28% of the mass of Earth as a whole, and is the third most common element in the universe.
Abscess	An abscess is a collection of pus collected in a cavity formed by the tissue on the basis of an infectious process (usually caused by bacteria or parasites) or other foreign materials (e.g. splinters or bullet wounds). It is a defensive reaction of the tissue to prevent the spread of infectious materials to other parts of the body.
Skull	Skull refers to a bony protective encasement of the brain and the organs of hearing and equilibrium; includes the facial bones. Also called the cranium.
Lymphocyte	A lymphocyte is a type of white blood cell involved in the human body's immune system. There are two broad categories, namely T cells and B cells.
Neutrophil	Neutrophil refers to a type of phagocytic leukocyte.
Osteomyelitis	Osteomyelitis is an infection of bone, usually caused by pyogenic bacteria or mycobacteria. It can be usefully subclassifed on the basis of the causative organism, the route, duration and anatomic location of the infection.
Heredity	Heredity refers to the transmission of genetic information from parent to offspring.
Autoimmunity	Autoimmunity is the failure of an organism to recognise its own constituent parts (down to the sub-molecular levels) as self, as a result of which it attempts to mount an immune response against its own cells and tissues.
Tremor	Tremor is the rhythmic, oscillating shaking movement of the whole body or just a certain part of it, caused by problems of the neurons responsible from muscle action.
Bladder	A hollow muscular storage organ for storing urine is a bladder.
Double vision	Diplopia, colloquially known as double vision, is the perception of two images from a single object. The images may be horizontal, vertical, or diagonal.
Exacerbation	Exacerbation is a period in an illness when the symptoms of the disease reappear.
Remission	Disappearance of the signs of a disease is called remission.
Magnetic resonance imaging	Magnetic resonance imaging refers to imaging technology that uses magnetism and radio waves to induce hydrogen nuclei in water molecules to emit faint radio signals. A computer creates images of the body from the radio signals.
Demyelination	Demyelination is a loss of myelin and is the root cause of symptoms experienced by patients with diseases such as multiple sclerosis and transverse myelitis.
Physical therapy	Physical therapy is a health profession concerned with the assessment, diagnosis, and treatment of disease and disability through physical means. It is based upon principles of medical science, and is generally held to be within the sphere of conventional medicine.
Organelle	Organelle refers to any structure within a cell that carries out one of its metabolic roles, such as mitochondria, centrioles, endoplasmic reticulum, and the nucleus.
Lysosome	Organelle that contains enzymes that degrade worn cell parts is called a lysosome.
Enzyme	An enzyme is a protein that catalyzes, or speeds up, a chemical reaction. They are essential

Chapter 16. Diseases of the Nervous System

Chapter 16. Diseases of the Nervous System

	to sustain life because most chemical reactions in biological cells would occur too slowly, or would lead to different products, without them.
Population	Population refers to all members of a well-defined group of organisms, events, or things.
Amyotrophic lateral sclerosis	Amyotrophic lateral sclerosis is a progressive, invariably fatal motor neurone disease. In ALS, both the upper motor neurons and the lower motor neurons degenerate or die, ceasing to send messages to muscles.
Motility	Motility is the ability to move spontaneously and independently. The term can apply to single cells, or to multicellular organisms.
Ventral	The surface or side of the body normally oriented upwards, away from the pull of gravity, is the dorsal side; the opposite side, typically the one closest to the ground when walking on all legs, swimming or flying, is the ventral side.
Atrophy	Atrophy is the partial or complete wasting away of a part of the body. Causes of atrophy include poor nourishment, poor circulation, loss of hormonal support, loss of nerve supply to the target organ, disuse or lack of exercise, or disease intrinsic to the tissue itself.
Motor unit	A motor neuron and all the muscle fibers it controls is called the motor unit.
Muscle contraction	A muscle contraction occurs when a muscle cell (called a muscle fiber) shortens. There are three general types: skeletal, heart, and smooth.
Electromyogram	Electromyography is a technique for measuring muscle response to nervous stimulation. It is performed using an instrument called an electromyograph, to produce a record called an electromyogram.
Aspiration	In medicine, aspiration is the entry of secretions or foreign material into the trachea and lungs.
Bradykinesia	Bradykinesia denotes "slow movement." It is a feature of a number of diseases, most notably Parkinson's disease and other disorders of the basal ganglia.
Dopamine	Dopamine is a chemical naturally produced in the body. In the brain, dopamine functions as a neurotransmitter, activating dopamine receptors. Dopamine is also a neurohormone released by the hypothalamus. Its main function as a hormone is to inhibit the release of prolactin from the anterior lobe of the pituitary.
Cardiovascular disease	Cardiovascular disease refers to afflictions in the mechanisms, including the heart, blood vessels, and their controllers, that are responsible for transporting blood to the body's tissues and organs. Psychological factors may play important roles in such diseases and their treatments.
Mental disorder	Mental disorder refers to a disturbance in a person's emotions, drives, thought processes, or behavior that involves serious and relatively prolonged distress and/or impairment in ability to function, is not simply a normal response to some event or set of events in the person's environment.
Alcohol	Alcohol is a general term, applied to any organic compound in which a hydroxyl group (-OH) is bound to a carbon atom, which in turn is bound to other hydrogen and/or carbon atoms. The general formula for a simple acyclic alcohol is $C_nH_{2n+1}OH$.
Cramp	A cramp is an unpleasant sensation caused by contraction, usually of a muscle. It can be caused by cold or overexertion.
Pulse	The rhythmic stretching of the arteries caused by the pressure of blood forced through the arteries by contractions of the ventricles during systole is a pulse.
Chorea	Chorea is the occurrence of continuous rapid, jerky, involuntary movements that may involve

Go to **Cram101.com** for the Practice Tests for this Chapter.

Chapter 16. Diseases of the Nervous System

Chapter 16. Diseases of the Nervous System

	the face and limb and result in an inability to maintain a posture. It is also known as St. Vitus Dance disease and is seen mostly in children.
Neurotransmitter	A neurotransmitter is a chemical that is used to relay, amplify and modulate electrical signals between a neuron and another cell.
Dementia	Dementia is progressive decline in cognitive function due to damage or disease in the brain beyond what might be expected from normal aging.
Genes	Genes are the units of heredity in living organisms. They are encoded in the organism's genetic material (usually DNA or RNA), and control the development and behavior of the organism.
Neuritic plaque	Neuritic plaque is a cluster of dead neurons often found in the brains of people with Alzheimer's disease.
Elderly	Old age consists of ages nearing the average life span of human beings, and thus the end of the human life cycle. Euphemisms for older people include advanced adult, elderly, and senior or senior citizen.
Toxemia	Toxemia is another term for blood poisoning, or the presence in the bloodstream of quantities of bacteria or bacterial toxins sufficient to cause serious illness.
Uremia	Uremia is a toxic condition resulting from renal failure, when kidney function is compromised and urea, a waste product normally excreted in the urine, is retained in the blood. Uremia can lead to disturbances in the platelets, among other effects.
Epilepsy	Epilepsy is a chronic neurological condition characterized by recurrent unprovoked neural discharges. It is commonly controlled with medication, although surgical methods are used as well.
Birth trauma	Birth trauma refers to injury or disturbing experiences sustained at the time of birth.
Alcoholism	A disorder that involves long-term, repeated, uncontrolled, compulsive, and excessive use of alcoholic beverages and that impairs the drinker's health and work and social relationships is called alcoholism.
Idiopathic	Idiopathic is a medical adjective that indicates that a recognized cause has not yet been established.
Predisposition	Predisposition refers to an inclination or diathesis to respond in a certain way, either inborn or acquired. In abnormal psychology, it is a factor that lowers the ability to withstand stress and inclines the individual toward pathology.
Consciousness	Consciousness refers to the ability to perceive, communicate, remember, understand, appreciate, and initiate voluntary movements; a functioning sensorium.
Eye	An eye is an organ that detects light. Different kinds of light-sensitive organs are found in a variety of creatures. The simplest eyes do nothing but detect whether the surroundings are light or dark, while more complex eyes can distinguish shapes and colors.
Urine	Concentrated filtrate produced by the kidneys and excreted via the bladder is called urine.
Health	Health is a term that refers to a combination of the absence of illness, the ability to cope with everyday activities, physical fitness, and high quality of life.
World Health Organization	The World Health Organization (WHO) is a specialized agency of the United Nations, acting as a coordinating authority on international public health, headquartered in Geneva, Switzerland.
Partial seizure	A partial seizure is a seizure which is characterized by consciousness, experiencing unusual feelings or sensations, sudden and unexplainable feelings of joy, anger, sadness or nausea,

Chapter 16. Diseases of the Nervous System

Chapter 16. Diseases of the Nervous System

	sensing things that are not real, having a change or loss of consciousness, and strange repetitive behaviors such as blinks, twitches, and mouth movements.
Electroencep-alogram	Electroencephalography is the neurophysiologic measurement of the electrical activity of the brain by recording from electrodes placed on the scalp, or in the special cases on the cortex. The resulting traces are known as an electroencephalogram and represent so-called brainwaves.
Anatomy	Anatomy is the branch of biology that deals with the structure and organization of living things. It can be divided into animal anatomy (zootomy) and plant anatomy (phytonomy).
Anticonvulsant	The anticonvulsant belong to a diverse group of pharmaceuticals used in prevention of the occurrence of epileptic seizures. The goal of an anticonvulsant is to suppress the rapid and excessive firing of neurons that start a seizure.
Spina bifida	Spina bifida are birth defects caused by an incomplete closure of one or more vertebral arches of the spine, resulting in malformations of the spinal cord. Spina bifida results in varying degrees of paralysis, absence of skin sensation, incontinence, and spine and limb problems depending on the severity and location of the lesion damage on the spine.
Vertebrae	Vertebrae are the individual bones that make up the vertebral column (aka spine) - a flexuous and flexible column.
Vertebral canal	The vertebral canal follows the different curves of the column; it is large and triangular in those parts of the column which enjoy the greatest freedom of movement, such as the cervical and lumbar regions; and is small and rounded in the thoracic region, where motion is more limited.
Cleft	Cleft is a congenital deformity caused by a failure in facial development during pregnancy.
Fetus	Fetus refers to a developing human from the ninth week of gestation until birth; has all the major structures of an adult.
Neural tube	The neural tube is the embryonal structure that gives rise to the brain and spinal cord. The neural tube is derived from a thickened area of ectoderm, the neural plate. The process of formation of the neural tube is called neurulation.
Strabismus	Strabismus is a lack of coordination between the extraocular muscles which prevents bringing the gaze of each eye to the same point in space, preventing proper binocular vision.
Intervertebral disk	Layer of cartilage located between adjacent vertebrae is referred to as intervertebral disk. Each disc forms a cartilaginous joint to allow slight movement of the vertebrae, and acts as a ligament to hold the vertebrae together.
Stenosis	A stenosis is an abnormal narrowing in a blood vessel or other tubular organ or structure. It is also sometimes called a "stricture" (as in urethral stricture).
Circulatory system	The circulatory system or cardiovascular system is the organ system which circulates blood around the body of most animals.
Suture	Suture refers to an immovable joint, such as that between flat bones of the skull. Also the stitches used to hold tissue together or to close a wound.
Veins	Blood vessels that return blood toward the heart from the circulation are referred to as veins.
Vein	Vein in animals, is a vessel that returns blood to the heart. In plants, a vascular bundle in a leaf, composed of xylem and phloem.
Absorption	Absorption is a physical or chemical phenomenon or a process in which atoms, molecules, or ions enter some bulk phase - gas, liquid or solid material. In nutrition, amino acids are

Chapter 16. Diseases of the Nervous System

Chapter 16. Diseases of the Nervous System

	broken down through digestion, which begins in the stomach.
Shunt	In medicine, a shunt is a hole or passage which moves, or allows movement of, fluid from one part of the body to another. The term may describe either congenital or acquired shunts; and acquired shunts may be either biological or mechanical.
Rubella	An infectious disease that, if contracted by the mother during the first three months of pregnancy, has a high risk of causing mental retardation and physical deformity in the child is called rubella.
Cerebral palsy	Cerebral palsy is a group of permanent disorders associated with developmental brain injuries that occur during fetal development, birth, or shortly after birth. It is characterized by a disruption of motor skills, with symptoms such as spasticity, paralysis, or seizures.
Hyperbilirub-nemia	With high doses of bilirubin (severe hyperbilirubinemia) there can be a complication known as kernicterus. This is the chief reason for neonatal jaundice to be treated.
Constant	A behavior or characteristic that does not vary from one observation to another is referred to as a constant.
Traction	Traction refers to the set of mechanisms for straightening broken bones or relieving pressure on the skeletal system. It is largely replaced now by more modern techniques, but certain approaches are still used today for hip fractures.
Stroke	A stroke or cerebrovascular accident (CVA) occurs when the blood supply to a part of the brain is suddenly interrupted.
Cerebrovascular accident	Cerebrovascular accident refers to a sudden stoppage of blood flow to a portion of the brain, leading to a loss of brain function.
Blood vessel	A blood vessel is a part of the circulatory system and function to transport blood throughout the body. The most important types, arteries and veins, are so termed because they carry blood away from or towards the heart, respectively.
Scar	A scar results from the biologic process of wound repair in the skin and other tissues of the body. It is a connective tissue that fills the wound.
Hypertension	Hypertension is a medical condition where the blood pressure in the arteries is chronically elevated. Persistent hypertension is one of the risk factors for strokes, heart attacks, heart failure and arterial aneurysm, and is a leading cause of chronic renal failure.
Aneurysm	An aneurysm is a localized dilation or ballooning of a blood vessel by more than 50% of the diameter of the vessel. Aneurysms most commonly occur in the arteries at the base of the brain and in the aorta (the main artery coming out of the heart) - this is an aortic aneurysm.
Descending aorta	Part of the aorta, further divided into the thoracic aorta and abdominal aorta is called the descending aorta.
Aorta	The largest artery in the human body, the aorta originates from the left ventricle of the heart and brings oxygenated blood to all parts of the body in the systemic circulation.
Aortic aneurysm	An aortic aneurysm is a general term for any swelling (dilatation or aneurysm) of the aorta, usually representing an underlying weakness in the wall of the aorta at that location. While the stretched vessel may occasionally cause discomfort, it is the risk of rupture causing severe pain, massive internal hemorrhage and, without prompt treatment, resulting in a quick death.
Infarction	The sudden death of tissue from a lack of blood perfusion is referred to as an infarction.
Thrombosis	Thrombosis is the formation of a clot inside a blood vessel, obstructing the flow of blood

Chapter 16. Diseases of the Nervous System

	through the circulatory system. A cerebral thrombosis can result in stroke.
Embolism	An embolism occurs when an object (the embolus) migrates from one part of the body and causes a blockage of a blood vessel in another part of the body.
Artery	Vessel that takes blood away from the heart to the tissues and organs of the body is called an artery.
Carotid artery	In human anatomy, the carotid artery refers to a number of major arteries in the head and neck.
Occlusion	The term occlusion is often used to refer to blood vessels, arteries or veins which have become totally blocked to any blood flow.
Base	The common definition of a base is a chemical compound that absorbs hydronium ions when dissolved in water (a proton acceptor). An alkali is a special example of a base, where in an aqueous environment, hydroxide ions are donated.
Posterior communicating artery	The posterior communicating artery is a blood vessel that connects the terminal end of the internal carotid artery and origin of the middle cerebral artery with the posterior cerebral artery.
Anterior communicating artery	The anterior communicating artery is a blood vessel of the brain that connects the left and right anterior cerebral arteries. It is part of the cerebral arterial circle, also known as the circle of Willis.
Posterior cerebral artery	The posterior cerebral artery is the blood vessel that supplies oxygenated blood to the posterior aspect of the brain (occipital lobe). It arises from the basilar artery and connects with the ipsilateral middle cerebral artery and internal carotid artery via the posterior communicating artery.
Anterior cerebral artery	The anterior cerebral artery supplies oxygen to most medial portions of frontal lobes and superior medial parietal lobes. It arises from the internal carotid artery and is part of the Circle of Willis.
Basilar artery	In human anatomy, the basilar artery is one of the arteries that supplies the brain with oxygen-rich blood. It arises from the confluence of the two vertebral arteries at the level of the medulla oblongata.
Activator	Activator (proteomics), is a type of effector that increases the rate of enzyme mediated reactions.
Aphasia	Aphasia is a loss or impairment of the ability to produce or comprehend language, due to brain damage. It is usually a result of damage to the language centers of the brain.
Angiography	Angiography is a medical imaging technique in which an X-Ray picture is taken to visualize the inner opening of blood filled structures, including arteries, veins and the heart chambers.
Transient ischemic attack	A transient ischemic attack (TIA, often colloquially referred to as "mini stroke") is caused by the temporary disturbance of blood supply to a restricted area of the brain, resulting in brief neurologic dysfunction that usually persists for less than 24 hours.
Critical period	A period of time when an instinctive response can be elicited by a particular stimulus is referred to as critical period.
Hemiparesis	Hemiparesis is the paralysis of one side of the body. It is caused by the lesions of the corticospinal tract, which runs down from the cortical neurons of the frontal lobe to the motor neurons of the spinal cord and is responsible for the movements of the muscles of the body and its limbs.

Chapter 16. Diseases of the Nervous System

Chapter 16. Diseases of the Nervous System

Concussion	Concussion, or mild traumatic brain injury (MTBI), is the most common and least serious type of brain injury. A milder type of diffuse axonal injury, concussion involves a transient loss of mental function. It can be caused by acceleration or deceleration forces, by a direct blow, or by penetrating injuries.
Contusion	Brain contusion, a form of traumatic brain injury, is a bruise of the brain tissue. Like bruises in other tissues, cerebral contusion can be caused by multiple microhemorrhages, small blood vessel leaks into brain tissue.
Epidural	The epidural space is a part of the human spine inside the spinal canal separated from the spinal cord and its surrounding cerebrospinal fluid (CSF) by a membrane called the dura mater or simply dura.
Alcoholic	An alcoholic is dependent on alcohol as characterized by craving, loss of control, physical dependence and withdrawal symptoms, and tolerance.
Subarachnoid space	Subarachnoid space is the interval between the arachnoid and pia mater. It is occupied by a spongy tissue consisting of trabeculæ of delicate connective tissue, and intercommunicating channels in which the subarachnoid fluid is contained.
Subarachnoid hemorrhage	A subarachnoid hemorrhage (SAH) is bleeding into the subarachnoid space surrounding the brain, i.e., the area between the arachnoid and the pia mater.
Benign tumor	A benign tumor does not invade neighboring tissues and do not seed metastases, but may locally grow to great size. They usually do not return after surgical removal.
Edema	Edema is swelling of any organ or tissue due to accumulation of excess fluid. Edema has many root causes, but its common mechanism is accumulation of fluid into the tissues.
Hematoma	A hematoma, or haematoma, is a collection of blood, generally the result of hemorrhage. Hematomas exist as bruises (ecchymoses), but can also develop in organs.
Middle meningeal artery	The middle meningeal artery is typically the first branch of the first part of the maxillary artery; one of the two terminal branches of the external carotid artery. After branching off the maxillary artery, it runs through the foramen spinosum to supply the dura and the calvaria.
Trigeminal nerve	The trigeminal nerve is the fifth (V) cranial nerve, and carries sensory information from most of the face, as well as motor supply to the muscles of mastication (the muscles enabling chewing), tensor tympani (in the middle ear) and other muscles in the floor of the mouth.
Facial nerve	The facial nerve is seventh of twelve paired cranial nerves. Its main function is motor control of most of the facial muscles and muscles of the inner ear.
Salivary gland	The salivary gland produces saliva, which keeps the mouth and other parts of the digestive system moist. It also helps break down carbohydrates and lubricates the passage of food down from the oro-pharynx to the esophagus to the stomach.
Distribution	Distribution in pharmacology is a branch of pharmacokinetics describing reversible transfer of drug from one location to another within the body.
Sensory division	The afferent neurons that convey information to the CNS from the sensory receptors that monitor the external and internal environment is referred to as the sensory division.
Electroencephalography	Electroencephalography is the neurophysiologic measurement of the electrical activity of the brain by recording from electrodes placed on the scalp, or in special cases on the cortex.
Microorganism	A microorganism or microbe is an organism that is so small that it is microscopic (invisible to the naked eye).
Hypoglycemia	An abnormally low level of glucose in the blood that results when the pancreas secretes too

Chapter 16. Diseases of the Nervous System

Chapter 16. Diseases of the Nervous System

	much insulin into the blood is called hypoglycemia.
Radiation	The emission of electromagnetic waves by all objects warmer than absolute zero is referred to as radiation.
Steroid	A steroid is a lipid characterized by a carbon skeleton with four fused rings. Different steroids vary in the functional groups attached to these rings. Hundreds of distinct steroids have been identified in plants and animals. Their most important role in most living systems is as hormones.
Liver	The liver is an organ in vertebrates, including humans. It plays a major role in metabolism and has a number of functions in the body including drug detoxification, glycogen storage, and plasma protein synthesis. It also produces bile, which is important for digestion.
Chemotherapy	Chemotherapy is the use of chemical substances to treat disease. In its modern-day use, it refers almost exclusively to cytostatic drugs used to treat cancer. In its non-oncological use, the term may also refer to antibiotics.
Angiogram	The X-ray film or image of the blood vessels is called an angiograph, or more commonly, an angiogram.
Ammonia	Ammonia is a compound of nitrogen and hydrogen with the formula NH_3. At standard temperature and pressure ammonia is a gas. It is toxic and corrosive to some materials, and has a characteristic pungent odor.
Aura	An aura is the perceptual disturbance experienced by some migraine sufferers before a migraine headache, and the telltale sensation experienced by some epileptics before a seizure. It often manifests as a strange light or an unpleasant smell.
Genetic counseling	Genetic counseling generally refers to prenatal counseling done when a genetic condition is suspected in a pregnancy. Genetic counseling is the process by which patients or relatives at risk of an inherited disorder are advised of the consequences and nature of the disorder, the probability of developing or transmitting it, and the options open to them in management and family planning in order to prevent, avoid or ameliorate it.
Critical thinking	Critical thinking consists of a mental process of analyzing or evaluating information, particularly statements or propositions that people have offered as true. It forms a process of reflecting upon the meaning of statements, examining the offered evidence and reasoning, and forming judgments about the facts.
Digestive tract	The digestive tract is the system of organs within multicellular animals which takes in food, digests it to extract energy and nutrients, and expels the remaining waste.
Joint	A joint (articulation) is the location at which two bones make contact (articulate). They are constructed to both allow movement and provide mechanical support.

Chapter 16. Diseases of the Nervous System

Chapter 17. Diseases of the Bones, Joints, and Muscles

Attachment	Attachment refers to the psychological tendency to seek closeness to another person, to feel secure when that person is present, and to feel anxious when that person is absent.
Muscle	Muscle is a contractile form of tissue. It is one of the four major tissue types, the other three being epithelium, connective tissue and nervous tissue. Muscle contraction is used to move parts of the body, as well as to move substances within the body.
Joint	A joint (articulation) is the location at which two bones make contact (articulate). They are constructed to both allow movement and provide mechanical support.
Medicine	Medicine is the branch of health science and the sector of public life concerned with maintaining or restoring human health through the study, diagnosis and treatment of disease and injury.
Nerve	A nerve is an enclosed, cable-like bundle of nerve fibers or axons, which includes the glia that ensheath the axons in myelin.
Muscle contraction	A muscle contraction occurs when a muscle cell (called a muscle fiber) shortens. There are three general types: skeletal, heart, and smooth.
Tissue	A collection of interconnected cells that perform a similar function within an organism is called tissue.
Minerals	Minerals refer to inorganic chemical compounds found in nature; salts.
Protein	A protein is a complex, high-molecular-weight organic compound that consists of amino acids joined by peptide bonds. They are essential to the structure and function of all living cells and viruses. Many are enzymes or subunits of enzymes.
Osteoblast	An osteoblast is a mononucleate cell that produces a protein that produces osteoid.
Skeletal system	Skeletal systems are commonly divided into three types - external (an exoskeleton), internal (an endoskeleton), and fluid based (a hydrostatic skeleton), though hydrostatic skeletal systems may be classified separately from the other two since they lack hardened support structures.
Compact bone	Type of bone that contains osteons consisting of concentric layers of matrix and osteocytes in lacunae is called compact bone. It forms the stout walls of the diaphysis of long bones and a thin wall of the epiphysis of long bones
Spongy bone	Type of bone that has an irregular meshlike arrangement of thin plates of bone filled with red marrow is spongy bone.
Bone marrow	Bone marrow is the tissue comprising the center of large bones. It is the place where new blood cells are produced. Bone marrow contains two types of stem cells: hemopoietic (which can produce blood cells) and stromal (which can produce fat, cartilage and bone).
Blood	Blood is a circulating tissue composed of fluid plasma and cells. The main function of blood is to supply nutrients (oxygen, glucose) and constitutional elements to tissues and to remove waste products.
Red bone marrow	A connective tissue located within spongy bone that contains the stem cells and their differentiated forms involved in blood cell formation is red bone marrow.
Yellow bone marrow	Yellow bone marrow refers to a tissue found within the central cavities of long bones in adults, consisting mostly of stored fat.
Growth plate	Cartilaginous layer within an epiphysis of a long bone that permits growth of bone to occur are growth plate.
Cartilage	Cartilage is a type of dense connective tissue. Cartilage is composed of cells called chondrocytes which are dispersed in a firm gel-like ground substance, called the matrix.

Go to Cram101.com for the Practice Tests for this Chapter.

Chapter 17. Diseases of the Bones, Joints, and Muscles

Chapter 17. Diseases of the Bones, Joints, and Muscles

	Cartilage is avascular (contains no blood vessels) and nutrients are diffused through the matrix.
Periosteum	The periosteum is an envelope of fibrous connective tissue that is wrapped around the bone in all places except at joints.
Connective tissue	Connective tissue is any type of biological tissue with an extensive extracellular matrix and often serves to support, bind together, and protect organs.
Fibrous connective tissue	Any connective tissue with a preponderance of fiber, such as areolar, reticular, dense regular, and dense irregular connective tissues is referred to as the fibrous connective tissue.
Tendon	A tendon or sinew is a tough band of fibrous connective tissue that connects muscle to bone. They are similar to ligaments except that ligaments join one bone to another.
Ligament	A ligament is a short band of tough fibrous connective tissue composed mainly of long, stringy collagen fibres. They connect bones to other bones to form a joint. (They do not connect muscles to bones.)
Joint capsule	The joint capsule or articular capsule form complete envelopes for the freely movable bone joints. Each capsule consists of two layers — a outer layer (stratum fibrosum) composed of white fibrous tissue, and an inner layer (stratum synoviale) which is a secreting layer.
Synovial membrane	Membrane that forms the inner lining of the capsule of a freely movable joint is called synovial membrane. The membrane contains a fibrous outer layer, as well as an inner layer that is responsible for the production of specific components of synovial fluid, which nourishes and lubricates the joint.
Friction	Friction is the force that opposes the relative motion or tendency of such motion of two surfaces in contact. The resulting injury to skin resembles an abrasion and can also damage superficial blood vessels directly under the skin.
Muscle fiber	Cell with myofibrils containing actin and myosin filaments arranged within sarcomeres is a muscle fiber.
Fiber	Fibers used by man come from a wide variety of sources: Natural fiber include those made out of plants, animal and mineral sources. Natural fibers can be classified according to their origin.
Organ	Organ refers to a structure consisting of several tissues adapted as a group to perform specific functions.
Smooth muscle	Smooth muscle is a type of non-striated muscle, found within the "walls" of hollow organs; such as blood vessels, the bladder, the uterus, and the gastrointestinal tract. Smooth muscle is used to move matter within the body, via contraction; it generally operates "involuntarily", without nerve stimulation.
Blood vessel	A blood vessel is a part of the circulatory system and function to transport blood throughout the body. The most important types, arteries and veins, are so termed because they carry blood away from or towards the heart, respectively.
Salt	Salt is a term used for ionic compounds composed of positively charged cations and negatively charged anions, so that the product is neutral and without a net charge.
Striated muscle	Striated muscle refers to contractile tissue characterized by multinucleated cells containing highly ordered arrangements of actin and myosin microfilaments. Also known as skeletal muscle.
Cardiac muscle	Cardiac muscle is a type of striated muscle found within the heart. Its function is to "pump" blood through the circulatory system. Unlike skeletal muscle, which contracts in response to

Chapter 17. Diseases of the Bones, Joints, and Muscles

Chapter 17. Diseases of the Bones, Joints, and Muscles

nerve stimulation, and like smooth muscle, cardiac muscle is myogenic, meaning that it stimulates its own contraction without a requisite electrical impulse.

Infection	The invasion and multiplication of microorganisms in body tissues is called an infection.
Extension	Movement increasing the angle between parts at a joint is referred to as extension.
Agent	Agent refers to an epidemiological term referring to the organism or object that transmits a disease from the environment to the host.
Vitamin	An organic compound other than a carbohydrate, lipid, or protein that is needed for normal metabolism but that the body cannot synthesize in adequate amounts is called a vitamin.
Atrophy	Atrophy is the partial or complete wasting away of a part of the body. Causes of atrophy include poor nourishment, poor circulation, loss of hormonal support, loss of nerve supply to the target organ, disuse or lack of exercise, or disease intrinsic to the tissue itself.
Antibiotic	Antibiotic refers to substance such as penicillin or streptomycin that is toxic to microorganisms. Usually a product of a particular microorvanism or plant.
Infectious disease	In medicine, infectious disease or communicable disease is disease caused by a biological agent such as by a virus, bacterium or parasite. This is contrasted to physical causes, such as burns or chemical ones such as through intoxication.
Inflammation	Inflammation is the first response of the immune system to infection or irritation and may be referred to as the innate cascade.
Osteomyelitis	Osteomyelitis is an infection of bone, usually caused by pyogenic bacteria or mycobacteria. It can be usefully subclassifed on the basis of the causative organism, the route, duration and anatomic location of the infection.
Affect	Affect is the scientific term used to describe a subject's externally displayed mood. This can be assesed by the nurse by observing facial expression, tone of voice, and body language.
Humerus	The humerus is a long bone in the arm or fore-legs (animals) that runs from the shoulder to the elbow. On a skeleton, it fits between the scapula and the radius and ulna.
Tibia	The Tibia or shin bone, in human anatomy, is the larger of the two bones in the leg below the knee. It is found medial (towards the middle) and anterior (towards the front) to the other such bone, the fibula. It is the second-longest bone in the human body.
Femur	The femur or thigh bone is the longest, most voluminous and strongest bone of the human body. It forms part of the hip and part of the knee.
Wound	A wound is type of physical trauma wherein the skin is torn, cut or punctured, or where blunt force trauma causes a contusion.
Microorganism	A microorganism or microbe is an organism that is so small that it is microscopic (invisible to the naked eye).
Abscess	An abscess is a collection of pus collected in a cavity formed by the tissue on the basis of an infectious process (usually caused by bacteria or parasites) or other foreign materials (e.g. splinters or bullet wounds). It is a defensive reaction of the tissue to prevent the spread of infectious materials to other parts of the body.
Pain	Pain is an unpleasant sensation which may be associated with actual or potential tissue damage and which may have physical and emotional components.
Necrosis	Necrosis is the name given to unprogrammed death of cells/living tissue. There are many causes of necrosis including injury, infection, cancer, infarction, and inflammation. Necrosis is caused by special enzymes that are released by lysosomes.

Go to Cram101.com for the Practice Tests for this Chapter.

Chapter 17. Diseases of the Bones, Joints, and Muscles

Chapter 17. Diseases of the Bones, Joints, and Muscles

Bacteria	The domain that contains procaryotic cells with primarily diacyl glycerol diesters in their membranes and with bacterial rRNA. Bacteria also is a general term for organisms that are composed of procaryotic cells and are not multicellular.
Systemic infection	Systemic infection is a generic term for infection caused by microorganisms in animals or plants, where the causal agent (the microbe) has spread actively or passively in the host's anatomy and is disseminated throughout several organs in different systems of the host.
Leukocytosis	Leukocytosis is an elevation of the white blood cell count above the normal range. The normal adult human leukocyte count in peripheral blood is 4.4-10.8 x 10^9/L. A white blood count of 11.0 or more suggests leukocytosis.
Lesion	A lesion is a non-specific term referring to abnormal tissue in the body. It can be caused by any disease process including trauma (physical, chemical, electrical), infection, neoplasm, metabolic and autoimmune.
Fever	Fever (also known as pyrexia, or a febrile response, and archaically known as ague) is a medical symptom that describes an increase in internal body temperature to levels that are above normal (37°C, 98.6°F).
Incidence	In epidemiological studies of a particular disorder, the rate at which new cases occur in a given place at a given time is called incidence.
Tuberculosis	Tuberculosis is an infection caused by the bacterium Mycobacterium tuberculosis, which most commonly affects the lungs but can also affect the central nervous system, lymphatic system, circulatory system, genitourinary system, bones and joints.
Lungs	Lungs are the essential organs of respiration in air-breathing vertebrates. Their principal function is to transport oxygen from the atmosphere into the bloodstream, and to excrete carbon dioxide from the bloodstream into the atmosphere.
Lead	Lead is a chemical element in the periodic table that has the symbol Pb and atomic number 82. A soft, heavy, toxic and malleable poor metal, lead is bluish white when freshly cut but tarnishes to dull gray when exposed to air. Lead is used in building construction, lead-acid batteries, bullets and shot, and is part of solder, pewter, and fusible alloys.
Vertebral column	In human anatomy, the vertebral column is a column of vertebrae situated in the dorsal aspect of the abdomen. It houses the spinal cord in its spinal canal.
Vertebrae	Vertebrae are the individual bones that make up the vertebral column (aka spine) - a flexuous and flexible column.
Spinal cord	The spinal cord is a part of the vertebrate nervous system that is enclosed in and protected by the vertebral column (it passes through the spinal canal). It consists of nerve cells. The spinal cord carries sensory signals and motor innervation to most of the skeletal muscles in the body.
Paralysis	Paralysis is the complete loss of muscle function for one or more muscle groups. Paralysis may be localized, or generalized, or it may follow a certain pattern.
Absorption	Absorption is a physical or chemical phenomenon or a process in which atoms, molecules, or ions enter some bulk phase - gas, liquid or solid material. In nutrition, amino acids are broken down through digestion, which begins in the stomach.
Rickets	Rickets is a disorder which most commonly relates directly to Vitamin D deficiency, which causes a lack of calcium being absorbed. It can also arise, however, from other etiologies such as rare mesenchymal tumors or any phosphate-wasting disease. It is a disorder which most commonly relates directly to Vitamin D deficiency, which causes a lack of calcium being absorbed.

Chapter 17. Diseases of the Bones, Joints, and Muscles

Chapter 17. Diseases of the Bones, Joints, and Muscles

Calcium	Calcium is the chemical element in the periodic table that has the symbol Ca and atomic number 20. Calcium is a soft grey alkaline earth metal that is used as a reducing agent in the extraction of thorium, zirconium and uranium. Calcium is also the fifth most abundant element in the Earth's crust.
Digestive tract	The digestive tract is the system of organs within multicellular animals which takes in food, digests it to extract energy and nutrients, and expels the remaining waste.
Phosphorus	Phosphorus is the chemical element in the periodic table that has the symbol P and atomic number 15.
Gastrointestnal tract	The gastrointestinal tract is the system of organs within multicellular animals which takes in food, digests it to extract energy and nutrients, and expels the remaining waste.
Sternum	Sternum or breastbone is a long, flat bone located in the center of the thorax (chest). It connects to the rib bones via cartilage, forming the rib cage with them, and thus helps to protect the lungs and heart from physical trauma.
Childbirth	Childbirth (also called labour, birth, partus or parturition) is the culmination of a human pregnancy with the emergence of a newborn infant from its mother's uterus.
Skin	Skin is an organ of the integumentary system composed of a layer of tissues that protect underlying muscles and organs.
Osteomalacia	Osteomalacia is also referred to as bow-leggedness or rickets. It is a disorder which most commonly relates directly to Vitamin D deficiency, which causes a lack of calcium being absorbed. It can also arise, however, from other etiologies such as rare mesenchymal tumors or any phosphate-wasting disease.
Liver	The liver is an organ in vertebrates, including humans. It plays a major role in metabolism and has a number of functions in the body including drug detoxification, glycogen storage, and plasma protein synthesis. It also produces bile, which is important for digestion.
Pelvis	The pelvis is the bony structure located at the base of the spine (properly known as the caudal end). The pelvis incorporates the socket portion of the hip joint for each leg (in bipeds) or hind leg (in quadrupeds). It forms the lower limb (or hind-limb) girdle of the skeleton.
Syndrome	Syndrome is the association of several clinically recognizable features, signs, symptoms, phenomena or characteristics which often occur together, so that the presence of one feature alerts the physician to the presence of the others
Immobilization	A mechanical action of preventing movement of a joint to allow for healing to occur is immobilization.
Hormone	A hormone is a chemical messenger from one cell to another. All multicellular organisms produce hormones. The best known hormones are those produced by endocrine glands of vertebrate animals, but hormones are produced by nearly every organ system and tissue type in a human or animal body. Hormone molecules are secreted directly into the bloodstream, they move by circulation or diffusion to their target cells, which may be nearby cells in the same tissue or cells of a distant organ of the body.
Parathyroid hormone	Parathyroid hormone is secreted by the parathyroid glands as a polypeptide containing 84 amino acids. It acts to increase the concentration of calcium in the blood, whereas calcitonin (a hormone produced by the thyroid gland) acts to decrease calcium concentration.
Hypercalcemia	Hypercalcemia refers to an excess of calcium ions in the blood.
Kidney	The kidney is a bean-shaped excretory organ in vertebrates. Part of the urinary system, the kidneys filter wastes (especially urea) from the blood and excrete them, along with water, as

Chapter 17. Diseases of the Bones, Joints, and Muscles

Chapter 17. Diseases of the Bones, Joints, and Muscles

	urine.
Renal	Pertaining to the kidney is referred to as renal.
Tumor	An abnormal mass of cells that forms within otherwise normal tissue is a tumor. This growth can be either malignant or benign
Osteoporosis	Osteoporosis is a disease of bone in which bone mineral density (BMD) is reduced, bone microarchitecture is disrupted, the amount and variety of non-collagenous proteins in bone is changed, and a concomitantly fracture risk is increased.
Osteopenia	Decreased bone mass caused by cancer, hyperthyroidism, or other reasons is called osteopenia.
Spinal nerve	The spinal nerve is usually a mixed nerve, formed from the dorsal and ventral roots that come out of the spinal cord.
Menopause	Menopause is the physiological cessation of menstrual cycles associated with advancing age in species that experience such cycles. Menopause is sometimes referred to as change of life or climacteric.
Estrogen	Estrogen is a steroid that functions as the primary female sex hormone. While present in both men and women, they are found in women in significantly higher quantities.
Value	Value is worth in general, and it is thought to be connected to reasons for certain practices, policies, actions, beliefs or emotions. Value is "that which one acts to gain and/or keep."
Skull	Skull refers to a bony protective encasement of the brain and the organs of hearing and equilibrium; includes the facial bones. Also called the cranium.
Optic nerve	The optic nerve is the nerve that transmits visual information from the retina to the brain. The blind spot of the eye is produced by the absence of retina where the optic nerve leaves the eye. This is because there are no photoreceptors in this area.
Auditory	Pertaining to the ear or to the sense of hearing is called auditory.
Cranial	In the limbs of most animals, the terms cranial and caudal are used in the regions proximal to the carpus (the wrist, in the forelimb) and the tarsus (the ankle in the hindlimb). Objects and surfaces closer to or facing towards the head are cranial; those facing away or further from the head are caudal.
Cranial nerves	Cranial nerves are nerves that emerge from the brainstem instead of the spinal cord. In human anatomy, there are exactly 12 pairs of them, traditionally abbreviated by the corresponding Roman numerals.
Auditory nerve	The nerve leading from the mammalian cochlea to the brain, carrying information about sound is the auditory nerve.
Cranial nerve	A cranial nerve is a nerve that emerges from the brainstem instead of the spinal cord. Nerves I and II are named as such, but are technically not nerves, as they are continuations of the central nervous system.
Sarcoma	Cancer of the supportive tissues, such as bone, cartilage, and muscle is referred to as sarcoma.
Trauma	Trauma refers to a severe physical injury or wound to the body caused by an external force, or a psychological shock having a lasting effect on mental life.
Scoliosis	Scoliosis is a condition that involves a lateral curvature of the spine; that is, the spine is bent sideways. Scoliosis is incurable, but its natural course can be affected with treatments such as surgery or bracing.

Go to **Cram101.com** for the Practice Tests for this Chapter.

Chapter 17. Diseases of the Bones, Joints, and Muscles

Chapter 17. Diseases of the Bones, Joints, and Muscles

Kyphosis	Kyphosis in the sense of a deformity is the pathologic curving of the spine, where parts of the spinal column lose some or all of their lordotic profile. This causes a bowing of the back, seen as a slouching posture.
Elderly	Old age consists of ages nearing the average life span of human beings, and thus the end of the human life cycle. Euphemisms for older people include advanced adult, elderly, and senior or senior citizen.
Benign tumor	A benign tumor does not invade neighboring tissues and do not seed metastases, but may locally grow to great size. They usually do not return after surgical removal.
Motility	Motility is the ability to move spontaneously and independently. The term can apply to single cells, or to multicellular organisms.
Chemotherapy	Chemotherapy is the use of chemical substances to treat disease. In its modern-day use, it refers almost exclusively to cytostatic drugs used to treat cancer. In its non-oncological use, the term may also refer to antibiotics.
Carcinoma	Cancer that originates in the coverings of the body, such as the skin or the lining of the intestinal tract is a carcinoma.
Stress	Stress refers to a condition that is a response to factors that change the human systems normal state.
Hip	In anatomy, the hip is the bony projection of the femur, known as the greater trochanter, and the overlying muscle and fat.
Arthritis	Arthritis is a group of conditions that affect the health of the bone joints in the body. Arthritis can be caused from strains and injuries caused by repetitive motion, sports, overexertion, and falls. Unlike the autoimmune diseases, it largely affects older people and results from the degeneration of joint cartilage.
Rheumatoid arthritis	Rheumatoid arthritis is a chronic, inflammatory autoimmune disorder that causes the immune system to attack the joints. It is a disabling and painful inflammatory condition, which can lead to substantial loss of mobility due to pain and joint destruction.
Diagnosis	In medicine, diagnosis is the process of identifying a medical condition or disease by its signs, symptoms, and from the results of various diagnostic procedures.
Young adult	An young adult is someone between the ages of 20 and 40 years old.
Exacerbation	Exacerbation is a period in an illness when the symptoms of the disease reappear.
Articular	The articular is a bone in the lower jaw of most tetrapods, including reptiles, birds, and amphibians, but has become a middle ear bone (the malleus) in mammals. It is the site of articulation between the lower jaw and the skull, and is connected to two other lower jaw bones, the suprangular and the angular.
Ankylosis	Ankylosis, or Anchylosis is a stiffness of a joint, the result of injury or disease. The rigidity may be complete or partial and may be due to inflammation of the tendinous or muscular structures outside the joint or of the tissues of the joint itself.
Sacrum	The sacrum is a large, triangular bone at the base of the vertebral column and at the upper and back part of the pelvic cavity, where it is inserted like a wedge between the two hip bones. Its upper part or base articulates with the last lumbar vertebra, its apex with the coccyx.
Scar	A scar results from the biologic process of wound repair in the skin and other tissues of the body. It is a connective tissue that fills the wound.
Fusion	Fusion refers to the combination of two atoms into a single atom as a result of a collision,

Go to **Cram101.com** for the Practice Tests for this Chapter.

Chapter 17. Diseases of the Bones, Joints, and Muscles

Chapter 17. Diseases of the Bones, Joints, and Muscles

	usually accompanied by the release of energy.
Eye	An eye is an organ that detects light. Different kinds of light-sensitive organs are found in a variety of creatures. The simplest eyes do nothing but detect whether the surroundings are light or dark, while more complex eyes can distinguish shapes and colors.
Autoimmune	Autoimmune refers to immune reactions against normal body cells; self against self.
Autoimmune disease	Disease that results when the immune system mistakenly attacks the body's own tissues is referred to as autoimmune disease.
Hypersensitivity	Hypersensitivity is an immune response that damages the body's own tissues. Four or five types of hypersensitivity are often described; immediate, antibody-dependent, immune complex, cell-mediated, and stimulatory.
Antibody	An antibody is a protein used by the immune system to identify and neutralize foreign objects like bacteria and viruses. Each antibody recognizes a specific antigen unique to its target.
Neutrophil	Neutrophil refers to a type of phagocytic leukocyte.
Predisposition	Predisposition refers to an inclination or diathesis to respond in a certain way, either inborn or acquired. In abnormal psychology, it is a factor that lowers the ability to withstand stress and inclines the individual toward pathology.
Acute	In medicine, an acute disease is a disease with either or both of: a rapid onset; and a short course (as opposed to a chronic course).
Steroid	A steroid is a lipid characterized by a carbon skeleton with four fused rings. Different steroids vary in the functional groups attached to these rings. Hundreds of distinct steroids have been identified in plants and animals. Their most important role in most living systems is as hormones.
Chronic disease	Disease of long duration often not detected in its early stages and from which the patient will not recover is referred to as a chronic disease.
Osteoarthritis	Osteoarthritis is a condition in which low-grade inflammation results in pain in the joints, caused by wearing of the cartilage that covers and acts as a cushion inside joints.
Range of motion	Range of motion is a measurement of movement through a particular joint or muscle range.
Base	The common definition of a base is a chemical compound that absorbs hydronium ions when dissolved in water (a proton acceptor). An alkali is a special example of a base, where in an aqueous environment, hydroxide ions are donated.
Heredity	Heredity refers to the transmission of genetic information from parent to offspring.
Uric acid	An insoluble precipitate of nitrogenous waste excreted by land snails, insects, birds, and some reptiles is called uric acid.
Crystal	Crystal is a solid in which the constituent atoms, molecules, or ions are packed in a regularly ordered, repeating pattern extending in all three spatial dimensions.
Acid	An acid is a water-soluble, sour-tasting chemical compound that when dissolved in water, gives a solution with a pH of less than 7.
Precipitation	The crystallization or suspension of particles that occurs due to the mixing of incompatible solutions or adding solutes to incompatible solutions is called precipitation. This results in the occlusion of an intravenous line.
Nucleic acid	A nucleic acid is a complex, high-molecular-weight biochemical macromolecule composed of nucleotide chains that convey genetic information.
Metabolism	Metabolism is the biochemical modification of chemical compounds in living organisms and

Go to Cram101.com for the Practice Tests for this Chapter.

Chapter 17. Diseases of the Bones, Joints, and Muscles

Chapter 17. Diseases of the Bones, Joints, and Muscles

	cells. This includes the biosynthesis of complex organic molecules (anabolism) and their breakdown (catabolism).
Purine	Purine refers to one of two families of nitrogenous bases found in nucleotides. Adenine and guanine are purines.
Bursitis	Bursitis is the inflammation of one or more bursae, or small sacks of oil, in the body. Bursitis is commonly caused by repetition of movement or excessive pressure.
Bursa	A bursa is a fluid filled sac located between a bone and tendon which normally serves to reduce friction between the two moving surfaces.
Inflammatory response	Inflammatory response refers to a complex sequence of events involving chemicals and immune cells that results in the isolation and destruction of antigens and tissues near the antigens.
Dislocation	Dislocation occurs when bones are forced out of their normal alignment at a joint.
Rotation	Movement turning a body part on its longitudinal axis is rotation.
Conditioning	Processes by which behaviors can be learned or modified through interaction with the environment are conditioning.
Carpal	In human anatomy, the carpal bones are the bones of the human wrist. There are eight of them altogether, and they can be thought of as forming two rows of four.
Repetitive strain injury	Repetitive strain injury is an occupational overuse syndrome affecting muscles, tendons and nerves in the arms and upper back. It occurs when muscles in these areas are kept tense for very long periods of time, due to poor posture and/or repetitive motions.
Carpal tunnel syndrome	Carpal tunnel syndrome (CTS) is a medical condition in which the median nerve is compressed at the wrist causing symptoms like tingling, pain, coldness, and sometimes weakness in parts of the hand.
Typing	Determining a patients blood type is called typing.
Median	The median is a number that separates the higher half of a sample, a population, or a probability distribution from the lower half. It is the middle value in a distribution, above and below which lie an equal number of values.
Motor nerve	A motor nerve enables the brain to stimulate muscle contraction. A motor nerve is an efferent nerve that exclusively contains the axons of motorneurons, which innervate skeletal muscle.
Injection	A method of rapid drug delivery that puts the substance directly in the bloodstream, in a muscle, or under the skin is called injection.
Transverse	A transverse (also known as axial or horizontal) plane is an X-Y plane, parallel to the ground, which (in humans) separates the superior from the inferior, or put another way, the head from the feet.
Skeletal muscle	Skeletal muscle is a type of striated muscle, attached to the skeleton. They are used to facilitate movement, by applying force to bones and joints; via contraction. They generally contract voluntarily (via nerve stimulation), although they can contract involuntarily.
Muscular dystrophy	Muscular dystrophy is a chronic disease characterized by progressive skeletal muscle weakness, defects in muscle proteins, and the death of muscle cells and tissue. In some forms of muscular dystrophy, cardiac and smooth muscles are affected. It is the most common hereditary diseases.
Mutation	A change in the structure of a gene is called a mutation.
Motor	The progression of muscular coordination required for physical activities is referred to as

Chapter 17. Diseases of the Bones, Joints, and Muscles

Chapter 17. Diseases of the Bones, Joints, and Muscles

development	motor development.
Phosphate	A phosphate is a polyatomic ion or radical consisting of one phosphorus atom and four oxygen. In the ionic form, it carries a -3 formal charge, and is denoted PO_4^{3-}.
Creatine phosphate	Compound unique to muscles that contains a high-energy phosphate bond is creatine phosphate or phosphocreatine.
Urine	Concentrated filtrate produced by the kidneys and excreted via the bladder is called urine.
Serum	Serum is the same as blood plasma except that clotting factors (such as fibrin) have been removed. Blood plasma contains fibrinogen.
Myasthenia gravis	Myasthenia gravis is a neuromuscular disease leading to fluctuating weakness and fatiguability.
Receptor	A receptor is a protein on the cell membrane or within the cytoplasm or cell nucleus that binds to a specific molecule (a ligand), such as a neurotransmitter, hormone, or other substance, and initiates the cellular response to the ligand. Receptor, in immunology, the region of an antibody which shows recognition of an antigen.
Neurotransmitter	A neurotransmitter is a chemical that is used to relay, amplify and modulate electrical signals between a neuron and another cell.
Acetylcholine	The chemical compound acetylcholine was the first neurotransmitter to be identified. It is a chemical transmitter in both the peripheral nervous system (PNS) and central nervous system (CNS) in many organisms including humans.
Thymus	The thymus is a ductless gland located in the upper anterior portion of the chest cavity. It is most active during puberty, after which it shrinks in size and activity in most individuals and is replaced with fat. The thymus plays an important role in the development of the immune system.
Gland	A gland is an organ in an animal's body that synthesizes a substance for release such as hormones, often into the bloodstream or into cavities inside the body or its outer surface.
Immune response	The body's defensive reaction to invasion by bacteria, viral agents, or other foreign substances is called immune response.
Remission	Disappearance of the signs of a disease is called remission.
Carbon	Carbon is a chemical element in the periodic table that has the symbol C and atomic number 6. An abundant nonmetallic, tetravalent element, carbon has several allotropic forms.
Oxygen	Oxygen is a chemical element in the periodic table. It has the symbol O and atomic number 8. Oxygen is the second most common element on Earth, composing around 46% of the mass of Earth's crust and 28% of the mass of Earth as a whole, and is the third most common element in the universe.
Carbon dioxide	Carbon dioxide is an atmospheric gas comprized of one carbon and two oxygen atoms. A very widely known chemical compound, it is frequently called by its formula CO_2. In its solid state, it is commonly known as dry ice.
Ventilation	Ventilation refers to a mechanism that provides contact between an animal's respiratory surface and the air or water to which it is exposed. It is also called breathing.
Prognosis	Prognosis refers to the prospects for the future or outcome of a disease.
Phosphatase	A phosphatase is an enzyme that hydrolyses phosphoric acid monoesters into a phosphate ion and a molecule with a free hydroxyl group.
Enzyme	An enzyme is a protein that catalyzes, or speeds up, a chemical reaction. They are essential

Chapter 17. Diseases of the Bones, Joints, and Muscles

Chapter 17. Diseases of the Bones, Joints, and Muscles

	to sustain life because most chemical reactions in biological cells would occur too slowly, or would lead to different products, without them.
Alkaline phosphatase	Alkaline phosphatase (ALP) (EC 3.1.3.1) is a hydrolase enzyme responsible for removing phosphate groups in the 5- and 3- positions from many types of molecules, including nucleotides, proteins, and alkaloids.
Erythrocyte	Red blood cells are the most common type of blood cell and are the vertebrate body's principal means of delivering oxygen from the lungs or gills to body tissues via the blood. Red blood cells are also known as erythrocyte.
Biopsy	Removal of small tissue sample from the body for microscopic examination is called biopsy.
Electromyography	Electromyography is a medical technique for measuring muscle response to nervous stimulation.
Skeleton	In biology, the skeleton or skeletal system is the biological system providing physical support in living organisms.
Critical thinking	Critical thinking consists of a mental process of analyzing or evaluating information, particularly statements or propositions that people have offered as true. It forms a process of reflecting upon the meaning of statements, examining the offered evidence and reasoning, and forming judgments about the facts.
Physical therapy	Physical therapy is a health profession concerned with the assessment, diagnosis, and treatment of disease and disability through physical means. It is based upon principles of medical science, and is generally held to be within the sphere of conventional medicine.
Axial skeleton	The axial skeleton consists of the bones in the head and trunk of a vertebrate body. It is composed of three major parts; the skull, the bony thorax (i.e. the ribs and sternum), and the vertebral column.
Synovial joint	Synovial joint refers to freely moving joint in which two bones are separated by a cavity.

Go to **Cram101.com** for the Practice Tests for this Chapter.

Chapter 17. Diseases of the Bones, Joints, and Muscles

Chapter 18. Diseases of the Skin

Organ	Organ refers to a structure consisting of several tissues adapted as a group to perform specific functions.
Skin	Skin is an organ of the integumentary system composed of a layer of tissues that protect underlying muscles and organs.
Pain	Pain is an unpleasant sensation which may be associated with actual or potential tissue damage and which may have physical and emotional components.
Microorganism	A microorganism or microbe is an organism that is so small that it is microscopic (invisible to the naked eye).
Cyanosis	Bluish skin coloration due to decreased blood oxygen concentration is called cyanosis.
Oxygen	Oxygen is a chemical element in the periodic table. It has the symbol O and atomic number 8. Oxygen is the second most common element on Earth, composing around 46% of the mass of Earth's crust and 28% of the mass of Earth as a whole, and is the third most common element in the universe.
Hemolysis	The rupture of red blood cells accompanied by the release of hemoglobin is called hemolysis.
Bilirubin	A bile pigment produced from hemoglobin breakdown is bilirubin.
Jaundice	Jaundice is yellowing of the skin, sclera (the white of the eyes) and mucous membranes caused by increased levels of bilirubin in the human body.
Liver	The liver is an organ in vertebrates, including humans. It plays a major role in metabolism and has a number of functions in the body including drug detoxification, glycogen storage, and plasma protein synthesis. It also produces bile, which is important for digestion.
Blood	Blood is a circulating tissue composed of fluid plasma and cells. The main function of blood is to supply nutrients (oxygen, glucose) and constitutional elements to tissues and to remove waste products.
Bile	Bile is a bitter, greenish-yellow alkaline fluid secreted by the liver of most vertebrates. In many species, it is stored in the gallbladder between meals and upon eating is discharged into the duodenum where it aids the process of digestion.
Red blood cells	Red blood cells are the most common type of blood cell and are the vertebrate body's principal means of delivering oxygen from the lungs or gills to body tissues via the blood.
Red blood cell	The red blood cell is the most common type of blood cell and is the vertebrate body's principal means of delivering oxygen from the lungs or gills to body tissues via the blood.
Polycythemia	Polycythemia is a condition in which there is a net increase in the total circulating red blood cell mass of the body.
Carbon	Carbon is a chemical element in the periodic table that has the symbol C and atomic number 6. An abundant nonmetallic, tetravalent element, carbon has several allotropic forms.
Fever	Fever (also known as pyrexia, or a febrile response, and archaically known as ague) is a medical symptom that describes an increase in internal body temperature to levels that are above normal (37°C, 98.6°F).
Anemia	Anemia is a deficiency of red blood cells and/or hemoglobin. This results in a reduced ability of blood to transfer oxygen to the tissues, and this causes hypoxia; since all human cells depend on oxygen for survival, varying degrees of anemia can have a wide range of clinical consequences.
Pallor	Pallor is an abnormal loss of skin or mucous membrane color. It can develop suddenly or gradually, depending of the cause.

Go to Cram101.com for the Practice Tests for this Chapter.

Chapter 18. Diseases of the Skin

Chapter 18. Diseases of the Skin

Health	Health is a term that refers to a combination of the absence of illness, the ability to cope with everyday activities, physical fitness, and high quality of life.
Mental health	Mental health refers to the 'thinking' part of psychosocial health; includes your values, attitudes, and beliefs.
Friction	Friction is the force that opposes the relative motion or tendency of such motion of two surfaces in contact. The resulting injury to skin resembles an abrasion and can also damage superficial blood vessels directly under the skin.
Tissue	A collection of interconnected cells that perform a similar function within an organism is called tissue.
Epithelium	Epithelium is a tissue composed of a layer of cells. Epithelium can be found lining internal (e.g. endothelium, which lines the inside of blood vessels) or external (e.g. skin) free surfaces of the body. Functions include secretion, absorption and protection.
Dermis	The dermis is the layer of skin beneath the epidermis that consists of connective tissue and cushions the body from stress and strain.
Keratin	Keratin is a family of fibrous structural proteins; tough and insoluble, they form the hard but nonmineralized structures found in reptiles, birds and mammals.
Stratum corneum	The stratum corneum ("the horny layer") is the outermost layer of the epidermis, and comprises the surface of the skin. It is composed mainly of dead cells that lack nuclei. As these dead cells slough off, they are continuously replaced by new cells from the stratum germinativum.
Keratinocyte	The keratinocyte is the major cell type of the epidermis, making up about 90% of epidermal cells. They are shed and replaced continuously from the stratum corneum.
Protein	A protein is a complex, high-molecular-weight organic compound that consists of amino acids joined by peptide bonds. They are essential to the structure and function of all living cells and viruses. Many are enzymes or subunits of enzymes.
Evaluation	The fifth step of the nursing process where nursing care and the patient's goal achievement are measured is the evaluation.
Epidermis	Epidermis is the outermost layer of the skin. It forms the waterproof, protective wrap over the body's surface and is made up of stratified squamous epithelium with an underlying basement membrane. It contains no blood vessels, and is nourished by diffusion from the dermis. In plants, the outermost layer of cells covering the leaves and young parts of a plant is the epidermis.
Affect	Affect is the scientific term used to describe a subject's externally displayed mood. This can be assesed by the nurse by observing facial expression, tone of voice, and body language.
Infection	The invasion and multiplication of microorganisms in body tissues is called an infection.
Subcutaneous	Subcutaneous injections are given by injecting a fluid into the subcutis. It is relatively painless and an effective way to administer particular types of medication.
Melanocyte	Melanocyte cells are located in the bottom layer of the skin's epidermis. With a process called melanogenesis, they produce melanin, a pigment in the skin, eyes, and hair.
Melanin	Broadly, melanin is any of the polyacetylene, polyaniline, and polypyrrole "blacks" or their mixed copolymers. The most common form of biological melanin is a polymer of either or both of two monomer molecules: indolequinone, and dihydroxyindole carboxylic acid.
Lymph vessel	Lymph vessel refers to one of the system of vessels carrying lymph from the lymph capillaries to the veins.

Chapter 18. Diseases of the Skin

Chapter 18. Diseases of the Skin

Sweat gland	Gland responsible for the loss of a watery fluid, consisting mainly of sodium chloride (commonly known as salt) and urea in solution, that is secreted through the skin is a sweat gland.
Sebaceous	The sebaceous glands are glands found in the skin of mammals. They secrete an oily substance called sebum that is made of fat (lipids) and the debris of dead fat-producing cells.
Nerve	A nerve is an enclosed, cable-like bundle of nerve fibers or axons, which includes the glia that ensheath the axons in myelin.
Lymph	Lymph originates as blood plasma lost from the circulatory system, which leaks out into the surrounding tissues. The lymphatic system collects this fluid by diffusion into lymph capillaries, and returns it to the circulatory system.
Gland	A gland is an organ in an animal's body that synthesizes a substance for release such as hormones, often into the bloodstream or into cavities inside the body or its outer surface.
Fiber	Fibers used by man come from a wide variety of sources: Natural fiber include those made out of plants, animal and mineral sources. Natural fibers can be classified according to their origin.
Connective tissue	Connective tissue is any type of biological tissue with an extensive extracellular matrix and often serves to support, bind together, and protect organs.
Elastic fiber	Elastic fiber is a bundles of proteins (elastin) found in connective tissue and produced by fibroblasts and smooth muscle cells in arteries.
Adipose tissue	Adipose tissue is an anatomical term for loose connective tissue composed of adipocytes. Its main role is to store energy in the form of fat, although it also cushions and insulates the body. It has an important endocrine function in producing recently-discovered hormones such as leptin, resistin and TNFalpha.
Lesion	A lesion is a non-specific term referring to abnormal tissue in the body. It can be caused by any disease process including trauma (physical, chemical, electrical), infection, neoplasm, metabolic and autoimmune.
Erythema	Abnormal redness of the skin due to such causes as burns, inflammation, and vasodilation is called erythema.
Inflammation	Inflammation is the first response of the immune system to infection or irritation and may be referred to as the innate cascade.
Diagnosis	In medicine, diagnosis is the process of identifying a medical condition or disease by its signs, symptoms, and from the results of various diagnostic procedures.
Edema	Edema is swelling of any organ or tissue due to accumulation of excess fluid. Edema has many root causes, but its common mechanism is accumulation of fluid into the tissues.
Vesicle	Membranous, cytoplasmic sac formed by an infolding of the cell membrane is called a vesicle.
Tumor	An abnormal mass of cells that forms within otherwise normal tissue is a tumor. This growth can be either malignant or benign
Blood vessel	A blood vessel is a part of the circulatory system and function to transport blood throughout the body. The most important types, arteries and veins, are so termed because they carry blood away from or towards the heart, respectively.
Pruritus	Pruritus is a sensation felt on an area of skin that makes a person or animal want to scratch it. Scratching may cause breaks in the skin that may result in infection. Pruritus can be related to anything from dry skin to undiagnosed cancer.
Chickenpox	Chickenpox refers to a highly contagious skin disease, usually affecting 2- to 7-year-old

Go to Cram101.com for the Practice Tests for this Chapter.

Chapter 18. Diseases of the Skin

Chapter 18. Diseases of the Skin

	children; it is caused by the varicellazoster virus, which is acquired by droplet inhalation into the respiratory system.
Urticaria	Urticaria or hives is a relatively common form of allergic reaction that causes raized red skin welts. Urticaria is also known as nettle rash or uredo. These welts can range in diameter from 5 mm (0.2 inches) or more, itch severely, and often have a pale border.
Elevation	Elevation refers to upward movement of a part of the body.
Serous	The term serous fluid is used for various bodily fluids that are typically pale yellow and transparent, and of a benign nature.
Ulcer	An ulcer is an open sore of the skin, eyes or mucous membrane, often caused by an initial abrasion and generally maintained by an inflammation and/or an infection.
Acne vulgaris	Acne Vulgaris is an inflammatory disease of the skin, caused by changes in the pilosebaceous units (skin structures consisting of a hair follicle and its associated sebaceous gland).
Impetigo	Impetigo superficial cutaneous disease, most commonly seen in children, is characterized by crusty lesions, usually located on the face; the lesions typically have vesicles surrounded by a red border. It is the most frequently diagnosed skin infection caused by S. pyogeoes.
Acute	In medicine, an acute disease is a disease with either or both of: a rapid onset; and a short course (as opposed to a chronic course).
Lymph node	A lymph node acts as a filter, with an internal honeycomb of connective tissue filled with lymphocytes that collect and destroy bacteria and viruses. When the body is fighting an infection, these lymphocytes multiply rapidly and produce a characteristic swelling of the lymph node.
Antibiotic	Antibiotic refers to substance such as penicillin or streptomycin that is toxic to microorganisms. Usually a product of a particular microorvanism or plant.
Erysipelas	Erysipelas is an acute streptococcus bacterial skin infection, resulting in inflammation and characteristically extending into underlying fat tissue.
Cellulitis	Cellulitis is an inflammation of the connective tissue underlying the skin, that can be caused by a bacterial infection. Cellulitis can be caused by normal skin flora or by exogenous bacteria, and often occurs where the skin has previously been broken.
Bacteria	The domain that contains procaryotic cells with primarily diacyl glycerol diesters in their membranes and with bacterial rRNA. Bacteria also is a general term for organisms that are composed of procaryotic cells and are not multicellular.
Follicle	Follicle refers to a cluster of cells surrounding, protecting, and nourishing a developing egg cell in the ovary; also secretes estrogen. In botany, a follicle is a type of simple dry fruit produced by certain flowering plants. It is regarded as one the most primitive types of fruits, and derives from a simple pistil or carpel.
Hair follicle	A hair follicle is part of the skin that grows hair by packing old cells together. Attached to the follicle is a sebaceous gland, a tiny sebum-producing gland found everywhere except on the palms and soles of the feet.
Antiseptic	An antiseptic is a substance that prevents the growth and reproduction of various microorganisms (such as bacteria, fungi, protozoa, and viruses) on the external surfaces of the body. Some are true germicides, capable of destroying the bacteria, whilst others merely prevent or inhibit their growth.
Viral	Viral phenomena are objects or patterns able to replicate themselves or convert other objects into copies of themselves when these objects are exposed to them.

Chapter 18. Diseases of the Skin

Chapter 18. Diseases of the Skin

Cold sore	Cold sore refers to a lesion caused by the herpes simplex virus; usually occurs on the border of the lips or nares. Also known as a fever blister or herpes labialis.
Wart	A wart is a generally small, rough, cauliflower-like growth, of viral origin, typically on hands and feet.
Virus	Obligate intracellular parasite of living cells consisting of an outer capsid and an inner core of nucleic acid is referred to as virus. The term virus usually refers to those particles that infect eukaryotes whilst the term bacteriophage or phage is used to describe those infecting prokaryotes.
Herpes simplex	Herpes simplex refers to two common types of viruses, herpes simplex virus 1 and herpes simplex virus 2. Herpes simplex virus 2 is responsible for the STD known as genital herpes.
Resistance	Resistance refers to a nonspecific ability to ward off infection or disease regardless of whether the body has been previously exposed to it. A force that opposes the flow of a fluid such as air or blood. Compare with immunity.
Stress	Stress refers to a condition that is a response to factors that change the human systems normal state.
Neoplasm	Neoplasm refers to abnormal growth of cells; often used to mean a tumor.
Young adult	An young adult is someone between the ages of 20 and 40 years old.
Plantar warts	Plantar warts are warts caused by the human papilloma virus (HPV). They are small lesions that appear on the sole of the foot and are cauliflower in appearance and may have small black specks within them which are abnormal capillaries.
Genital warts	A sexually transmitted disease, caused by a virus, that forms growths or bumps on the external genitalia, in or around the vagina or anus, or on the cervix in females or penis, scrotum, groin, or thigh in males are called genital warts.
Dermatophyte	A dermatophyte is a fungus parasitic upon the skin.
Fungi	Fungi refers to simple parasitic life forms, including molds, mildews, yeasts, and mushrooms. They live on dead or decaying organic matter. Fungi can grow as single cells, like yeast, or as multicellular colonies, as seen with molds.
Solution	Solution refers to homogenous mixture formed when a solute is dissolved in a solvent.
Candidiasis	Candidiasis, commonly called yeast infection, is a fungal infection of any of the Candida species. Yeast organisms are always present in all people, but are usually prevented from "overgrowth" by naturally occurring microorganisms.
Tinea cruris	Tinea cruris refers to a fungal infection of the groin caused by either Epidermophytonfloccosusn, Trichophyton mentagrophytes, or T rubrum; also known as jock itch.
Tinea	A name applied to many different kinds of superficial fungal infections of the skin, nails, and hair, the specific type usually designated by a modifying term is referred to as tinea.
Vagina	The vagina is the tubular tract leading from the uterus to the exterior of the body in female placental mammals and marsupials, or to the cloaca in female birds, monotremes, and some reptiles. Female insects and other invertebrates also have a vagina, which is the terminal part of the oviduct.
Thrush	Thrush is an infection of the oral mucous membrane by the fungus Candida albicans; also known as oral candidiasis.
Agent	Agent refers to an epidemiological term referring to the organism or object that transmits a disease from the environment to the host.

Chapter 18. Diseases of the Skin

Chapter 18. Diseases of the Skin

Epidemic	An epidemic is a disease that appears as new cases in a given human population, during a given period, at a rate that substantially exceeds what is "expected", based on recent experience.
Saliva	Saliva is the moist, clear, and usually somewhat frothy substance produced in the mouths of some animals, including humans.
Egg	An egg is the zygote, resulting from fertilization of the ovum. It nourishes and protects the embryo.
Sexually transmitted disease	Infection transmitted from one individual to another by direct contact during sexual activity is referred to as a sexually transmitted disease.
Hypersensitivity	Hypersensitivity is an immune response that damages the body's own tissues. Four or five types of hypersensitivity are often described; immediate, antibody-dependent, immune complex, cell-mediated, and stimulatory.
Allergy	An allergy or Type I hypersensitivity is an immune malfunction whereby a person's body is hypersensitized to react immunologically to typically nonimmunogenic substances. When a person is hypersensitized, these substances are known as allergens.
Predisposition	Predisposition refers to an inclination or diathesis to respond in a certain way, either inborn or acquired. In abnormal psychology, it is a factor that lowers the ability to withstand stress and inclines the individual toward pathology.
Allergen	An allergen is any substance (antigen), most often eaten or inhaled, that is recognized by the immune system and causes an allergic reaction.
Capillaries	Capillaries refer to the smallest of the blood vessels and the sites of exchange between the blood and tissue cells.
Capillary	A capillary is the smallest of a body's blood vessels, measuring 5-10 micro meters. They connect arteries and veins, and most closely interact with tissues. Their walls are composed of a single layer of cells, the endothelium. This layer is so thin that molecules such as oxygen, water and lipids can pass through them by diffusion and enter the tissues.
Steroid	A steroid is a lipid characterized by a carbon skeleton with four fused rings. Different steroids vary in the functional groups attached to these rings. Hundreds of distinct steroids have been identified in plants and animals. Their most important role in most living systems is as hormones.
Antihistamine	An antihistamine is a drug which serves to reduce or eliminate effects mediated by histamine, an endogenous chemical mediator released during allergic reactions, through action at the histamine receptor.
Sensitization	Sensitization refers to the type of sensory adaptation in which we become more sensitive to stimuli that are low in magnitude. Also called positive adaptation. The first exposure of the body to an allergen.
Lymphocyte	A lymphocyte is a type of white blood cell involved in the human body's immune system. There are two broad categories, namely T cells and B cells.
Antigen	An antigen is a substance that stimulates an immune response, especially the production of antibodies. They are usually proteins or polysaccharides, but can be any type of molecule, including small molecules (haptens) coupled to a protein (carrier).
Corticosteroid	Any steroid hormone secreted by the adrenal cortex, such as aldosterone, cortisol, and sex steroids is called a corticosteroid.
Allergic	Allergic contact dermatitis refers to an allergic reaction caused by haptens that combine

Chapter 18. Diseases of the Skin

Chapter 18. Diseases of the Skin

contact dermatitis	with proteins in the skin to form the allergen that produces the immune response.
Anaphylaxis	Anaphylaxis refers to an immediate hypersensitivity reaction following exposure of a sensitized individual to the appropriate antigen.
Shock	Circulatory shock, a state of cardiac output that is insufficient to meet the body's physiological needs, with consequences ranging from fainting to death is referred to as shock. Insulin shock, a state of severe hypoglycemia caused by administration of insulin.
Tetracycline	Tetracycline is an antibiotic produced by the streptomyces bacterium, indicated for use against many bacterial infections. It is commonly used to treat acne.
Penicillin	Penicillin refers to a group of β-lactam antibiotics used in the treatment of bacterial infections caused by susceptible, usually Gram-positive, organisms.
Morphine	Morphine, the principal active agent in opium, is a powerful opioid analgesic drug. According to recent research, it may also be produced naturally by the human brain. Morphine is usually highly addictive, and tolerance and physical and psychological dependence develop quickly.
Codeine	Codeine is an opioid used for its analgesic, antitussive and antidiarrheal properties
Anticonvulsant	The anticonvulsant belong to a diverse group of pharmaceuticals used in prevention of the occurrence of epileptic seizures. The goal of an anticonvulsant is to suppress the rapid and excessive firing of neurons that start a seizure.
Incidence	In epidemiological studies of a particular disorder, the rate at which new cases occur in a given place at a given time is called incidence.
Melanoma	Melanoma is a malignant tumor of melanocytes. Melanocytes predominantly occur in the skin but can be found elsewhere, especially the eye. The vast majority of melanomas originate in the skin.
Cancer	Cancer is a class of diseases or disorders characterized by uncontrolled division of cells and the ability of these cells to invade other tissues, either by direct growth into adjacent tissue through invasion or by implantation into distant sites by metastasis.
Carcinogen	A carcinogen is any substance or agent that promotes cancer. A carcinogen is often, but not necessarily, a mutagen or teratogen.
Carcinoma	Cancer that originates in the coverings of the body, such as the skin or the lining of the intestinal tract is a carcinoma.
Basal cell carcinoma	Basal cell carcinoma refers to the most common form of skin cancer that forms in the innermost skin layer.
Channel	Channel, in communications (sometimes called communications channel), refers to the medium used to convey information from a sender (or transmitter) to a receiver.
Squamous cell carcinoma	In medicine, squamous cell carcinoma is a form of cancer of the carcinoma type that may occur in many different organs, including the skin, the esophagus, the lungs, and the cervix.
Radiation	The emission of electromagnetic waves by all objects warmer than absolute zero is referred to as radiation.
Sarcoma	Cancer of the supportive tissues, such as bone, cartilage, and muscle is referred to as sarcoma.
Metastasis	The spread of cancer cells beyond their original site are called metastasis.
Infiltration	Infiltration is the diffusion or accumulation (in a tissue or cells) of substances not normal to it or in amounts in excess of the normal. The material collected in those tissues or cells

Chapter 18. Diseases of the Skin

Chapter 18. Diseases of the Skin

	is also called infiltration.
Prognosis	Prognosis refers to the prospects for the future or outcome of a disease.
Sebaceous gland	The sebaceous gland is found in the skin of mammals. They secrete an oily substance called sebum that is made of fat and the debris of dead fat-producing cells. These glands exist in humans througout the skin except in the palms and soles.
Hyperactivity	Hyperactivity can be described as a state in which a individual is abnormally easily excitable and exuberant. Strong emotional reactions and a very short span of attention is also typical for the individual.
Population	Population refers to all members of a well-defined group of organisms, events, or things.
Constant	A behavior or characteristic that does not vary from one observation to another is referred to as a constant.
Brain	The part of the central nervous system involved in regulating and controlling body activity and interpreting information from the senses transmitted through the nervous system is referred to as the brain.
Cyst	A cyst is a closed sac having a distinct membrane and developing abnormally in a cavity or structure of the body. They may occur as a result of a developmental error in the embryo during pregnancy or they may be caused by infections.
Puberty	A time in the life of a developing individual characterized by the increasing production of sex hormones, which cause it to reach sexual maturity is called puberty.
Estrogen	Estrogen is a steroid that functions as the primary female sex hormone. While present in both men and women, they are found in women in significantly higher quantities.
Sebum	Oily secretion of the sebaceous glands is sebum.
Lead	Lead is a chemical element in the periodic table that has the symbol Pb and atomic number 82. A soft, heavy, toxic and malleable poor metal, lead is bluish white when freshly cut but tarnishes to dull gray when exposed to air. Lead is used in building construction, lead-acid batteries, bullets and shot, and is part of solder, pewter, and fusible alloys.
Rosacea	Rosacea is a common but often misunderstood condition that is estimated to affect over 45 million people worldwide. It begins as flushing and redness on the central face and across the cheeks, nose, or forehead but can also less commonly affect the neck, chest, scalp or ears.
Idiopathic	Idiopathic is a medical adjective that indicates that a recognized cause has not yet been established.
Older adult	Older adult is an adult over the age of 65.
Exacerbation	Exacerbation is a period in an illness when the symptoms of the disease reappear.
Albinism	Albinism is a lack of pigmentation in the eyes, skin and hair. Albinism is an inherited condition resulting from the combination of recessive alleles passed from both parents of an individual. This condition is known to affect mammals, fish, birds, reptiles, and amphibians.
Eye	An eye is an organ that detects light. Different kinds of light-sensitive organs are found in a variety of creatures. The simplest eyes do nothing but detect whether the surroundings are light or dark, while more complex eyes can distinguish shapes and colors.
Purulent	Anything that creates or contains pus is purulent.
Culture	Culture, generally refers to patterns of human activity and the symbolic structures that give such activity significance.

Chapter 18. Diseases of the Skin

Chapter 18. Diseases of the Skin

Microscope	A microscope is an instrument for viewing objects that are too small to be seen by the naked or unaided eye.
Neoplastic	The least common and most severe type of pemphigus is the neoplastic variety. This disorder is usually found in conjunction with an already-existing malignancy. Very painful sores appear on the mouth, lips, and the esophagus.
Biopsy	Removal of small tissue sample from the body for microscopic examination is called biopsy.
Neoplasia	Neoplasia refers to abnormal, disorganized growth in a tissue or organ; often used to mean formation of cancer.
Benign tumor	A benign tumor does not invade neighboring tissues and do not seed metastases, but may locally grow to great size. They usually do not return after surgical removal.
Ringworm	Ringworm is a contagious fungal infection of the skin. Ringworm is very common, especially among children, and may be spread by skin-to-skin contact, as well as via contact with contaminated items such as hairbrushes.
Outpatient	Outpatient refers to a patient who requires treatment but does not need to be admitted into the institution for those sevices.
Complaint	Complaint refers to report made by the police or some other agency to the court that initiates the intake process.
Chemotherapy	Chemotherapy is the use of chemical substances to treat disease. In its modern-day use, it refers almost exclusively to cytostatic drugs used to treat cancer. In its non-oncological use, the term may also refer to antibiotics.
Penis	The penis is the male reproductive organ and for mammals additionally serves as the external male organ of urination.
Antipsychotic	The term antipsychotic is applied to a group of drugs used to treat psychosis.
Systemic infection	Systemic infection is a generic term for infection caused by microorganisms in animals or plants, where the causal agent (the microbe) has spread actively or passively in the host's anatomy and is disseminated throughout several organs in different systems of the host.
Wellness	A dimension of health beyond the absence of disease or infirmity, including social, emotional, and spiritual aspects of health is called wellness.

Chapter 18. Diseases of the Skin

Chapter 19. Stress and Aging

Dehydration	Dehydration is the removal of water from an object. Medically, dehydration is a serious and potentially life-threatening condition in which the body contains an insufficient volume of water for normal functioning.
Tissue	A collection of interconnected cells that perform a similar function within an organism is called tissue.
Overhydration	An excess of water in the body is overhydration.
Hypothalamus	Located below the thalamus, the hypothalamus links the nervous system to the endocrine system by synthesizing and secreting neurohormones often called releasing hormones because they function by stimulating the secretion of hormones from the anterior pituitary gland.
Gland	A gland is an organ in an animal's body that synthesizes a substance for release such as hormones, often into the bloodstream or into cavities inside the body or its outer surface.
Brain	The part of the central nervous system involved in regulating and controlling body activity and interpreting information from the senses transmitted through the nervous system is referred to as the brain.
Pituitary gland	The pituitary gland or hypophysis is an endocrine gland about the size of a pea that sits in the small, bony cavity (sella turcica) at the base of the brain. Its posterior lobe is connected to a part of the brain called the hypothalamus via the infundibulum (or stalk), giving rise to the tuberoinfundibular pathway.
Homeostasis	Homeostasis is the property of an open system, especially living organisms, to regulate its internal environment to maintain a stable, constant condition, by means of multiple dynamic equilibrium adjustments, controlled by interrelated regulation mechanisms.
Hormone	A hormone is a chemical messenger from one cell to another. All multicellular organisms produce hormones. The best known hormones are those produced by endocrine glands of vertebrate animals, but hormones are produced by nearly every organ system and tissue type in a human or animal body. Hormone molecules are secreted directly into the bloodstream, they move by circulation or diffusion to their target cells, which may be nearby cells in the same tissue or cells of a distant organ of the body.
Stress	Stress refers to a condition that is a response to factors that change the human systems normal state.
Nervous system	The nervous system of an animal coordinates the activity of the muscles, monitors the organs, constructs and processes input from the senses, and initiates actions.
Health	Health is a term that refers to a combination of the absence of illness, the ability to cope with everyday activities, physical fitness, and high quality of life.
Autonomic nervous system	The autonomic nervous system is the part of the nervous system that is not consciously controlled. It is commonly divided into two usually antagonistic subsystems: the sympathetic and parasympathetic nervous system.
Sympathetic	The sympathetic nervous system activates what is often termed the "fight or flight response". It is an automatic regulation system, that is, one that operates without the intervention of conscious thought.
Parasympathetic division	Parasympathetic division refers to one of two sets of neurons in the autonomic nervous system. It generally promotes body activities that gain and conserve energy, such as digestion and reduced heart rate.
Sympathetic division	Sympathetic division refers to one of two sets of neurons in the autonomic nervous system. It generally prepares the body for energy-consuming activities, such as fleeing or fighting. It also is a subdivision of the autonomic nervous system.

Chapter 19. Stress and Aging

Chapter 19. Stress and Aging

Blood	Blood is a circulating tissue composed of fluid plasma and cells. The main function of blood is to supply nutrients (oxygen, glucose) and constitutional elements to tissues and to remove waste products.
Blood pressure	Blood pressure is the pressure exerted by the blood on the walls of the blood vessels.
Digestion	Digestion refers to the mechanical and chemical breakdown of food into molecules small enough for the body to absorb; the second main stage of food processing, following ingestion.
Muscle	Muscle is a contractile form of tissue. It is one of the four major tissue types, the other three being epithelium, connective tissue and nervous tissue. Muscle contraction is used to move parts of the body, as well as to move substances within the body.
Digestive tract	The digestive tract is the system of organs within multicellular animals which takes in food, digests it to extract energy and nutrients, and expels the remaining waste.
Glucose	Glucose, a simple monosaccharide sugar, is one of the most important carbohydrates and is used as a source of energy in animals and plants. Glucose is one of the main products of photosynthesis and starts respiration.
Liver	The liver is an organ in vertebrates, including humans. It plays a major role in metabolism and has a number of functions in the body including drug detoxification, glycogen storage, and plasma protein synthesis. It also produces bile, which is important for digestion.
Metabolism	Metabolism is the biochemical modification of chemical compounds in living organisms and cells. This includes the biosynthesis of complex organic molecules (anabolism) and their breakdown (catabolism).
Thyroxine	The thyroid hormone thyroxine is a tyrosine-based hormone produced by the thyroid gland. An important component in the synthesis is iodine. It acts on the body to increase the basal metabolic rate, affect protein synthesis and increase the body's sensitivity to catecholamines.
Thyroid	The thyroid is one of the larger endocrine glands in the body. It is located in the neck and produces hormones, principally thyroxine and triiodothyronine, that regulate the rate of metabolism and affect the growth and rate of function of many other systems in the body.
Cortisol	Cortisol is a corticosteroid hormone that is involved in the response to stress; it increases blood pressure and blood sugar levels and suppresses the immune system.
Adrenal	In mammals, the adrenal glands are the triangle-shaped endocrine glands that sit atop the kidneys. They are chiefly responsible for regulating the stress response through the synthesis of corticosteroids and catecholamines, including cortisol and adrenaline.
Adrenocortic-tropic hormone	Adrenocorticotropic hormone is a polypeptide hormone synthesised and secreted from corticotropes in the anterior lobe of the pituitary gland in response to the hormone corticotropin-releasing factor released by the hypothalamus. It stimulates the cortex of the adrenal gland and boosts the synthesis of corticosteroids, mainly glucocorticoids but also mineralcorticoids and sex steroids.
Corticosteroid	Any steroid hormone secreted by the adrenal cortex, such as aldosterone, cortisol, and sex steroids is called a corticosteroid.
Alarm reaction	The first stage of the general adaptation syndrome, which is triggered by the impact of a stressor and characterized by sympathetic activity is called the alarm reaction.
Adrenal gland	In mammals, the adrenal gland (also known as suprarenal glands or colloquially as kidney hats) are the triangle-shaped endocrine glands that sit atop the kidneys; their name indicates that position.
Immune response	The body's defensive reaction to invasion by bacteria, viral agents, or other foreign

Chapter 19. Stress and Aging

Chapter 19. Stress and Aging

	substances is called immune response.
Vitamin	An organic compound other than a carbohydrate, lipid, or protein that is needed for normal metabolism but that the body cannot synthesize in adequate amounts is called a vitamin.
Stress hormones	Group of hormones including cortico steroids, that are involved in the body's physiological stress response are referred to as stress hormones.
Epinephrine	Epinephrine is a hormone and a neurotransmitter. Epinephrine plays a central role in the short-term stress reaction—the physiological response to threatening or exciting conditions (fight-or-flight response). It is secreted by the adrenal medulla.
Sympathetic nervous system	The sympathetic nervous system activates what is often termed the "fight or flight response". Messages travel through in a bidirectional flow. Efferent messages can trigger changes in different parts of the body simultaneously.
Neurotransmitter	A neurotransmitter is a chemical that is used to relay, amplify and modulate electrical signals between a neuron and another cell.
Cardiac output	Cardiac output is the volume of blood being pumped by the heart in a minute. It is equal to the heart rate multiplied by the stroke volume.
Arthritis	Arthritis is a group of conditions that affect the health of the bone joints in the body. Arthritis can be caused from strains and injuries caused by repetitive motion, sports, overexertion, and falls. Unlike the autoimmune diseases, it largely affects older people and results from the degeneration of joint cartilage.
Allergy	An allergy or Type I hypersensitivity is an immune malfunction whereby a person's body is hypersensitized to react immunologically to typically nonimmunogenic substances. When a person is hypersensitized, these substances are known as allergens.
Rheumatoid arthritis	Rheumatoid arthritis is a chronic, inflammatory autoimmune disorder that causes the immune system to attack the joints. It is a disabling and painful inflammatory condition, which can lead to substantial loss of mobility due to pain and joint destruction.
Infection	The invasion and multiplication of microorganisms in body tissues is called an infection.
Edema	Edema is swelling of any organ or tissue due to accumulation of excess fluid. Edema has many root causes, but its common mechanism is accumulation of fluid into the tissues.
Cardiovascular system	The circulatory system or cardiovascular system is the organ system which circulates blood around the body of most animals.
Blood vessel	A blood vessel is a part of the circulatory system and function to transport blood throughout the body. The most important types, arteries and veins, are so termed because they carry blood away from or towards the heart, respectively.
Aldosterone	Aldosterone is a steroid hormone synthesized from cholesterol by the enzyme aldosterone synthase. It helps regulate the body's electrolyte balance by acting on the mineralocorticoid receptor. It diminishes the secretion of sodium ions and therefore, water and stimulates the secretion of potassium ions through the kidneys.
Sodium	Sodium is the chemical element in the periodic table that has the symbol Na (Natrium in Latin) and atomic number 11. Sodium is a soft, waxy, silvery reactive metal belonging to the alkali metals that is abundant in natural compounds (especially halite). It is highly reactive.
Hypertension	Hypertension is a medical condition where the blood pressure in the arteries is chronically elevated. Persistent hypertension is one of the risk factors for strokes, heart attacks, heart failure and arterial aneurysm, and is a leading cause of chronic renal failure.

Chapter 19. Stress and Aging

Chapter 19. Stress and Aging

Wellness	A dimension of health beyond the absence of disease or infirmity, including social, emotional, and spiritual aspects of health is called wellness.
Releasing hormone	A releasing hormone is a hormone whose main purpose is to stimulate the release of another hormone.
Respiratory system	The respiratory system is the biological system of any organism that engages in gas exchange.In humans and other mammals, the respiratory system consists of the airways, the lungs, and the respiratory muscles that mediate the movement of air into and out of the body.
Common cold	An acute, self-limiting, and highly contagious virus infection of the upper respiratory tract that produces inflammation, profuse discharge, and other symptoms is referred to as the common cold.
Asthma	Asthma is a complex disease characterized by bronchial hyperresponsiveness (BHR), inflammation, mucus production and intermittent airway obstruction.
Hyperactivity	Hyperactivity can be described as a state in which a individual is abnormally easily excitable and exuberant. Strong emotional reactions and a very short span of attention is also typical for the individual.
Tuberculosis	Tuberculosis is an infection caused by the bacterium Mycobacterium tuberculosis, which most commonly affects the lungs but can also affect the central nervous system, lymphatic system, circulatory system, genitourinary system, bones and joints.
Skin	Skin is an organ of the integumentary system composed of a layer of tissues that protect underlying muscles and organs.
Integumentary system	Integumentary system is often the largest organ system of an animal, comprising skin, hair, feathers, scales, nails, skin glands and their products (sweat, slime). It separates, protects, and informs the animal with regard to its surroundings.
Immune system	The immune system is the system of specialized cells and organs that protect an organism from outside biological influences. When the immune system is functioning properly, it protects the body against bacteria and viral infections, destroying cancer cells and foreign substances.
Resistance	Resistance refers to a nonspecific ability to ward off infection or disease regardless of whether the body has been previously exposed to it. A force that opposes the flow of a fluid such as air or blood. Compare with immunity.
Cold sore	Cold sore refers to a lesion caused by the herpes simplex virus; usually occurs on the border of the lips or nares. Also known as a fever blister or herpes labialis.
Viral	Viral phenomena are objects or patterns able to replicate themselves or convert other objects into copies of themselves when these objects are exposed to them.
Virus	Obligate intracellular parasite of living cells consisting of an outer capsid and an inner core of nucleic acid is referred to as virus. The term virus usually refers to those particles that infect eukaryotes whilst the term bacteriophage or phage is used to describe those infecting prokaryotes.
Inflammatory response	Inflammatory response refers to a complex sequence of events involving chemicals and immune cells that results in the isolation and destruction of antigens and tissues near the antigens.
Lesion	A lesion is a non-specific term referring to abnormal tissue in the body. It can be caused by any disease process including trauma (physical, chemical, electrical), infection, neoplasm, metabolic and autoimmune.
Diarrhea	Diarrhea or diarrhoea is a condition in which the sufferer has frequent and watery, chunky,

Chapter 19. Stress and Aging

Chapter 19. Stress and Aging

	or loose bowel movements.
Constipation	Constipation is a condition of the digestive system where a person (or other animal) experiences hard feces that are difficult to eliminate; it may be extremely painful, and in severe cases (fecal impaction) lead to symptoms of bowel obstruction.
Trauma	Trauma refers to a severe physical injury or wound to the body caused by an external force, or a psychological shock having a lasting effect on mental life.
Ulcer	An ulcer is an open sore of the skin, eyes or mucous membrane, often caused by an initial abrasion and generally maintained by an inflammation and/or an infection.
Shock	Circulatory shock, a state of cardiac output that is insufficient to meet the body's physiological needs, with consequences ranging from fainting to death is referred to as shock. Insulin shock, a state of severe hypoglycemia caused by administration of insulin.
Inflammation	Inflammation is the first response of the immune system to infection or irritation and may be referred to as the innate cascade.
Colon	The colon is the part of the intestine from the cecum to the rectum. Its primary purpose is to extract water from feces.
Ulcerative colitis	Ulcerative colitis (UC) is a form of inflammatory bowel disease (IBD) featuring systemic inflammation specifically causing episodic mucosal inflammation of the colon (large bowel).
Mucus	Mucus is a slippery secretion of the lining of various membranes in the body (mucous membranes). Mucus aids in the protection of the lungs by trapping foreign particles that enter the nose during normal breathing. Additionally, it prevents tissues from drying out.
Antibiotic	Antibiotic refers to substance such as penicillin or streptomycin that is toxic to microorganisms. Usually a product of a particular microorvanism or plant.
Anxiety	Anxiety is a complex combination of the feeling of fear, apprehension and worry often accompanied by physical sensations such as palpitations, chest pain and/or shortness of breath.
Pain	Pain is an unpleasant sensation which may be associated with actual or potential tissue damage and which may have physical and emotional components.
Migraine	Migraine is a neurologic disease, of which the most common symptom is an intense and disabling headache. Migraine is the most common type of vascular headache.
Photophobia	Photophobia is a symptom of excessive sensitivity to light and the aversion to sunlight or well-lit places.
Alcohol	Alcohol is a general term, applied to any organic compound in which a hydroxyl group (-OH) is bound to a carbon atom, which in turn is bound to other hydrogen and/or carbon atoms. The general formula for a simple acyclic alcohol is $C_nH_{2n+1}OH$.
Flushing	For a person to flush is to become markedly red in the face and often other areas of the skin, from various physiological conditions. Flushing is generally distinguished, despite a close physiological relation between them, from blushing, which is milder, generally restricted to the face or cheeks, and generally assumed to reflect embarrassment.
Aura	An aura is the perceptual disturbance experienced by some migraine sufferers before a migraine headache, and the telltale sensation experienced by some epileptics before a seizure. It often manifests as a strange light or an unpleasant smell.
Vasodilation	An increase in the diameter of superficial blood vessels triggered by nerve signals that relax the smooth muscles of the vessel walls is referred to as vasodilation.
Cranial	In the limbs of most animals, the terms cranial and caudal are used in the regions proximal

Go to **Cram101.com** for the Practice Tests for this Chapter.

Chapter 19. Stress and Aging

Chapter 19. Stress and Aging

	to the carpus (the wrist, in the forelimb) and the tarsus (the ankle in the hindlimb). Objects and surfaces closer to or facing towards the head are cranial; those facing away or further from the head are caudal.
Artery	Vessel that takes blood away from the heart to the tissues and organs of the body is called an artery.
Vasoconstriction	Vasoconstriction refers to a decrease in the diameter of a blood vessel.
Eye	An eye is an organ that detects light. Different kinds of light-sensitive organs are found in a variety of creatures. The simplest eyes do nothing but detect whether the surroundings are light or dark, while more complex eyes can distinguish shapes and colors.
Nerve	A nerve is an enclosed, cable-like bundle of nerve fibers or axons, which includes the glia that ensheath the axons in myelin.
Serotonin	Serotonin is a monoamine neurotransmitter synthesized in serotonergic neurons in the central nervous system and enterochromaffin cells in the gastrointestinal tract. It is believed to play an important part of the biochemistry of depression, migraine, bipolar disorder and anxiety.
Vasoconstrictor	A vasoconstrictor is any substance that acts to constrict blood vessels. Many act on specific receptors, such as vasopressin receptors or adrenoreceptors. They are are also used clinically to increase blood pressure or to reduce local blood flow.
Analgesic	An analgesic is any member of the diverse group of drugs used to relieve pain and to achieve analgesia. Analgesic drugs act in various ways on the peripheral and central nervous system.
Affect	Affect is the scientific term used to describe a subject's externally displayed mood. This can be assesed by the nurse by observing facial expression, tone of voice, and body language.
Antidepressants	Antidepressants are medications used primarily in the treatment of clinical depression. Antidepressants create little if any immediate change in mood and require between several days and several weeks to take effect.
Antidepressant	An antidepressant is a medication used primarily in the treatment of clinical depression. They are not thought to produce tolerance, although sudden withdrawal may produce adverse effects. They create little if any immediate change in mood and require between several days and several weeks to take effect.
Cluster headache	Cluster headache sufferers typically experience very severe headaches of a piercing quality near one eye or temple that last for between 15 minutes and three hours. The headaches are unilateral and occasionally change sides.
Sleep deprivation	Sleep deprivation is an overall lack of the necessary amount of sleep. A person can be deprived of sleep by their own body and mind, insomnia, or actively deprived by another individual.
Sexuality	Sexuality refers to the expression of sexual sensation and related intimacy between human beings, as well as the expression of identity through sex and as influenced by or based on
Organ	Organ refers to a structure consisting of several tissues adapted as a group to perform specific functions.
Ovaries	Ovaries are egg-producing reproductive organs found in female organisms.
Testes	The testes are the male generative glands in animals. Male mammals have two testes, which are often contained within an extension of the abdomen called the scrotum.
Ovary	The primary reproductive organ of a female is called an ovary.
Menstruation	Loss of blood and tissue from the uterine lining at the end of a female reproductive cycle

Chapter 19. Stress and Aging

Chapter 19. Stress and Aging

	are referred to as menstruation.
Libido	Libido in its common usage means sexual desire, however more technical definitions, such as found in the work of Carl Jung, are more general, referring to libido as the free creative, or psychic, energy an individual has to put toward personal development, or individuation.
Sperm	Sperm refers to the male sex cell with three distinct parts at maturity: head, middle piece, and tail.
Gonad	Gonad refers to a sex organ in an animal; an ovary or a testis. It is the organ that makes gametes.
Gonadotropic hormone	Substance secreted by anterior pituitary that regulates the activity of the ovaries and testes is referred to as gonadotropic hormone.
Gonadotropin	A hormone that stimulates the gonads is gonadotropin. They are protein hormones secreted by gonadotrope cells of the pituitary gland of vertebrates.
Biofeedback	Biofeedback is the process of measuring and quantifying an aspect of a subject's physiology, analyzing the data, and then feeding back the information to the subject in a form that allows the subject to enact physiological change.
Free radicals	Free radicals are atomic or molecular species with unpaired electrons on an otherwise open shell configuration.
Endocrine gland	An endocrine gland is one of a set of internal organs involved in the secretion of hormones into the blood. These glands are known as ductless, which means they do not have tubes inside them.
Follicle	Follicle refers to a cluster of cells surrounding, protecting, and nourishing a developing egg cell in the ovary; also secretes estrogen. In botany, a follicle is a type of simple dry fruit produced by certain flowering plants. It is regarded as one the most primitive types of fruits, and derives from a simple pistil or carpel.
Melanin	Broadly, melanin is any of the polyacetylene, polyaniline, and polypyrrole "blacks" or their mixed copolymers. The most common form of biological melanin is a polymer of either or both of two monomer molecules: indolequinone, and dihydroxyindole carboxylic acid.
Hair follicle	A hair follicle is part of the skin that grows hair by packing old cells together. Attached to the follicle is a sebaceous gland, a tiny sebum-producing gland found everywhere except on the palms and soles of the feet.
Heredity	Heredity refers to the transmission of genetic information from parent to offspring.
Diagnosis	In medicine, diagnosis is the process of identifying a medical condition or disease by its signs, symptoms, and from the results of various diagnostic procedures.
Diabetes	Diabetes is a medical disorder characterized by varying or persistent elevated blood sugar levels, especially after eating. All types of diabetes share similar symptoms and complications at advanced stages: dehydration and ketoacidosis, cardiovascular disease, chronic renal failure, retinal damage which can lead to blindness, nerve damage which can lead to erectile dysfunction, gangrene with risk of amputation of toes, feet, and even legs.
Course	Pattern of development and change of a disorder over time is a course.
Elderly	Old age consists of ages nearing the average life span of human beings, and thus the end of the human life cycle. Euphemisms for older people include advanced adult, elderly, and senior or senior citizen.
Osteoporosis	Osteoporosis is a disease of bone in which bone mineral density (BMD) is reduced, bone microarchitecture is disrupted, the amount and variety of non-collagenous proteins in bone is

Chapter 19. Stress and Aging

Chapter 19. Stress and Aging

	changed, and a concomitantly fracture risk is increased.
Lead	Lead is a chemical element in the periodic table that has the symbol Pb and atomic number 82. A soft, heavy, toxic and malleable poor metal, lead is bluish white when freshly cut but tarnishes to dull gray when exposed to air. Lead is used in building construction, lead-acid batteries, bullets and shot, and is part of solder, pewter, and fusible alloys.
Hip	In anatomy, the hip is the bony projection of the femur, known as the greater trochanter, and the overlying muscle and fat.
Heart attack	A heart attack, is a serious, sudden heart condition usually characterized by varying degrees of chest pain or discomfort, weakness, sweating, nausea, vomiting, and arrhythmias, sometimes causing loss of consciousness. It occurs when the blood supply to a part of the heart is interrupted, causing death and scarring of the local heart tissue.
Infarction	The sudden death of tissue from a lack of blood perfusion is referred to as an infarction.
Coronary	Referring to the heart or the blood vessels of the heart is referred to as coronary.
Myocardial infarction	Acute myocardial infarction, commonly known as a heart attack, is a serious, sudden heart condition usually characterized by varying degrees of chest pain or discomfort, weakness, sweating, nausea, vomiting, and arrhythmias, sometimes causing loss of consciousness.
Coronary arteries	Arteries that directly supply the heart with blood are referred to as coronary arteries.
Coronary artery	An artery that supplies blood to the wall of the heart is called a coronary artery.
Stroke	A stroke or cerebrovascular accident (CVA) occurs when the blood supply to a part of the brain is suddenly interrupted.
Joint	A joint (articulation) is the location at which two bones make contact (articulate). They are constructed to both allow movement and provide mechanical support.
Range of motion	Range of motion is a measurement of movement through a particular joint or muscle range.
Osteoarthritis	Osteoarthritis is a condition in which low-grade inflammation results in pain in the joints, caused by wearing of the cartilage that covers and acts as a cushion inside joints.
Thrombosis	Thrombosis is the formation of a clot inside a blood vessel, obstructing the flow of blood through the circulatory system. A cerebral thrombosis can result in stroke.
Embolism	An embolism occurs when an object (the embolus) migrates from one part of the body and causes a blockage of a blood vessel in another part of the body.
Atrophy	Atrophy is the partial or complete wasting away of a part of the body. Causes of atrophy include poor nourishment, poor circulation, loss of hormonal support, loss of nerve supply to the target organ, disuse or lack of exercise, or disease intrinsic to the tissue itself.
Gallbladder	The gallbladder is a pear-shaped organ that stores bile until the body needs it for digestion. It is connected to the liver and the duodenum by the biliary tract.
Complaint	Complaint refers to report made by the police or some other agency to the court that initiates the intake process.
Hyperplasia	Hyperplasia is a general term for an increase in the number of the cells of an organ or tissue causing it to increase in size.
Cystitis	Cystitis is the inflammation of the bladder. The condition primarily affects women, but can affect all age groups from either sex.
Bladder	A hollow muscular storage organ for storing urine is a bladder.

Chapter 19. Stress and Aging

Chapter 19. Stress and Aging

Urine	Concentrated filtrate produced by the kidneys and excreted via the bladder is called urine.
Urinary tract infection	A urinary tract infection is an infection anywhere from the kidneys to the ureters to the bladder to the urethra.
Urination	Urination is the process of disposing urine from the urinary bladder through the urethra to the outside of the body. The process of urination is usually under voluntary control.
Urinary incontinence	Urinary incontinence is the involuntary excretion of urine from one's body. It is often temporary, and it almost always results from an underlying medical condition.
Cancer	Cancer is a class of diseases or disorders characterized by uncontrolled division of cells and the ability of these cells to invade other tissues, either by direct growth into adjacent tissue through invasion or by implantation into distant sites by metastasis.
Agent	Agent refers to an epidemiological term referring to the organism or object that transmits a disease from the environment to the host.
Cataract	Opaqueness of the lens of the eye, making the lens incapable of transmitting light is called a cataract.
Visual acuity	The ability of the eyes to distinguish fine detail is visual acuity.
Lens	The lens or crystalline lens is a transparent, biconvex structure in the eye that, along with the cornea, helps to refract light to focus on the retina. Its function is thus similar to a man-made optical lens.
Outpatient	Outpatient refers to a patient who requires treatment but does not need to be admitted into the institution for those sevices.
Intraocular	Intraocular describes anything of or related to the inside of the eyeball.
Disorientation	A state of mental confusion with respect to time, place, identity of self, other persons, and objects is disorientation.
Delusion	A false belief, not generally shared by others, and that cannot be changed despite strong evidence to the contrary is a delusion.
Apathy	Apathy is the lack of emotion, motivation, or enthusiasm. Apathy is a psychological term for a state of indifference — where an individual is unresponsive or "indifferent" to aspects of emotional, social, or physical life.
Anesthesia	Anesthesia is the process of blocking the perception of pain and other sensations. This allows patients to undergo surgery and other procedures without the distress and pain they would otherwise experience.
Local anesthesia	Local anesthesia is any technique to render part of the body insensitive to pain without affecting consciousness.
Epidemiology	Epidemiology is the study of the distribution and determinants of disease and disorders in human populations, and the use of its knowledge to control health problems.Epidemiology is considered the cornerstone methodology in all of public health research, and is highly regarded in evidence-based clinical medicine for identifying risk factors for disease and determining optimal treatment approaches to clinical practice.
Syndrome	Syndrome is the association of several clinically recognizable features, signs, symptoms, phenomena or characteristics which often occur together, so that the presence of one feature alerts the physician to the presence of the others
Irritability	Irritability is an excessive response to stimuli. Irritability takes many forms, from the contraction of a unicellular organism when touched to complex reactions involving all the senses of higher animals.

Chapter 19. Stress and Aging

Chapter 19. Stress and Aging

Depression	In everyday language depression refers to any downturn in mood, which may be relatively transitory and perhaps due to something trivial. This is differentiated from Clinical depression which is marked by symptoms that last two weeks or more and are so severe that they interfere with daily living.
Hallucination	Hallucination refers to a perception in the absence of sensory stimulation that is confused with reality.
Nerve cell	A cell specialized to originate or transmit nerve impulses is referred to as nerve cell.
Cortex	In anatomy and zoology the cortex is the outermost or superficial layer of an organ or the outer portion of the stem or root of a plant.
Neuron	The neuron is a major class of cells in the nervous system. In vertebrates, they are found in the brain, the spinal cord and in the nerves and ganglia of the peripheral nervous system, and their primary role is to process and transmit neural information.
Protein	A protein is a complex, high-molecular-weight organic compound that consists of amino acids joined by peptide bonds. They are essential to the structure and function of all living cells and viruses. Many are enzymes or subunits of enzymes.
Enzyme	An enzyme is a protein that catalyzes, or speeds up, a chemical reaction. They are essential to sustain life because most chemical reactions in biological cells would occur too slowly, or would lead to different products, without them.
Median	The median is a number that separates the higher half of a sample, a population, or a probability distribution from the lower half. It is the middle value in a distribution, above and below which lie an equal number of values.
Geriatrics	Geriatrics is the branch of medicine that focuses on health promotion and the prevention and treatment of disease and disability in later life.
Medicine	Medicine is the branch of health science and the sector of public life concerned with maintaining or restoring human health through the study, diagnosis and treatment of disease and injury.
Gerontology	The interdisciplinary study of aging and of the special problems of the elderly is referred to as gerontology.
Minerals	Minerals refer to inorganic chemical compounds found in nature; salts.
Anemia	Anemia is a deficiency of red blood cells and/or hemoglobin. This results in a reduced ability of blood to transfer oxygen to the tissues, and this causes hypoxia; since all human cells depend on oxygen for survival, varying degrees of anemia can have a wide range of clinical consequences.
Red blood cell	The red blood cell is the most common type of blood cell and is the vertebrate body's principal means of delivering oxygen from the lungs or gills to body tissues via the blood.
Pneumonia	Pneumonia is an illness of the lungs and respiratory system in which the microscopic, air-filled sacs (alveoli) responsible for absorbing oxygen from the atmosphere become inflamed and flooded with fluid.
Vaccine	A harmless variant or derivative of a pathogen used to stimulate a host organism's immune system to mount a long-term defense against the pathogen is referred to as vaccine.
Oxygen	Oxygen is a chemical element in the periodic table. It has the symbol O and atomic number 8. Oxygen is the second most common element on Earth, composing around 46% of the mass of Earth's crust and 28% of the mass of Earth as a whole, and is the third most common element in the universe.

Chapter 19. Stress and Aging

Chapter 19. Stress and Aging

Medulla	Medulla in general means the inner part, and derives from the Latin word for 'marrow'. In medicine it is contrasted to the cortex.
Adrenal medulla	Composed mainly of hormone-producing chromaffin cells, the adrenal medulla is the principal site of the conversion of the amino acid tyrosine into the catecholamines epinephrine and norepinephrine.
Adrenal cortex	Situated along the perimeter of the adrenal gland, the adrenal cortex mediates the stress response through the production of mineralocorticoids and glucocorticoids, including aldosterone and cortisol respectively. It is also a secondary site of androgen synthesis.
Glucocorticoid	Glucocorticoid is a class of steroid hormones characterized by the ability to bind with the cortisol receptor and trigger similar effects. They are distinguished from mineralocorticoids and sex steroids by the specific receptors, target cells, and effects.
Digestive system	The organ system that ingests food, breaks it down into smaller chemical units, and absorbs the nutrient molecules is referred to as the digestive system.
Incidence	In epidemiological studies of a particular disorder, the rate at which new cases occur in a given place at a given time is called incidence.
Critical thinking	Critical thinking consists of a mental process of analyzing or evaluating information, particularly statements or propositions that people have offered as true. It forms a process of reflecting upon the meaning of statements, examining the offered evidence and reasoning, and forming judgments about the facts.
Parasympathetic nervous system	The parasympathetic nervous system is one of two divisions of the autonomic nervous system. It conserves energy as it slows the heart rate, increases intestinal and gland activity, and relaxes sphincter muscles in the gastro-intestinal tract. In other words, it acts to reverse the effects of the sympathetic nervous system.
Peripheral nervous system	The peripheral nervous system consists of the nerves and neurons that reside or extend outside the central nervous system--to serve the limbs and organs. The peripheral nervous system is divided into the somatic nervous system and the autonomic nervous system.
Sugar	A sugar is the simplest molecule that can be identified as a carbohydrate. These include monosaccharides and disaccharides, trisaccharides and the oligosaccharides. The term "glyco-" indicates the presence of a sugar in an otherwise non-carbohydrate substance.

Chapter 19. Stress and Aging

Chapter 20. Wellness

Health	Health is a term that refers to a combination of the absence of illness, the ability to cope with everyday activities, physical fitness, and high quality of life.
Organ	Organ refers to a structure consisting of several tissues adapted as a group to perform specific functions.
Wellness	A dimension of health beyond the absence of disease or infirmity, including social, emotional, and spiritual aspects of health is called wellness.
Mental health	Mental health refers to the 'thinking' part of psychosocial health; includes your values, attitudes, and beliefs.
Cholesterol	Cholesterol is a steroid, a lipid, and an alcohol, found in the cell membranes of all body tissues, and transported in the blood plasma of all animals. It is an important component of the membranes of cells, providing stability; it makes the membrane's fluidity stable over a bigger temperature interval.
Blood	Blood is a circulating tissue composed of fluid plasma and cells. The main function of blood is to supply nutrients (oxygen, glucose) and constitutional elements to tissues and to remove waste products.
Blood pressure	Blood pressure is the pressure exerted by the blood on the walls of the blood vessels.
Sugar	A sugar is the simplest molecule that can be identified as a carbohydrate. These include monosaccharides and disaccharides, trisaccharides and the oligosaccharides. The term "glyco-" indicates the presence of a sugar in an otherwise non-carbohydrate substance.
Nicotine	Nicotine is an organic compound, an alkaloid found naturally throughout the tobacco plant, with a high concentration in the leaves. It is a potent nerve poison and is included in many insecticides. In lower concentrations, the substance is a stimulant and is one of the main factors leading to the pleasure and habit-forming qualities of tobacco smoking.
Skin	Skin is an organ of the integumentary system composed of a layer of tissues that protect underlying muscles and organs.
Craving	Craving refers to the powerful desire to use a psychoactive drug or engage in a compulsive behavior. It is manifested in physiological changes, such as raised heart rate, sweating, anxiety, drop in body temperature, pupil dilation, and stomach muscle movements.
Withdrawal symptoms	Withdrawal symptoms are physiological changes that occur when the use of a drug is stopped or dosage decreased.
Affect	Affect is the scientific term used to describe a subject's externally displayed mood. This can be assesed by the nurse by observing facial expression, tone of voice, and body language.
Diabetes	Diabetes is a medical disorder characterized by varying or persistent elevated blood sugar levels, especially after eating. All types of diabetes share similar symptoms and complications at advanced stages: dehydration and ketoacidosis, cardiovascular disease, chronic renal failure, retinal damage which can lead to blindness, nerve damage which can lead to erectile dysfunction, gangrene with risk of amputation of toes, feet, and even legs.
Cancer	Cancer is a class of diseases or disorders characterized by uncontrolled division of cells and the ability of these cells to invade other tissues, either by direct growth into adjacent tissue through invasion or by implantation into distant sites by metastasis.
Chronic disease	Disease of long duration often not detected in its early stages and from which the patient will not recover is referred to as a chronic disease.
Egg	An egg is the zygote, resulting from fertilization of the ovum. It nourishes and protects the embryo.

Chapter 20. Wellness

Chapter 20. Wellness

Fiber	Fibers used by man come from a wide variety of sources: Natural fiber include those made out of plants, animal and mineral sources. Natural fibers can be classified according to their origin.
Lipid	Lipid is one class of aliphatic hydrocarbon-containing organic compounds essential for the structure and function of living cells. They are characterized by being water-insoluble but soluble in nonpolar organic solvents.
Triglyceride	Triglyceride is a glyceride in which the glycerol is esterified with three fatty acids. They are the main constituent of vegetable oil and animal fats and play an important role in metabolism as energy sources. They contain a bit more than twice as much energy as carbohydrates and proteins.
Triglycerides	Triglycerides refer to fats and oils composed of fatty acids and glycerol; are the body's most concentrated source of energy fuel; also known as neutral fats.
Fatty acid	A fatty acid is a carboxylic acid (or organic acid), often with a long aliphatic tail (long chains), either saturated or unsaturated.
Glycerol	Glycerol is a three-carbon substance that forms the backbone of fatty acids in fats. When the body uses stored fat as a source of energy, glycerol and fatty acids are released into the bloodstream. The glycerol component can be converted to glucose by the liver and provides energy for cellular metabolism.
Acid	An acid is a water-soluble, sour-tasting chemical compound that when dissolved in water, gives a solution with a pH of less than 7.
Hydrogen	Hydrogen is a chemical element in the periodic table that has the symbol H and atomic number 1. At standard temperature and pressure it is a colorless, odorless, nonmetallic, univalent, tasteless, highly flammable diatomic gas.
Carbon	Carbon is a chemical element in the periodic table that has the symbol C and atomic number 6. An abundant nonmetallic, tetravalent element, carbon has several allotropic forms.
Atom	An atom is the smallest possible particle of a chemical element that retains its chemical properties.
Saturated fat	Saturated fat is fat that consists of triglycerides containing only fatty acids that have no double bonds between the carbon atoms of the fatty acid chain (hence, they are fully saturated with hydrogen atoms).
Epidemiology	Epidemiology is the study of the distribution and determinants of disease and disorders in human populations, and the use of its knowledge to control health problems. Epidemiology is considered the cornerstone methodology in all of public health research, and is highly regarded in evidence-based clinical medicine for identifying risk factors for disease and determining optimal treatment approaches to clinical practice.
Stress	Stress refers to a condition that is a response to factors that change the human systems normal state.
Dietary fiber	Dietary fiber is the indigestible portion of plant foods that move food through the digestive system and absorb water.
Carbohydrate	Carbohydrate is a chemical compound that contains oxygen, hydrogen, and carbon atoms. They consist of monosaccharide sugars of varying chain lengths and that have the general chemical formula $C_n(H_2O)_n$ or are derivatives of such.
Intestine	The intestine is the portion of the alimentary canal extending from the stomach to the anus and, in humans and mammals, consists of two segments, the small intestine and the large intestine. The intestine is the part of the body responsible for extracting nutrition from

Chapter 20. Wellness

Chapter 20. Wellness

	food.
Bacteria	The domain that contains procaryotic cells with primarily diacyl glycerol diesters in their membranes and with bacterial rRNA. Bacteria also is a general term for organisms that are composed of procaryotic cells and are not multicellular.
Lead	Lead is a chemical element in the periodic table that has the symbol Pb and atomic number 82. A soft, heavy, toxic and malleable poor metal, lead is bluish white when freshly cut but tarnishes to dull gray when exposed to air. Lead is used in building construction, lead-acid batteries, bullets and shot, and is part of solder, pewter, and fusible alloys.
Large intestine	In anatomy of the digestive system, the colon, also called the large intestine or large bowel, is the part of the intestine from the cecum ('caecum' in British English) to the rectum. Its primary purpose is to extract water from feces.
Diarrhea	Diarrhea or diarrhoea is a condition in which the sufferer has frequent and watery, chunky, or loose bowel movements.
Colon	The colon is the part of the intestine from the cecum to the rectum. Its primary purpose is to extract water from feces.
Constipation	Constipation is a condition of the digestive system where a person (or other animal) experiences hard feces that are difficult to eliminate; it may be extremely painful, and in severe cases (fecal impaction) lead to symptoms of bowel obstruction.
Carotene	Carotene is an orange photosynthetic pigment important for photosynthesis. It is responsible for the orange color of the carrot and many other fruits and vegetables. It contributes to photosynthesis by transmitting the light energy it absorbs to chlorophyll.
Vitamin	An organic compound other than a carbohydrate, lipid, or protein that is needed for normal metabolism but that the body cannot synthesize in adequate amounts is called a vitamin.
Free radicals	Free radicals are atomic or molecular species with unpaired electrons on an otherwise open shell configuration.
Absorption	Absorption is a physical or chemical phenomenon or a process in which atoms, molecules, or ions enter some bulk phase - gas, liquid or solid material. In nutrition, amino acids are broken down through digestion, which begins in the stomach.
Phosphorus	Phosphorus is the chemical element in the periodic table that has the symbol P and atomic number 15.
Calcium	Calcium is the chemical element in the periodic table that has the symbol Ca and atomic number 20. Calcium is a soft grey alkaline earth metal that is used as a reducing agent in the extraction of thorium, zirconium and uranium. Calcium is also the fifth most abundant element in the Earth's crust.
Sterol	A sterol, or steroid alcohols are a subgroup of steroids with a hydroxyl group in the 3-position of the A-ring. They are amphipathic lipids synthetized from Acetyl coenzyme A.
Folic acid	Folic acid and folate (the anion form) are forms of a water-soluble B vitamin. These occur naturally in food and can also be taken as supplements.
Riboflavin	Riboflavin is an easily absorbed, water-soluble micronutrient with a key role in maintaining human health. Like the other B vitamins, it supports energy production by aiding in the metabolising of fats, carbohydrates, and proteins.
Thiamine	Thiamine, also known as vitamin B_1, is a colorless compound with chemical formula $C_{12}H_{17}ClN_4OS$. Systemic thiamine deficiency can lead to myriad problems including neurodegeneration, wasting, and death. Well-known syndromes caused by lack of thiamine due to malnutrition or a diet high in thiaminase-rich foods include Wernicke-Korsakoff syndrome and

Go to **Cram101.com** for the Practice Tests for this Chapter.

Chapter 20. Wellness

Chapter 20. Wellness

	beriberi, diseases also common in chronic abusers of alcohol.
Niacin	Niacin, also known as vitamin B3, is a water-soluble vitamin whose derivatives such as NADH play essential roles in energy metabolism in the living cell and DNA repair. The designation vitamin B3 also includes the amide form, nicotinamide or niacinamide.
Red blood cells	Red blood cells are the most common type of blood cell and are the vertebrate body's principal means of delivering oxygen from the lungs or gills to body tissues via the blood.
Red blood cell	The red blood cell is the most common type of blood cell and is the vertebrate body's principal means of delivering oxygen from the lungs or gills to body tissues via the blood.
Anemia	Anemia is a deficiency of red blood cells and/or hemoglobin. This results in a reduced ability of blood to transfer oxygen to the tissues, and this causes hypoxia; since all human cells depend on oxygen for survival, varying degrees of anemia can have a wide range of clinical consequences.
Alcoholic	An alcoholic is dependent on alcohol as characterized by craving, loss of control, physical dependence and withdrawal symptoms, and tolerance.
Elderly	Old age consists of ages nearing the average life span of human beings, and thus the end of the human life cycle. Euphemisms for older people include advanced adult, elderly, and senior or senior citizen.
Addict	A person with an overpowering physical or psychological need to continue taking a particular substance or drug is referred to as an addict.
Nervous system	The nervous system of an animal coordinates the activity of the muscles, monitors the organs, constructs and processes input from the senses, and initiates actions.
Brain	The part of the central nervous system involved in regulating and controlling body activity and interpreting information from the senses transmitted through the nervous system is referred to as the brain.
Acute	In medicine, an acute disease is a disease with either or both of: a rapid onset; and a short course (as opposed to a chronic course).
Cirrhosis	Cirrhosis is a chronic disease of the liver in which liver tissue is replaced by connective tissue, resulting in the loss of liver function. Cirrhosis is caused by damage from toxins (including alcohol), metabolic problems, chronic viral hepatitis or other causes
Liver	The liver is an organ in vertebrates, including humans. It plays a major role in metabolism and has a number of functions in the body including drug detoxification, glycogen storage, and plasma protein synthesis. It also produces bile, which is important for digestion.
International unit	International unit refers to a crude measure of vitamin activity, often based on the growth rate of animals. Today these units have generally been replaced by precise measurement of actual quantities in milligrams or micrograms.
Heart attack	A heart attack, is a serious, sudden heart condition usually characterized by varying degrees of chest pain or discomfort, weakness, sweating, nausea, vomiting, and arrhythmias, sometimes causing loss of consciousness. It occurs when the blood supply to a part of the heart is interrupted, causing death and scarring of the local heart tissue.
Potassium	Potassium is a chemical element in the periodic table. It has the symbol K (L. kalium) and atomic number 19. Potassium is a soft silvery-white metallic alkali metal that occurs naturally bound to other elements in seawater and many minerals.
Magnesium	Magnesium is the chemical element in the periodic table that has the symbol Mg and atomic number 12 and an atomic mass of 24.31.

Chapter 20. Wellness

Chapter 20. Wellness

Minerals	Minerals refer to inorganic chemical compounds found in nature; salts.
Alcohol	Alcohol is a general term, applied to any organic compound in which a hydroxyl group (-OH) is bound to a carbon atom, which in turn is bound to other hydrogen and/or carbon atoms. The general formula for a simple acyclic alcohol is $C_nH_{2n+1}OH$.
Artery	Vessel that takes blood away from the heart to the tissues and organs of the body is called an artery.
Bile	Bile is a bitter, greenish-yellow alkaline fluid secreted by the liver of most vertebrates. In many species, it is stored in the gallbladder between meals and upon eating is discharged into the duodenum where it aids the process of digestion.
Plasma	Fluid portion of circulating blood is called plasma.
Value	Value is worth in general, and it is thought to be connected to reasons for certain practices, policies, actions, beliefs or emotions. Value is "that which one acts to gain and/or keep."
Serum	Serum is the same as blood plasma except that clotting factors (such as fibrin) have been removed. Blood plasma contains fibrinogen.
Stroke	A stroke or cerebrovascular accident (CVA) occurs when the blood supply to a part of the brain is suddenly interrupted.
Blood plasma	Blood plasma is the liquid component of blood, in which the blood cells are suspended. Serum is the same as blood plasma except that clotting factors (such as fibrin) have been removed.
Protein	A protein is a complex, high-molecular-weight organic compound that consists of amino acids joined by peptide bonds. They are essential to the structure and function of all living cells and viruses. Many are enzymes or subunits of enzymes.
Lipoprotein	A lipoprotein is a biochemical assembly that contains both proteins and lipids and may be structural or catalytic in function. They may be enzymes, proton pumps, ion pumps, or some combination of these functions.
Coronary	Referring to the heart or the blood vessels of the heart is referred to as coronary.
Coronary artery disease	Coronary artery disease (CAD) is the end result of the accumulation of atheromatous plaques within the walls of the arteries that supply the myocardium (the muscle of the heart).
Coronary artery	An artery that supplies blood to the wall of the heart is called a coronary artery.
Elimination	Elimination refers to the physiologic excretion of drugs and other substances from the body.
Risk factor	A risk factor is a variable associated with an increased risk of disease or infection but risk factors are not necessarily causal.
Calorie	Calorie refers to a unit used to measure heat energy and the energy contents of foods.
Aerobic	An aerobic organism is an organism that has an oxygen based metabolism. Aerobes, in a process known as cellular respiration, use oxygen to oxidize substrates (for example sugars and fats) in order to obtain energy.
Oxygen	Oxygen is a chemical element in the periodic table. It has the symbol O and atomic number 8. Oxygen is the second most common element on Earth, composing around 46% of the mass of Earth's crust and 28% of the mass of Earth as a whole, and is the third most common element in the universe.
Aerobic exercise	Exercise in which oxygen is used to produce ATP is aerobic exercise.
Heart rate	Heart rate is a term used to describe the frequency of the cardiac cycle. It is considered one of the four vital signs. Usually it is calculated as the number of contractions of the

Chapter 20. Wellness

Chapter 20. Wellness

	heart in one minute and expressed as "beats per minute".
Lungs	Lungs are the essential organs of respiration in air-breathing vertebrates. Their principal function is to transport oxygen from the atmosphere into the bloodstream, and to excrete carbon dioxide from the bloodstream into the atmosphere.
Muscle	Muscle is a contractile form of tissue. It is one of the four major tissue types, the other three being epithelium, connective tissue and nervous tissue. Muscle contraction is used to move parts of the body, as well as to move substances within the body.
Blood vessel	A blood vessel is a part of the circulatory system and function to transport blood throughout the body. The most important types, arteries and veins, are so termed because they carry blood away from or towards the heart, respectively.
Conditioning	Processes by which behaviors can be learned or modified through interaction with the environment are conditioning.
Anaerobic exercise	Anaerobic exercise is one where anaerobic metabolism is taking place. In a long exercise the glycogen supply local to the muscle runs out and the body converts to aerobic metabolism; when aerobic metabolism is sustaining the workout it is an aerobic exercise.
Osteoporosis	Osteoporosis is a disease of bone in which bone mineral density (BMD) is reduced, bone microarchitecture is disrupted, the amount and variety of non-collagenous proteins in bone is changed, and a concomitantly fracture risk is increased.
Digestive tract	The digestive tract is the system of organs within multicellular animals which takes in food, digests it to extract energy and nutrients, and expels the remaining waste.

Chapter 20. Wellness